Clinical Applications of Artificial Intelligence in Real-World Data

Folkert W. Asselbergs · Spiros Denaxas ·
Daniel L. Oberski · Jason H. Moore
Editors

Clinical Applications of Artificial Intelligence in Real-World Data

Springer

Editors
Folkert W. Asselbergs
Amsterdam University Medical Center
University of Amsterdam
Amsterdam, The Netherlands

Institute of Health Informatics
University College London
London, UK

Daniel L. Oberski
Department of Data Science and Biostatistics
University Medical Center Utrecht (UMCU)
Utrecht, The Netherlands

Spiros Denaxas
Institute of Health Informatics
University College London
London, UK

Jason H. Moore
Cedars-Sinai Medical Center
Los Angeles, CA, USA

ISBN 978-3-031-36677-2 ISBN 978-3-031-36678-9 (eBook)
https://doi.org/10.1007/978-3-031-36678-9

This Springer imprint is published by the registered company Springer Nature Switzerland AG
The registered company address is: Gewerbestrasse 11, 6330 Cham, Switzerland

Paper in this product is recyclable.

Contents

Data Processing, Storage, Regulations

Biomedical Big Data: Opportunities and Challenges (Overview)

Folkert W. Asselbergs, Spiros Denaxas and Jason H. Moore

Abstract

Artificial Intelligence (AI) in medicine stands at the cusp of revolutionizing clinician reasoning and decision-making. Since its foundational years in the mid-20th century, the progression of medical AI has seen considerable advancements, concurrently grappling with various challenges. Early attempts of AI showcased immense potential, yet faced hurdles from data integration to machine-driven clinical decisions. Modern deep learning neural networks, particularly in image analysis, represent promising advancements. Ensuring the trustworthiness of AI systems is paramount for stakeholders to fully embrace its potential in healthcare. To safeguard patient care and guarantee effective outcomes, a rigorous evaluation of AI applications is essential before wide-scale adoption. This textbook illuminates the multifaceted journey of AI in healthcare, emphasizing its challenges, opportunities, and the pressing need for a rigorous, informed evaluation to ensure AI's responsible and impactful integration.

Keywords

Artificial intelligence · Data science · Healthcare · Medicine

Artificial intelligence (AI) has many definitions and means different things to different people. However, a common theme is to develop computer systems and software that can solve problems as well or better than humans. This is a good starting definition for AI in medicine as we strive to augment, or in some cases replace, clinician reasoning and decision making. The phrase artificial intelligence was solidified as a descriptor and name for the field at summer workshop held at Dartmouth College in the United States in 1956. Prior to that time, a variety of other names such as cybernetics and automata were inconsistently used.

The 1950s was a period of excitement for AI as computers and the first programming languages became available to implement some of the first AI methods. For example, the FORmula TRANslation (FORTRAN) and Lisp

F. W. Asselbergs (✉)
Department of Cardiology, Amsterdam University Medical Centers, University of Amsterdam, Amsterdam, The Netherlands
e-mail: f.w.asselbergs@amsterdamumc.nl

F. W. Asselbergs · S. Denaxas
Health Data Research UK and Institute of Health Informatics, University College London, London, UK

J. H. Moore
Department of Computational Biomedicine, Cedars-Sinai Medical Center, West Hollywood, CA, USA

F. W. Asselbergs et al. (eds.), *Clinical Applications of Artificial Intelligence in Real-World Data*,
https://doi.org/10.1007/978-3-031-36678-9_1

programming language were developed in the mid-1950s and became widely used in AI program development for decades. Prior to this time AI was the subject of science fiction and speculation by researchers. The development of AI in medicine paralleled the development and adoption of electronic health records (EHR) in the 1960s and beyond for storing and managing patient data.

One of the earliest and most notable examples of AI in medicine was the MYCIN expert system for prescribing antibiotics for treating intensive care unit patients presenting with infection [9]. Expert systems such as MYCIN have several key components. First, a database of facts about each patient is needed. Second, a database of knowledge about the clinical problem is needed. Third, an inference engine is needed to combine the facts with the knowledge (often represented by rules) to arrive at a decision. Interestingly, the MYCIN system was demonstrated to be clinically effective [13]. However, it was never used in clinical practice due to data entry challenges and concerns about how patients and their families would react to the involvement of a computer in making healthcare decisions.

Early successes in AI, and the continued evolution of computers and programming languages, led to a lot of hype about what AI could do through the 1980s. Unfortunately, the technology could not keep up with the promises leading to what many refer to as an "AI winter" in the 1990s and early 2000s when both government and industry funding for AI dried up. This all changed in 2011 when IBM Watson AI competed on the TV quiz show Jeopardy and beat the top human champion. This was a monumental feat and convinced many that the AI winter was over. Watson used natural language processing, machine learning, information retrieval, knowledge engineering, and high-performance computing to be able to rapidly formulate the right questions to the answers presented in real time on the TV show. This was truly a human-competitive AI. The challenges faced by the Watson team has been previously reviewed [3].

Building on the success of Watson, IBM decided to enter the healthcare market with Watson Oncology to assist with prescribing chemotherapy to cancer patients. Several prominent cancer centers in the United States licensed Watson and put it to the test. Unfortunately, Watson did not perform as well as oncologists leading to some negative headlines. The rollout, evaluation, and consequences of IBM Watson in the healthcare space has been reviewed by Strickland [10]. The underwhelming performance of Watson is likely more a statement about the complexities associated with modeling and predicting health outcomes than the technology itself. The Watson experience is important to understand as we continue to develop and deploy AI in the clinic.

AI approaches, and particularly deep learning algorithms, are particularly well suited in combining multiple data modalities together and making statistical inferences from large, complex, multidimensional input. In healthcare, when individuals interact with care providers, a wealth of metadata and data are generated and captured electronically in EHR systems. These systems contain pieces of information on healthcare utilization and interactions as well as clinically-meaningful information such as diagnoses, symptoms, interventions and procedures, laboratory measurements, and prescriptions of medications. This rapid and increasing availability of data, combined with advances in AI-driven analytical methods has fueled the expectations of applying AI approaches in the context of healthcare, but, as illustrated by the Watson experience, challenges exist regarding accessibility, interoperability and information governance.

EHR data can broadly be classified in four categories: structured, unstructured, imaging and signal data. Structured data are the fundamental building blocks of creating a patients longitudinal health snapshot and are the most popular data modality used in healthcare at the moment, They are recorded using controlled clinical terminologies which are structured medical ontologies that contains terms related to healthcare. For example, SNOMED-CT contains over 500,000 unique concepts organized in a hierarchy and enables healthcare professionals to record information about patient interactions. Likewise, the International Statistical Classification of Diseases (ICD-10) which is maintained by the WHO contains approximately 10,000 unique terms that can be used to record information on diagnoses, symptoms and other parameters of interaction with the healthcare system. Semi-structured information, such as physical examination measurements (e.g. systolic blood pressure, HbA1C values) are also recorded using a combination of terminologies and data fields.

Unstructured data capture clinical narrative which is often, but not always, found in medical notes or care reports. Medical notes can contain important information (e.g. signs or symptoms) that supplement the data found in the structured part of the record but often can contain information that is not coded at all. Text data requires the application of specialized methods, such as Natural Language Processing (NLP) approaches, for processing and extracting clinically important pieces of information and converting the data into a machine-readable structure. Imaging data includes data that are generated for example by radiologists such as CT or MRI scans and which often combine both imaging information and unstructured data (e.g. a report from a radiologist that accompanies a MRI scan). Finally, signaling data captures electrophysiological measurements such as ECGs or EKGs that are also often accompanied by a text report.

In most use cases, AI-driven algorithms are trained on large datasets of multimodal data. This wealth of information however that is captured during healthcare interactions is primarily collected for clinical care or billing/reimbursements. As a result, the data have a number of challenges associated with them such as data quality, bias, consistency. The data itself are influenced by numerous factors such as clinical practice guidelines which could influence the underlying healthcare processes and pathways while the information systems utilized to record the information has also been shown to affect data completeness. Certain sub-populations, such as particular ethnical minorities or people experiencing homelessness, might be significantly underrepresented in the data. Healthcare utilization itself is associated with socioeconomic status and data might reflect this as recently shown in an American study that demonstrated racial bias within a commercial algorithm that incorrectly classified black patients at lower risk due to health expenditure [8]. In order to create accurate, safe, and fair healthcare analytics, these challenges have to be addressed prior to including the data in any AI algorithm for clinical use. For this purpose, a multi-disciplinary team of researchers, clinicians, patient representatives, editors, industry have developed a pragmatic framework, CODE-EHR, to guide researchers with step-by-step approach to provide clarity on how the dataset was constructed, the details on the used coding systems, analytical methods, information governance and patient-public involvement to have confidence in the reported results and enable others to validate and improve the findings [5].

Equally important, the standardized reporting of biases and the relevant features that are associated with them in the analyses is required in order to assess diversity and inclusiveness in AI research. Examples of standardized reporting is the reporting protocol Transparent Reporting of a multivariable prediction model of Individual Prognosis Or Diagnosis (TRIPOD) and its recent AI extension TRIPOD-AI [2]. Furthermore, the evaluation of AI models need to be robust similar to medicine approval processes before they can be widely adopted in healthcare. Randomized clinical trials are still the gold standard and much needed in this space to prove the added value of AI interventions in comparison to current care. CONSORT-AI has developed a reporting guideline specifically for AI interventions [7].

Despite all these challenges, progress has been made in the last few years. A modern success story of AI in medicine is deep learning neural networks for the analysis of images [6, 11]. Deep learning is a type of neural network with a large number of inputs and hidden layer nodes that facilitate the processing of lots of data and their relationships. This approach has been very effective for image analysis through the use of 'convolutions' that are able to decompose and model images as a series of layers each providing different information. The best example of deep learning in medicine is the use of convolutional neural networks for diagnosing diabetic retinopathy from images of the fundus [1, 4]. In 2018, the U.S. Food and Drug Administration approved this deep learning approach for commercial use and it is increasingly approving novel AI and ML enabled medical devices in recent years [12]. These applications are predominantly in imaging and cardiac rhythm monitoring. However, AI algorithms that uses all multi-modal data within routine healthcare including EHR unstructured data, laboratory measurements, imaging, wearable data are still in their infancy and only available within a research setting and limited to specific vendors or networks. More importantly, no international consensus has yet been reached regarding the definition of trustworthy AI, including technical robustness, clinical utility and applicability, transparency and explainability, fairness and non-discrimination, transferability and generalizability, as well as ethical and legal compliance.

In this textbook, background information on the most commonly used AI methods will be discussed including its opportunities and challenges for use in routine clinical care. As novel AI enabled will be increasingly entering the clinical arena, it is of eminent importance that healthcare workforce and clinical researchers are educated and well informed to ensure responsible implementation and evaluation of AI in healthcare to maximize its potential for patients.

References

1. Abràmoff MD, Lou Y, Erginay A, Clarida W, Amelon R, Folk JC, Niemeijer M. Improved automated detection of diabetic retinopathy on a publicly available dataset through integration of deep learning. Invest Ophthalmol Vis Sci. 2016;57(13):5200–6.
2. Collins GS, Dhiman P, Andaur Navarro CL, et al. Protocol for development of a reporting guideline (TRIPOD-AI) and risk of bias tool (PROBAST-AI) for diagnostic and prognostic prediction model studies based on artificial intelligence. BMJ Open. 2021;11:e048008.
3. Ferrucci DA, Brown EW, Chu-Carroll J, Fan J, Gondek D, Kalyanpur A, Lally A, Murdock JW, Nyberg E, Prager JM, Schlaefer N, Welty CA. Building Watson: an overview of the DeepQA project. AI Mag. 2010;31:59–79.
4. Grzybowski A, Brona P, Lim G, Ruamviboonsuk P, Tan GSW, Abramoff M, Ting DSW. Artificial intelligence for diabetic retinopathy screening: a review. Eye (Lond). 2020;34(3):451–60.
5. Kotecha D, Asselbergs FW, Achenbach S, et al. CODE-EHR best practice framework for the use of structured electronic healthcare records in clinical research. BMJ. 2022;29(378): e069048.
6. LeCun Y, Bengio Y, Hinton G. Deep learning. Nature. 2015;521:436.
7. Liu X, Rivera SC, Moher D, Calvert MJ, Denniston AK. SPIRIT-AI and CONSORT-AI working group. Reporting guidelines for clinical trial reports for interventions involving artificial intelligence: the CONSORT-AI Extension. BMJ. 2020;370:m3164.
8. Obermeyer Z, Powers B, Vogeli C, Mullainathan S. Dissecting racial bias in an algorithm used to manage the health of populations. Science. 2019;366(6464):447–53.
9. Shortliffe EH, Axline SG, Buchanan BG, Merigan TC, Cohen SN. An artificial intelligence program to advise physicians regarding antimicrobial therapy. Comput Biomed Res. 1973;6(6):544–60.
10. Strickland EK. IBM Watson, heal thyself: how IBM overpromised and underdelivered on AI health care IEEE Spectrum 2019;56:24–31.
11. Topol EJ. High-performance medicine: the convergence of human and artificial intelligence. Nat Med. 2019;25(1):44–56.
12. Wu E, Wu K, Daneshjou R, et al. How medical AI devices are evaluated: limitations and recommendations from an analysis of FDA approvals. Nat Med. 2021;27:582–4.
13. Yu VL, Fagan LM, Wraith SM, Clancey WJ, Scott AC, Hannigan J, Blum RL, Buchanan BG, Cohen SN. Antimicrobial selection by a computer. A blinded evaluation by infectious diseases experts. JAMA. 1979;242(12):1279–82.

Quality Control, Data Cleaning, Imputation

Dawei Liu, Hanne I. Oberman, Johanna Muñoz, Jeroen Hoogland and Thomas P. A. Debray

Abstract

This chapter addresses important steps during the quality assurance and control of RWD, with particular emphasis on the identification and handling of missing values. A gentle introduction is provided on common statistical and machine learning methods for imputation. We discuss the main strengths and weaknesses of each method, and compare their performance in a literature review. We motivate why the imputation of RWD may require additional efforts to avoid bias, and highlight recent advances that account for informative missingness and repeated observations. Finally, we introduce alternative methods to address incomplete data without the need for imputation.

Keywords

Missing data · Imputation · Missing at random · Missing not at random · Missing completely at random · Informative missingness · Sporadically missing · Systematically missing · Joint modelling imputation · Conditional modelling imputation · Machine learning imputation · Nearest neighbor · Matrix completion · Tree-based ensembles · Support vector machines · Neural networks · Rubin's rules · Pattern submodels · Surrogate splits · Missing indicator · Heckman selection model

1 Introduction

1.1 Quality Control

Increasingly often, researchers have access to data collected from the routine clinical practice with information on patient health or the delivery of health care from a variety of sources other than traditional clinical trials [1, 2]. These data are also known as Real World Data (RWD).

D. Liu
Biogen Digital Health, Biogen, 225 Binney Street, Cambridge, MA 02142, USA

H. I. Oberman
Utrecht University, Padualaan 14, 3584 CH Utrecht, The Netherlands

J. Muñoz · J. Hoogland · T. P. A. Debray
Julius Center for Health Sciences and Primary Care, University Medical Center Utrecht, Utrecht University, Heidelberglaan 100, Utrecht, The Netherlands

T. P. A. Debray
Health Data Research UK and Institute of Health Informatics, University College London, Gibbs Building, 215 Euston Road, London NW1 2BE, UK

T. P. A. Debray (✉)
Smart Data Analysis and Statistics, Utrecht, The Netherlands
e-mail: tdebray@fromdatatowisdom.com

F. W. Asselbergs et al. (eds.), *Clinical Applications of Artificial Intelligence in Real-World Data*,
https://doi.org/10.1007/978-3-031-36678-9_2

Some examples of RWD include administrative databases or clinical registries with electronic healthcare records (EHR), which contain information on patient characteristics, admission details, treatment procedures and clinical outcomes [3].

The generation and collection of RWD is often pragmatic, and limited efforts are made to control the data collection scheme or information flow. The quality of RWD thus can vary dramatically across clinical domains and individual databases [4–8]. For example, health care records are often incomplete and may contain information that is inaccurate or even inconsistent with other data sources [9, 10]. It is therefore imperative that studies involving RWD investigate the nature of recorded information to improve their quality, raise awareness on their strengths and weaknesses, and take these into account to facilitate valid inference on the research question at hand.

Although there is no formal framework to assess the quality of RWD, it is common to focus on at least three domains: accuracy, timeliness and completeness [11]. Data accuracy relates to the validity of individual data entries [12]. It is typically assessed by examining distributional properties of the observed data (e.g., mean, standard deviation, range) and comparing this information with other sources (e.g., previously published population characteristics). Timeliness refers to the degree to which the available data represent reality from the required point in time. Problems can arise when recorded observations (e.g. taken after surgery) do not adequately reflect the patient's health state at the intended measurement time (e.g. before surgery). Finally, completeness represents the existence and amount of missing data.

In this chapter, we first briefly discuss important preprocessing steps in data quality assurance and quality control (QA/QC). Subsequently, we focus on the handling of missing data. As RWD is typically incomplete when missing values are not handled properly, straightforward analysis will very likely lead to misleading conclusions. As such, there is a strong justification to consider and select appropriate analytical methods for handling missing data.

1.2 Data Preparation

The analysis of RWD often necessitates multiple preprocessing steps to create a meaningful and analyzable dataset from the raw data. In general, we can distinguish between three types of preprocessing steps: data integration, data cleaning, and data transformation.

The first step is to identify and integrate relevant sources of data (e.g. hospital registries, administrative databases) such that all information of interest becomes available for the studied individuals. These data may, for instance, include information on signs and symptoms, diseases, test results, diagnoses, referrals, and mortality. Sometimes, it is also possible to retrieve information from unstructured data sources including texts, audio recordings, and/or images (Ref Chap. 8 on text mining). When multiple sources of data are available, it is possible to check for duplicate or inconsistent information across data sources, and thus the accuracy of the data can be assessed. Strategies for data integration are discussed in Ref Chap. 7 on data integration. Once all relevant data sources have been integrated, it is important to select those individuals that are eligible for the intended analysis. The selection requires the identification of the target population, and is often based on disease status or combinations of information (e.g. morbidity code with relevant prescription or results from a diagnostic test). In addition, it is helpful to define relevant time points, including the starting time (also known as index date or baseline) and endpoint (e.g., the outcome of interest) of the study. Although measurements at other time points can be discarded from the dataset, this information can sometimes be used to facilitate risk prediction or missing data imputation (Sect. 6.2). When repeated measurements are available for one or more variables, they can be formatted using two approaches [13]. One approach is to code observations made at different time points as separate columns, leading to a so-called "wide format". This approach works well when the repeated measurements occur at regular time intervals, which is rather uncommon for RWD. A second approach is to record repeated information as separate rows, and to include a "time" variable that indicates when the measurements were taken. This approach is also known as the "long format".

As a second step in data preprocessing, it is recommended to inspect the constructed dataset and to generate descriptive summaries such as the mean, standard deviation, range and amount of missing values for each variable [14]. This information can be used to assess completeness of the data and to identify outliers with impossible or extreme values. When invalid measurements or recordings are detected, corresponding values can be treated as missing data and subsequently be recovered using imputation methods. Alternatively, in case of extreme but valid values, the analysis may be rendered more robust to outliers by windsorizing (i.e., observations are transformed by limiting extreme values) or trimming (i.e., simply discarding extreme observations). Such methods always cause a loss of information, and their use should be guided by good reasons to reduce the influence of such observations. This will heavily depends on the analysis of interest. For instance, mean and variance measures are heavily affected by outliers, but the median is not affected at all. Unfortunately, it is often difficult to assess the validity of individual measurements. For this reason, researchers may sometimes consider analysis methods that directly account for the (potential) presence of measurement error in the entire dataset during model estimation (Ref Chap. 9 on measurement error).

Finally, in the last step, data transformations can be performed. For instance, it is sometimes helpful to transform continuous variables (e.g., in line with model assumptions or to improve numerical stability), to re-code categorical variables (e.g., dummy coding to allow unordered and non-equidistant steps between categories), or to collapse multiple variables into an aggregate measure (i.e., data reduction). Further, when the focus of a study is on the development of a prediction model, it is necessary to set up a training and validation set. Although it is common to randomly split the data into two parts, resampling methods have been recommended to make better use of the data in terms of bias and efficiency (Ref Chap. 15 on model evaluation).

2 Missing Data

Pre-processing often brings to light that records in some data fields are missing. This requires careful consideration since it may indicate loss of information and almost surely affects the analysis and the subsequent interpretation of findings. The degree to which this is the case primarily relates to the type of missing data. Therefore, first and foremost, it is important to try to understand why data are missing, as this will guide any further processing.

2.1 Types of Missing Data Mechanisms

In the broadest sense, there two large groups of missing data mechanisms.

The first group relates to situations where data cannot or should not be measured. For example, it is not possible to assess tumor characteristics or disease severity for healthy patients. Although the absence of any measurements could here be identified and treated as a missing data problem, this strategy should be avoided because it fails to address the fact that no information is actually missing.

The second group arises when variables could have been measured but were not recorded (i.e., information is actually missing). It is, for instance, possible that observations are missing because no measurements were taken or because available measurements were considered invalid or not correctly recorded. Alternatively, it is possible that data collection is complete for individual patients. However, when data are combined across patients or clinical centers, key variables may become incomplete. When trying to understand the consequences of these missing data and to guide the best way forward, it is helpful to distinguish between three mechanisms by which missing data can arise [15]: Missing Completely At Random (MCAR), Missing At Random (MAR), and Missing Not At Random (MNAR).

Briefly, MCAR occurs when the probability that a certain type of measurement is missing does not depend on the values of either observed or missing data. This directly implies that missingness is not related to any of the recorded data and that records with missing data do not form any special group. As an example, physical examination records can be lost due to an administrative computer error. There are no measures, either observed or unobserved, that explain missingness for these particular cases: missingness is said to be *completely* at random.[1]

In MAR, the probability that a variable is missing differs across records based on the values of observed data. For example, a particular type of diagnostic measure may be ordered more often upon certain blood sample deviations. If these data are indeed missing at random (MAR), this means that the probability that a value is missing is again completely at random *within* subgroups with the same blood sample analysis. That is, after taking observed blood sample measures into account, there is no further information that predicts missingness.

Lastly, MNAR describes the situation that the probability that a certain type of measurement is missing is associated with *un*observed data. For instance, if certain measures are more often performed in those with a high suspicion of an unfavorable outcome, but this suspicion cannot be derived from other measures that were observed and recorded in the database. An important particular case is where missingness depends on the value of the measure being missing itself. For instance, alcoholics might be less likely to respond to a questionnaire on alcohol intake.

The distinction between these types of missing data mechanisms is helpful when thinking about the inferences one can make based on the observed data only, without modelling the missing data mechanism itself. As it turns out, several methods can obtain unbiased inference when the MAR assumption holds without explicitly modelling the missing data mechanism[2] (See Sect. 4). Although MAR is often a useful and sometimes convenient assumption from a statistical point of view, the analysis of incomplete data will often need to be supplemented by sensitivity analyses that allow for a more complex missingness mechanism [16]. Methods for this purpose are discussed in more detail in Sect. 6.

2.2 Types of Missing Data Patterns

The manifestation of missing values (regardless of their cause) can be classified into different patterns, each of which requires a different analysis approach. We here focus on common patterns that arise when analyzing RWD.

Real world data are often collected over a period of time and may therefore contain multiple observations for one or more variables. When data are incomplete, it is helpful to distinguish between monotone (e.g., dropout) and non-monotone (intermittent) patterns of missingness (Fig. 1). The dropout pattern occurs when a variable is observed up to a certain

[1] The notion of 'completely at random' is intended to mean: not depending on any observed or missing values out of the measures analyzed. Therefore, is does not have to imply that the missing data pattern is totally unsystematic; it may for instance relate to a measure that is not measured and not of interest for the final analysis. Therefore, the definition of MCAR (and equivalently MAR and MNAR) depends on the set of variables of interest.

[2] In the likelihood and Bayesian paradigm, and when mild regularity conditions are satisfied, the MCAR and MAR mechanisms are ignorable, in the sense that inferences an proceed by analyzing the observed data only, without explicitly addressing the missing data mechanism. In this situation, MNAR mechanisms are nonignorable. Note that in frequentist inference the missingness is generally ignorable only under MCAR [92].

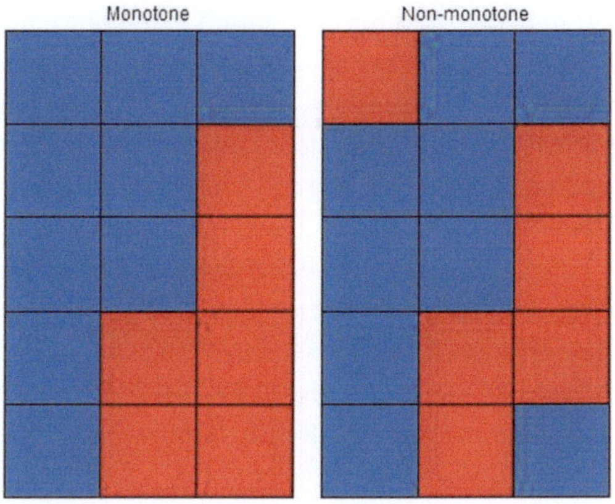

Fig. 1 Illustration of missing data patterns in multivariable data. Each row represents the measurements for a unique patient or timepoint. Columns represent individual variables. Missing values are displayed in red, observed values are displayed in blue

time-point, and missing thereafter [17]. This situation may, for instance, occur when an individual leaves the study prematurely or dies. More generally, a missing data pattern is said to be monotone if the variables can be sorted conveniently according to the percentage of missing data [18]. Univariate missing data form a special monotone pattern. The presence of monotone missingness offers important computational savings and can sometimes be addressed using likelihood-based methods (Sect. 5.2). Conversely, the intermittent pattern occurs when an observed value occurs after a missing value. Because the collection of RWD is often driven by local healthcare demands, measurements tend to be unavailable for time points that are of primary interest to researchers. Intermittent patterns of missingness are therefore relatively common for variables that were measured at multiple occasions. In Sect. 6.2, we discuss dedicated imputation methods to address these non-monotone patterns of missingness.

Real-world data originating from multiple sources (e.g., hospitals, or even countries) tend to be clustered, with distributions and effects that may differ between clusters. In this context, one can distinguish between data values that are sporadically missing (at least some values available in each cluster) and those that are systematically missing (not measured at all in a particular cluster) [18–20]. Systematically missing data are more common when combining routinely collected data from multiple different sources, such as in claims databases. Also, in a pharmacoepidemiologic multi-database studies, there is a high likelihood of missing data because the multiple databases involved may record different variables [21, 22]. Sporadically missing values often occur and are just the within cluster counterpart of usual missing data. This also leads to the main advantage of dealing with just sporadically missing data. Since at least some information on the joint distribution of the data is available in each cluster, regular missing data methods can be implemented *within* clusters if they have sufficient size. In contrast, more evolved missing data methods that accommodate the clustered nature of the data are necessary to handle systematically missing data. A detailed account of missing data methods designed for clustered data is available elsewhere [18–20].

2.3 A Bird's Eye View on Missing Data Methods

Datasets that are collected in real-world settings are typically large and complex. They are large not only in the sense of the number of individuals, but also in terms of the number of collected variables. At the same time, the structure of RWD also tends to be very complicated. It generally has mixed variable types, containing continuous, categorical and time-to-event variables, some of which could have very sophisticated relationships. It is also common that many variables have missing values and that some variables are incomplete for most individuals. Moreover, when missingness occurs, it is often difficult to determine whether the missing data mechanism is MCAR, MAR or MNAR. Instead, it is very likely that all three missing data mechanisms co-exist in the dataset. The validity of analyses involving RWD will therefore often depend highly on whether missing data were handled appropriately.

Fortunately, several strategies exist to address the presence of missing data. In this chapter, we focus on imputation methods which can address many of the aforementioned challenges. These methods replace the missing values by one (single imputation, see Sect. 3) or more (multiple imputation, see Sect. 4) plausible values. Imputation avoids the need to discard patient records and separates the missing data problem from the substantive analysis problem (e.g., estimation of a causal effect or predictive model). This implies that imputed data can be analysed using standard methods and software, and as such be directly available for inference (e.g., parameter estimation or hypothesis testing) and the generation of risk predictions. However, as we discuss later in this chapter, single imputation methods are best avoided in most settings because they are not capable of preserving uncertainty about the missing values and their imputation [23]. We therefore recommend more advanced approaches that are based on multiple imputation (Sect. 4) or avoid imputation altogether (Sect. 5). These methods can mainly be applied when data are MCAR or MAR. When the missingness mechanism is MNAR or unknown, additional methods need to be employed (Sect. 6.1).

Traditional methods for multiple imputation have been studied extensively in the literature, and are briefly summarized in Sects. 4.1 and 4.2. More recently, numerous imputation methods have also been proposed in the field of machine learning [24]. Although these methods tend to be relatively data hungry, they offer increased flexibility and may therefore improve the quality of subsequent analyses (Sect. 4.3). To evaluate the potential merit of advanced imputation methods, we embarked on a literature review and focused on imputation methods that are well-suited to handle mixed data types, a large number of both cases and variables, and different types of missing data mechanisms. Briefly, we searched relevant publications on PubMed and ArXiv that describe quantitative evaluations of missing data methods. Initially, we identified 15 relevant papers based on our own experience in the field. These papers compared several statistical and machine learning imputation techniques and were used to inform an active learning literature review. To this purpose, we used the software ASReview, a machine-learning framework that facilitates the screening of titles and abstracts [25, 26]. To achieve full merit of the framework, a 'stopping criterion' is required–in our case when the software had selected all 15 priory identified publications. A flow diagram of the review methods is presented in Fig. 2. We made use of the following eligibility criteria:

- Inclusion criteria: the paper concerns an evaluation of missing data methods through simulation; the paper matches the search query "(simulation[Title/Abstract]) AND ((missing[Title/Abstract]) OR (incomplete[Title/Abstract]))"; the paper is selected by ASReview before the stopping criterion is reached.
- Exclusion criteria during abstract screening: the paper does not concern an evaluation of missing data methods through simulation; the paper concerns a datatype that deviates from typical EHR data (e.g., imaging data, free text data, traffic sensor data); the paper only concerns (variations of) the *analysis* model, not the *imputation* model; the paper only concerns (variations of) one missing data method.
- Exclusion criteria during full text screening (all of the above, plus): the paper only concerns two missing data methods, one of which is complete case analysis; the paper only concerns single-patient data; the paper only concerns a MCAR missingness mechanism (equivalently, the paper does not concern MAR, MNAR or empirical missingness mechanisms).

After omitting duplicates and removing papers that did not meet the eligibility criteria, we obtained 67 publications. These are listed on zotero.org/groups/4418459/clinical-applications-of-ai/library.

Based on the aforementioned considerations, we decided to focus on five types of machine learning methods that can be used for imputation: nearest neighbour methods, matrix

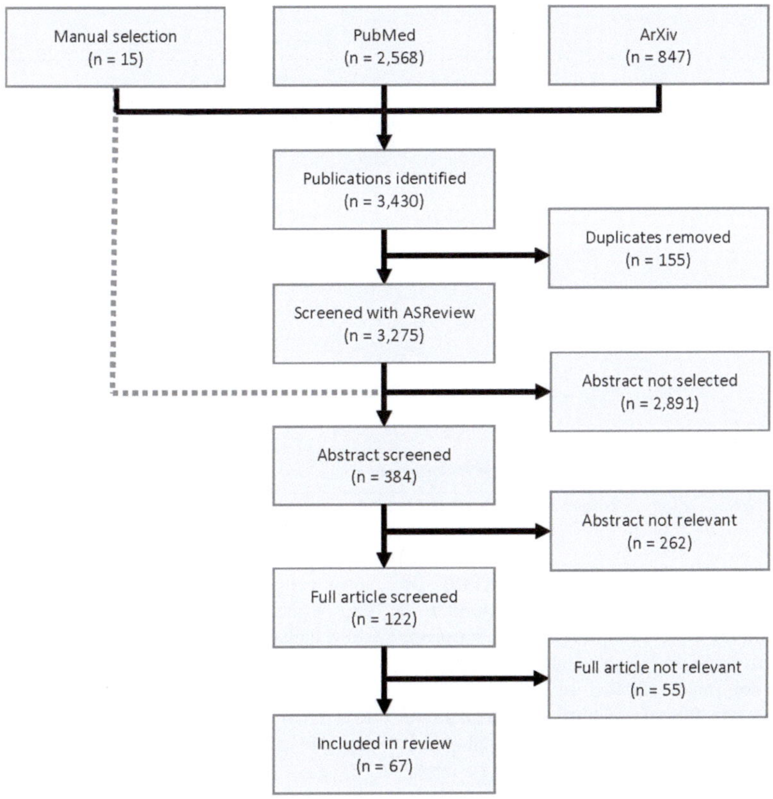

Fig. 2 Flow chart of the literature review to identify quantitative evaluations of missing data methods

completion, support vector machines, tree-based ensembles, and neural networks. In the following sections, we briefly introduce each method, discuss its strengths and weaknesses, and provide software implementations. We summarize the main findings from our review in Sect. 6.3, offering also a list of recommendations.

2.4 Introduction of Case Study Data (MIMIC-III)

The Medical Information Mart for Intensive Care (MIMIC)-III database contains information on 38,597 adults and 7870 neonates that were admitted to critical care units at Beth Israel Deaconess Medical Center [27, 28]. Various types of patient-level data are available, including vital signs, laboratory measurements, imaging reports, received treatments, hospital length of stay, and survival. Although many variables were only measured upon admission, temporal data are also available. For instance, there are 753 types of laboratory measurements in MIMIC-III, each with on average 8.13 observations per patient. As illustrated in Fig. 3, the missingness rate in MIMIC-III greatly varies between variables and can be as high as 96%.

3 Single Imputation Methods

A common approach to address the presence of missing values is to simply replace them by a plausible value or prediction [30]. This approach is adopted by many software packages that implement contemporary machine learning methods. Below, we outline and illustrate three single imputation methods to recover missing systolic blood pressure levels in MIMIC-III.

In single value imputation (SVI), it is widespread to replace missing values of a variable

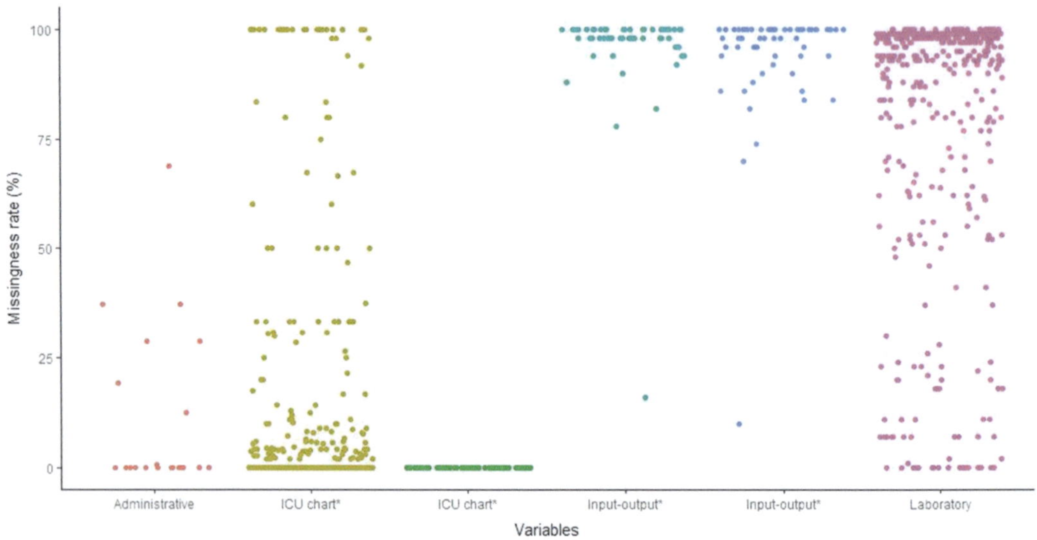

Fig. 3 Visualization of missing data in MIMIC-III [29]. Missingness rate is calculated as the proportion of individuals that do not have any observation for a given variable. Administrative variables include demographic data and were not much affected by missing values (e.g., missingness rate for date of birth = 0%). Intensive Care Unit (ICU) chart variables include patient monitoring variables. Input–output variables relate to intake substances (e.g., liquids, medication) and excretions (e.g., urine, fluid from the lungs).Finally, laboratory variables include microbiology results. * Two different critical care information systems were in place over the data collection period. For this reason, missingness rates for ICU chart and input–output variables are presented as separate categories

by a convenient summary statistic, such as the mean, median, or mode of the corresponding variable. For example, patients without follow-up data are sometimes assumed to be alive. Similarly, when blood oxygenation levels are incomplete, it is possible to assume that corresponding patients are in perfect health and simply impute a constant that reflects this condition (e.g., 100%). Alternatively, when the health conditions of included patients are suboptimal, it is possible to impute the average of the observed blood oxygenation levels (left graph in Fig. 4).

A more advanced approach to generate imputations is to adopt multivariable (e.g., regression or machine learning) models that replace each missing value by a prediction [18]. For instance, it is possible to predict blood oxygenation levels in the MIMIC-III database using information on patient age by adopting a regression model (middle graph in Fig. 4). As more (auxiliary) variables are used to predict the missing values, the accuracy of imputed values tends to increase [31].

Unfortunately, single imputation methods tend to distort the data distribution because they do not account for sampling variability and model uncertainty [17, 18]. Because this usually leads to biased inference, single imputation methods are best avoided [30]. Their implementation can, however, be acceptable in some circumstances [18]. For example, it is possible to add noise to imputed values in order to account for sampling variability (right graph in Fig. 4). Also, when applying a prediction model in clinical practice, single imputation methods can greatly facilitate real-time handling of missing values on a case-by-case basis [31, 32].

4 Multiple Imputation Methods

In general, the preferred approach to address the presence of missing data is to adopt multiple imputation [18, 30]. In this approach, each missing value in the original dataset is replaced by a set of $m > 1$ simulated values, leading to

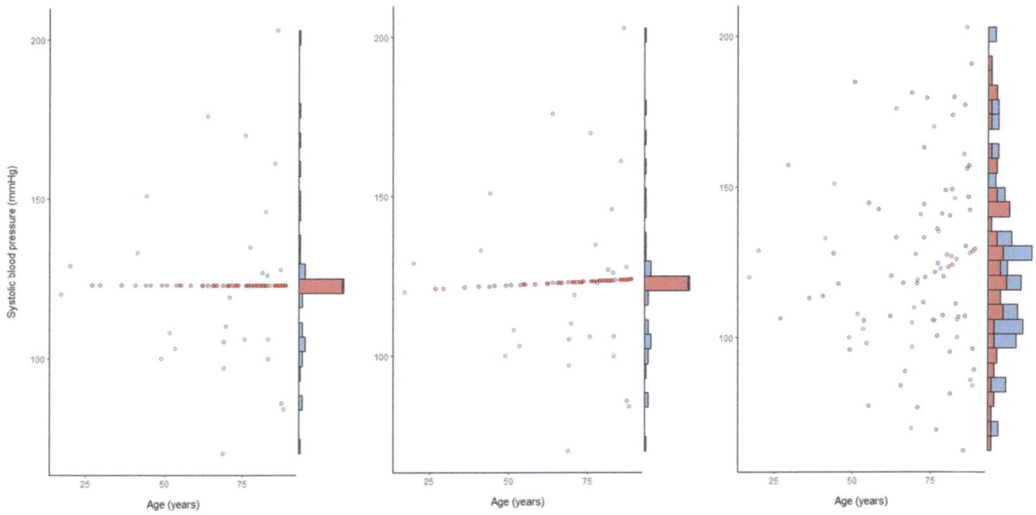

Fig. 4 Illustration of imputation strategies using 100 patients from MIMIC-III. The observed data are displayed in blue and represent the first available measurement for systolic blood pressure after hospital admission. Imputed data are displayed in red, and were generated using mean imputation (left), regression imputation (middle), stochastic regression imputation (right)

multiple completed datasets. The entire procedure is illustrated in Fig. 5.

The generation of plausible values typically involves modelling the observed data distribution and imposing corresponding parameters on the missing data. A major advantage of multiple imputation is that the extent to which the missing values can accurately be recovered becomes more transparent. The variability of imputed values will be large for variables that cannot adequately be retrieved from the observed data (and vice versa). For example, when temperature measurements are missing for a patient diagnosed with COVID-19 and having symptoms that often coexist with fever, imputed values will have a high probability to indicate the presence of fever. In contrast, fever imputations for a patient with a positive COVID-19 test and only mild disease can be expected to be more variable.

A key challenge in multiple imputation is to generate random samples that are plausible and

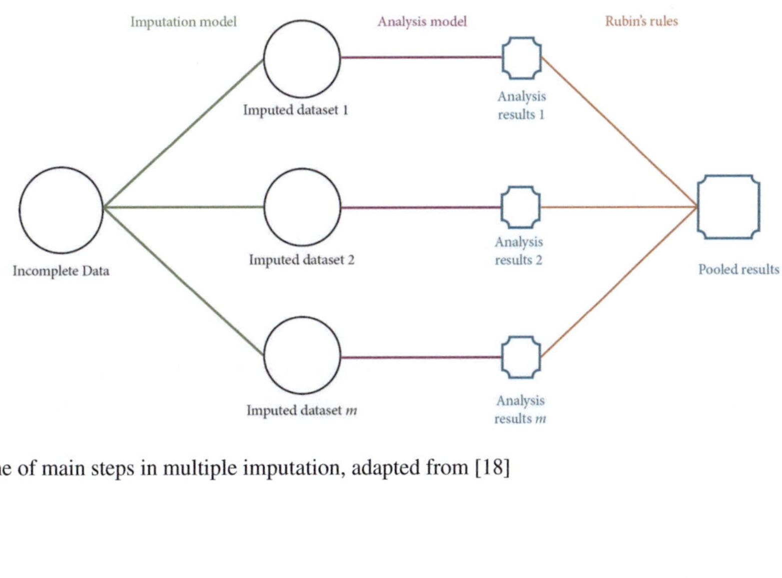

Fig. 5 Scheme of main steps in multiple imputation, adapted from [18]

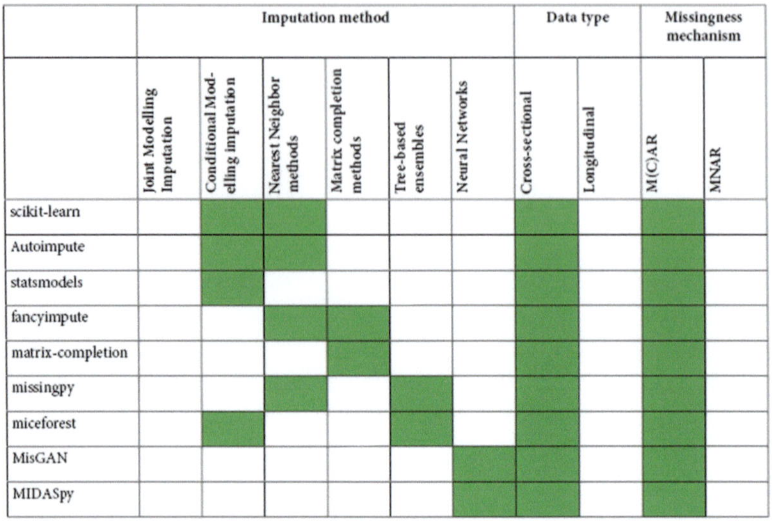

Fig. 6 Python modules for multiple imputation. If an analyst decides to use SVM for imputation, they may need to manually incorporate the algorithm into the imputation procedure. In Python, SVM can be implemented using the scikit-learn library, or using GitHub repositories such as SVMAlgorithm and SupportVectorMachine

exhibit an appropriate amount of variability. Conceptually, this can be achieved by generating imputations from a probability distribution. For instance, consider that some patients in MIMIC-III have missing values for age. A simple solution is to approximate the empirical (observed) age distribution, which has a mean value of 65.8 years and a standard deviation of 18.5 years, with a suitable well-known distribution. New values for patient age could then be generated from a normal distribution with the aforementioned characteristics. It may be clear that the aforementioned (univariate) approach does not account for any relation with other variables in the dataset, and thus leads to imputations that are not very plausible. A better approach is to consider the entire (multivariate) distribution of the available data and draw imputations tailored to each patient [33]. Here, we discuss two broad strategies to generate personalized imputations: joint modelling imputation and conditional modelling imputation. For the latter, both statistical and machine learning methods can be used. Software implementations are summarized in Fig. 6 (Python) and Fig. 7 (R).

4.1 Joint Modelling Imputation

A direct approach to consider the entire data distribution is to explicitly specify a parametric joint model for the observed data [34]. The parameters of this (imputation) model are estimated from the observed data, and subsequently used to generate imputed values. It is, for instance, common to assume that the observed patient characteristics arise from a multivariate normal model. The mean and covariance can be estimated using Markov Chain Monte Carlo (MCMC) methods and directly be used to draw imputed values that account for individual patient characteristics [32]. This approach is also known as multivariate normal imputation [35]. Recent work shows that multiple imputation based on more flexible joint models of the data (e.g. allowing for variables of different types, hierarchical structure of the data, or interaction effects) can also be achieved within the Bayesian framework [36, 37]. Often, it is difficult to identify an appropriate joint model that describes the observed data. Many datasets contain a combination of binary, continuous,

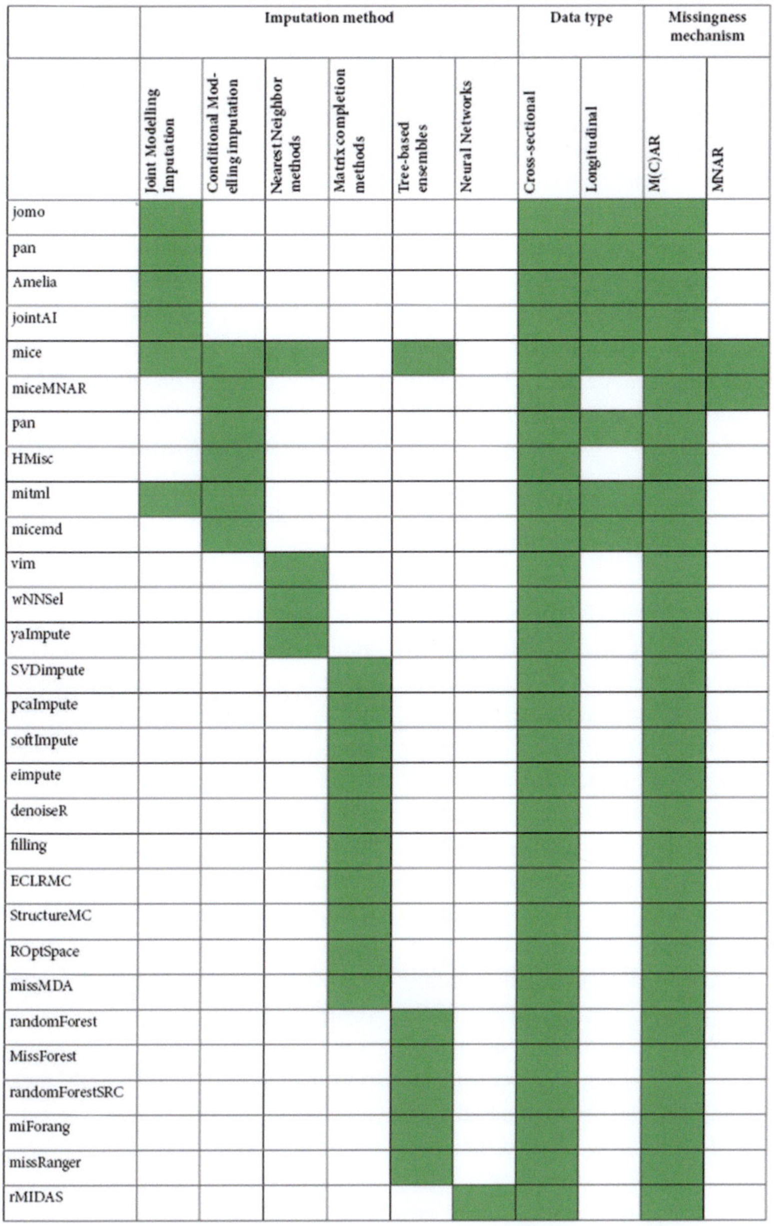

Fig. 7 Software packages in R for multiple imputation. More detailed information for R packages is available from https://cran.r-project.org/web/views/MissingData.html

categorical, and other data types. These mixed data types usually cannot be described using a multivariate distribution with a well-known density. A common strategy to relax this limitation is to approximate the (multivariate) data distribution by a series of conditional (univariate) distributions which is the focus of the next section.

4.2 Conditional Modelling Imputation

Conditional modelling imputation implies that a separate imputation model is estimated for each incomplete variable [38]. For instance, a logistic regression model can be used to describe the conditional distribution of a binary variable (e.g., current smoker). Conversely, a linear regression model can be used to describe the conditional distribution of a continuous variable (e.g., systolic blood pressure). As discussed in Sect. 4.3, it is also possible to adopt machine learning models to describe these conditional distributions. Imputed values are then generated by sampling successively from each of the conditional models, which requires an iterative Monte Carlo procedure. This approach is also known as conditional modelling imputation [32], chained equations imputation [39], or fully conditional specification.

4.3 Machine Learning Imputation

Multiple imputation methods often require explicit assumptions about the distribution(s) of the data, including consideration of the potential presence of interactive and non-linear effects. If the imputation model(s) are based on invalid distributional assumptions or fail to incorporate important covariate effects, subsequent analyses can lead to substantial bias [40]. For instance, consider that an interaction exists between the age of a patient and their blood test results (which contains missing values). If this interaction is not explicitly accommodated during imputation, its magnitude will be attenuated in the imputed data. Thus, constructing an appropriate imputation model requires consideration of how the imputed data will eventually be used [23]. Unfortunately, it is often difficult to predetermine how data will be analyzed, especially when the available data sources were not designed for the intended analysis. It is therefore helpful for imputation models to anticipate certain features of the data (such as interactions, nonlinearities, and complex distributions) without making any specific commitments. Such flexibility can be realized by non-parametric (e.g., nearest neighbor) or semi-parametric models (e.g., neural networks, random forests, or support vector machines) that avoid making distributional assumptions about the observed data. Below, we discuss a selection of common approaches that yield multiple imputed datasets. In general, machine learning methods can be used in two different contexts. One approach is to embed machine learning models in conditional modelling imputation to describe the conditional distribution of a certain variable. For example, missing blood pressure levels could be imputed using a random forest. A second approach is to generate imputed values directly using a dedicated machine learning method, such as matrix completion or adversarial networks.

4.3.1 Nearest Neighbor Methods

Nearest neighbor (NN) methods offer a non-parametric approach to generate imputations without making distributional assumptions. To this purpose, a distance metric is used to determine the relatedness between any two individuals and to identify *neighbors* with complete information for each individual with one or more missing values. Imputation is then achieved by simply copying the observed values from the nearest neighbor (1-NN) or by combining the observed values from *k* nearest neighbors (kNN) into a weighted average [41]. Since NN methods generate imputations by (re)sampling from observed data, no special efforts are required to address complex data types. Accordingly, they are often used with incomplete variables that are restricted to a certain range (e.g., due to truncation), skewed, or semi-continuous. To allow for multiple imputed values, NN methods typically determine the distance between two individuals using a random subset of variables, rather than all observed variables [42]. Although NN methods can directly be used as a non-parametric imputation approach, they can also serve as an intermediate step in semi-parametric imputation procedures [43]. For instance, predictive mean matching combines conditional modelling imputation with NN methods to draw imputations from the observed data [44]. It has been demonstrated that NN methods perform well when data are MCAR or MAR [45–47]. Although NN methods are simple and easy to implement [48], they strongly depend on the specification of a suitable multivariate distance measure and a reasonably small dimension (since there are fewer near neighbors in high dimensional space). Consequently, the performance of NN methods tends to suffer from high dimensionality problems [49] and declines when k is too small or too large. Finally, NN methods do not facilitate the incorporation of MNAR mechanisms, and therefore appear less suitable in RWD.

4.3.2 Matrix Completion Methods

Matrix completion methods aim to recover an intact matrix from the dataset with incomplete observations. To this purpose, they decompose the original (high-dimensional) matrix into a product of lower dimensional matrices [50]. Missing data are then imputed by identifying an appropriate low-rank approximation to the original data matrix.

For instance, singular value decomposition (SVD) can be used to describe a dataset X with n rows (e.g., patients) and k columns (e.g., variables) by a matrix product $X = UDV\prime$. In this expression, D is a diagonal matrix with k singular values, U is an $n \times k$ matrix of left singular vectors, and V is an $k \times k$ matrix of right singular vectors. The entries of D are used to scale U and V, and therefore describe how much information each singular vector provides to the original data matrix. Recall that the rank of a matrix is the maximal number of linearly independent column vectors or row vectors in the matrix, which is also equal to the number of non-zero singular values of the matrix. By omitting singular values that are close to 0 from D (and omitting the corresponding vectors from U and V), the rank of a matrix can be reduced without much loss of information. This, in turn, gives a lower-rank approximation to the original matrix. In case of missing data, the key idea is to find a low-rank approximation that closely fits the observed entries in X from a lower-rank approximation, with the rank sufficiently reduced to fill in the missing parts of X.

Other methods that apply matrix completion include (robust) principle component analysis (PCA) and nuclear-norm regularization [50, 51]. In the latter, the singular values are summarized into a nuclear norm that is optimized using expectation maximization. Matrix completion methods do not make any assumptions about the distribution of the observed data, and can handle high-dimensional data in a straightforward manner. Although their implementation is mainly justified when data are MCAR or MAR, several extensions exist for MNAR situations [52, 53]. Unfortunately, matrix completion is primarily used for numerical data. For categorical data, mode imputation is generally used. Another limitation is related to the implicit linearity assumption. As rank is a concept for the linear relationship between rows or columns of a matrix, the method does not preserve nonlinear relationships between rows or columns.

4.3.3 Tree-Based Ensembles

Tree-based ensemble methods estimate multiple decision trees on the available data and adopt boosting (e.g., XGBoost) or bagging (e.g., random forests) to combine their predictions. Tree-based ensembles can be applied to mixed data types, do not require distributional assumptions, and naturally allow for variable selection. Moreover, their recursive partitioning operation predisposes to capture nonlinear effects and interactions between variables. Several simulation studies have shown that tree-based ensemble methods can outperform commonly used multiple imputation methods [54–56]. We here focus on the use of random forests to generate imputed values, for which at least four different implementations are available [57]. In Sect. 5.3, we discuss additional approaches for developing random forests without the need for imputation.

The first tree-based approach to handle missing data was proposed by Breiman and is implemented in the R package *randomForest* with the function "rfImpute" [58]. It relies on the concept of "proximity" for missing data imputation. Missing values are initially replaced by a simple summary such as their mean or mode, then a forest is constructed and the proximity matrix is calculated. The proximity matrix is a square matrix where each row and column represents a specific individual. Each matrix entry then quantifies the probability that the individuals from the corresponding row and column fall in the same leaf node. The missing value of a particular variable for a specific individual is imputed using an average over the non-missing values of the variable or the most frequent non-missing value where the average or frequency is weighted by the proximities between the case and the non-missing value cases. The process is repeated for each imputed dataset [58].

A second approach termed "on-the-fly-imputation method" was proposed by Ishwara et al. and is implemented in the R package *randomForestSRC* [59]. In this method, only observed values are used to calculate the split-statistic when growing a tree. At each node of a tree, when a split decision needs to be made, missing values will be replaced by random observed values within the corresponding subtree. After each node split, imputed values are set back to missing and the process continues until no more splits can be made. Missing data in terminal nodes are then imputed using the mean or mode of out-of-bag non-missing terminal node data from all the trees.

A third approach was proposed by Stekhoven and Buehlmann and is implemented in the R packages *MissForest and missRanger* [54]. In this method, missing values are initially imputed using simple methods such as mean or mode. The completed data is then used to construct a forest, which in turn is used to predict the missing values. In contrast to the approach proposed by Breiman, this process of training and predicting iterates until a stopping criterion is met, or until a maximum number of user-specified iterations is reached.

Finally, a fourth approach is to use random forests to approximate the conditional (univariate) distribution of the observed data [60]. The chained equations framework is then used to iteratively replace the missing values for each incomplete variable (Sect 4.2). Conditional modeling imputation using random forests has, for instance, been implemented by the function *mice.impute.rf* in the R package *mice* and tends to yield better performance than the three approaches mentioned above [55, 61]. A major advantage of this approach is that imputed data can be analyzed using any method of choice.

4.3.4 Support Vector Machines

Support Vector Machines (SVM) were developed more than thirty years ago [62, 63] and have been successfully used in many real-world applications focusing on classification or prediction. A key building block and also the driving force behind SVM's success is the employment of a kernel function. The kernel function implicitly defines a high-dimensional, or even infinite dimensional feature space (hyperplane), in which data points from different classes could be linearly separated or a continuous response variable could be linearly related to the feature vector. The kernel function needs to be carefully selected, and often takes the form of a Gaussian or polynomial (e.g., when the model should allow for non-linear relations). The most typical scenario for the application of SVM is when all predictors are continuous and when the outcome is binary or continuous. When a predictor variable is categorical, dummy coding needs to be applied. Extensions of SVM are available that can handle categorical or survival outcome data. After the completion of the training process, an SVM generally depends only on a small subset of the original data points, called "support vectors". Although SVM are very powerful in handling high-dimensional data, they are not commonly used for missing data imputation. Possibly, this is because SVM algorithms are very sensitive to noise and less suitable when the sample size is large. For the application of SVM for missing data imputation, no formal statistical software packages were found.

4.3.5 Neural Networks

Neural networks are emerging methods in the field of machine learning and are commonly applied for data generation, feature extraction and dimension reduction. We here discuss two main categories of neural networks that can be used for missing data imputation: autoencoders (AEs) and generative adversarial nets (GANs).

An AE is an artificial neural network specifically designed to learn a representation of the observed data. It typically contains an encoder and a decoder. The encoder maps the original input data to a lower-dimensional representation through successive hidden layers of a neural network. The final layer of an encoder is the output layer, which simply describes the original input layer in a lower dimension [64, 65]. The decoder then maps the output from the encoder to reconstruct the original input, again through successive hidden layers of a neural network. Unfortunately, standard implementations of AEs require data to be complete, and they may end up learning an identity map (hence perfectly reconstructing the input data when an identity map is used instead of successfully reducing the complexity). To address these problems, several AE variants have been proposed. One approach is to adopt denoising autoencoders (DAE) that corrupt the input data with noise [66]. The most common way of adding noise is to randomly set some of the observed input values to zero. This approach can also be applied to incomplete input data, by simply replacing missing values by zero. To facilitate multiple imputation, missing values can be replaced by random samples [67]. Further, it is also possible to treat missing values as an additional type of corrupted data, and to draw imputations from an AE trained to minimize the reconstruction error on the originally observed data. This approach has, for instance, been implemented by Multiple Imputation with Denoising Autoencoders (MIDAS) [68]. A second extension of AE is to adopt variational autoencoders (VAEs) that learn to encode the input using a latent vector from a probabilistic distribution [69–71]. The original data can then be imputed by sampling from the latent posterior distribution.

GANs are another type of neural network that consists of two parts; a generator and a discriminator [72]. In an adversarial process, the generator learns to generate samples that resemble the original data distribution, and the discriminator learns to distinguish whether a presented example is original or artificial. The GAN procedure can be extended to allow for the imputation of missing data [73–75]. Generative Adversarial Imputation Nets (GAIN) adapt the original GAN architecture as follows [75]. The generator learns to model the distribution of the data and to impute missing values accurately. The discriminator then learns to distinguish which values were observed or imputed. The generator's input combines the original input data and a mask matrix that indicates the presence of missing values. Conversely, the input of the discriminator is given by the output of the generator and a hint matrix, which reveals partial information about the missingness of the original data. The discriminator then learns to reconstruct the mask matrix.

4.4 Analyzing and Combining the Imputed Datasets

Once multiple imputed datasets have been generated, they can be analyzed separately using the procedure that would have been followed if all data were complete (Fig. 5). For example, studies aiming to evaluate a relative treatment effect can perform a regression analysis in the imputed data to estimate an odds ratio adjusted for confounders. From each analysis, one or more parameter estimates (and corresponding estimates of uncertainty) are then obtained and need to be combined. Pooling results across multiple imputed datasets is not trivial and typically requires to consider three sources of uncertainty. In particular, there is estimation error within each imputed dataset (e.g., reflected by the estimated standard errors in each completed dataset), variation due to missing data (reflected by the between-imputation variance of parameter estimates), and uncertainty arising from a finite number of imputations. Although point estimates (e.g., regression coefficients) can simply be averaged across the imputed datasets, the pooling of standard errors requires adopting a series of equations that account for aforementioned sources of uncertainty. These equations are also known as Rubin's rules [33, 76, 77] and have been implemented in most contemporary software packages.

If pooling is done appropriately, multiple imputation methods yield valid parameter estimates with appropriate confidence intervals. In some situations, however, the implementation of Rubin's rules cannot be justified. For example, an exception arises when data are available for the entire population [78]. The application of Rubin's rules also becomes more complicated when imputed datasets are analyzed using non-parametric approaches (e.g., recursive partitioning) or approaches that do not result in the same number of parameters across imputations (e.g., variable selection algorithms) [79–81]. In such situations, it may be helpful to avoid imputation altogether.

5 Non-imputation Methods

5.1 Complete Case Analysis

A simple approach to address missing data is to simply remove incomplete records from the dataset. This approach, also known as complete case analysis (CCA), is generally valid but needlessly inefficient under the usually unrealistic MCAR assumption. The adoption of CCA is therefore more appealing when conducting likelihood-based inference under MAR conditions or in datasets where only the outcome is missing (Sect. 5.2). Unfortunately, CCA does not offer a solution when estimated models (e.g., for risk prediction or classification) are applied to new patients with incomplete data.

5.2 Likelihood-Based Methods

More advanced approaches to address missing values define a model for the observed data only. For example, survival models can be used to analyze binary outcome variables that are affected by censoring (e.g., due to drop-out). Similarly, multilevel models can be used to analyze repeated outcomes that were measured at arbitrary follow-up times. A special situation arises when missing values only occur for the outcome, as multiple imputation then requires auxiliary variables that are not part of the analysis model to offer an advantage over likelihood-based methods. The adoption of likelihood-based methods is therefore particularly appealing when missingness only depends on covariates that are included in the analysis model (such that missingness is ignorable) [82].

Likelihood-based methods can also be used to address missing covariate values, and often require advanced procedures for parameter estimation [83, 84]. Although likelihood-based methods tend to be much faster and produce more accurate results than multiple imputation, their applicability is limited to very specific analytical scenarios. Likelihood-based methods may therefore have limited usefulness in RWD, where patterns of missingness can be very complex and additional adjustments may be required to account for other sources of bias (e.g., time-varying confounding).

5.3 Pattern Submodels

A straightforward alternative to imputation methods is to develop separate models for each missingness pattern. For instance, those individuals for which c-reactive protein (CRP) has been observed contribute to a different model than those individuals for which CRP was not observed. This idea has also been referred to as a pattern submodel approach [85]. This type of approach is particularly helpful when the number of missingness patterns is fairly limited with respect to the number of observations, since model development occurs in partitions of the original data. Nonetheless, this is a setting that can be expected to occur quite often RWD. For instance, a whole array of venous blood results, genetics, or imaging data will often be entirely missing or entirely observed. Key benefits of patterns submodels include ease of use (both during development and application) and the fact that it does not rely on assumptions about the missingness pattern. Clear costs include loss of information due to partitioning of the data into missingness patterns (this can be relaxed to allow borrowing of information between patterns, but this invokes the MAR assumption across the patterns for which it is relaxed), and the fact that many models are developed instead of just one. As already noted by Mercaldo and Blume [85], different methods can be envisioned to allow borrowing of information between missingness patterns while retaining some of the robustness with respect to missing data mechanisms, but this is still ongoing research.

5.4 Surrogate Splits

Surrogate splits is a missing data method that is specific to tree-based methods and was proposed in the context of classification and regression trees [86]. The key idea is to not only find the optimal split point when building a tree, but also find second best (or more) split points on variables other than the one providing the optimal split point. This allows using an alternative (surrogate) split variable when the optimal variable is missing. Similar ideas have been proposed throughout tree-based methods research. For instance, instead of finding surrogate splits, the popular XGBoost method [87] finds a default direction for each split point in case the variable to split on is missing. While these methods are easy to apply on any data set with missing values, they have important limitations. For instance, surrogate splits are not able to use information from observed data to infer something about the missing variable. Instead, imputed values are generated conditionally on their position in the tree, which roughly correspond to conditional mean imputation. A more robust approach would be to apply the tree-based methods in multiple imputed data based on flexible methods that preserve more of the data complexities, and subsequently bag the results.

5.5 Missing Indicator

The indicator method replaces missing values by a fixed value (zero or the mean value for the variable) and the indicators are used as dummy variables in analytical models to indicate that a value was missing. The procedure is applied to each incomplete variable, and can be implemented in any analysis method (e.g., regression, decision trees, neural network). The indicator method allows for systematic differences between the observed and the unobserved data by including the response indicator, and thus to address MNAR. However, its implementation usually leads to biased model parameters and can create peculiar feedback mechanisms between the user of the model (e.g. a clinician) and the model itself [88]. For this reason, it is generally discouraged to adopt the missing indicator method for addressing missing data.[3]

6 Imputation of Real-World Data

Although the principles and methods outlined in Sect. 4 are primarily designed for imputing missing data in medical studies a clear sampling or data collection design (e.g., an observational cohort study or clinical trial), they can also be applied to incomplete sources of RWD that were not generated under a specific research design. In this section, we discuss two common characteristics of RWD that require more advanced imputation methods and software packages that were discussed in Sect. 4. A first challenge is the presence of informative missingness and typically arises when missing data mechanisms are complex and partially unknown. A second challenge is the presence of repeated observations, which occurs when patients are followed for a period of time. Below, we discuss methods that are well suited to address these challenges.

6.1 Informative Missingness

It is often difficult to determine the exact mechanisms by which missing values occur in RWD.

[3] While the details are beyond the scope of this chapter, Mercaldo and Blume [85] describe the implementation of missing indicator methodology in the context of multiple imputation, which does provide unbiased inference and has an interesting relation to the pattern submodels described above.

In fact, the distinction between MCAR, MAR and MNAR is a theoretical exercise and all these missingness mechanisms could co-exist in RWD. It is not uncommon that important causes of missingness are not recorded, and missingness in routine healthcare data is often informative [9, 21]. Unfortunately, traditional imputation methods are not well equipped to address this situation, as they do not distinguish between the observed and missing data distribution.

For example, the CRP test is often ordered when there is suspicion of an infection or an inflammation. Lab results may therefore be missing when elevated levels are deemed unlikely. Although multiple imputation could be used to recover these missing test results from information recorded in the EHR database, this approach is problematic when data on signs and symptoms are unavailable. Similar problems arise when test results are directly linked to their missingness. For instance, it is possible that some patients were referred from another hospital based on their lab results, and therefore did not undergo further testing. In general, when missing data mechanisms depend on unobserved information, the presence of missing values becomes informative about the patient, their physician or even the health care center [89, 90].

The plausibility of the MAR assumption (and thus the validity of "traditional" imputation methods) can often be increased by implementing imputation models with auxiliary variables that explain the reasons of missingness during imputation [91]. As more patient characteristics are recorded, it becomes less likely that the presence of missing values depends on unobserved information. For instance, when hospital registries only record information on patient age, sex, and blood test results, CRP levels are highly likely to be MNAR when unavailable. Conversely, when information on signs, symptoms, diagnostic suspicions, and other laboratory markers are also recorded, it becomes more likely that these observations explain why CRP is missing. At the very least, it will decrease the influence of MNAR mechanisms.

Unfortunately, the use of auxiliary variables becomes problematic when they are substantially affected by missing values or when they do not strongly predict the presence of missingness. Unfortunately, EHR databases are notoriously prone to prominent levels of missingness, often caused by complex recording processes. For this reason, the imputation of RWD may benefit from more advanced imputation methods that explicitly account for different missing data mechanisms [92]. When data are MNAR, it is necessary to model the joint distribution of the data and the missingness through selection, pattern-mixture or shared parameter models [93, 94]. Selection models factorize the joint distribution into the marginal distribution of the complete data and the distribution of the missingness. As an example, we discuss the Heckman selection model in more detail below [95, 96]. Conversely, pattern-mixture models separate the marginal distribution for the missingness mechanism and the data distribution conditional on the type of missingness. Essentially, this requires to estimate separate (pattern sub) models for each missingness pattern and to combine their inferences by means of integration. Finally, shared parameter models assume that the data distribution and the missingness indicator are conditionally independent after conditioning on a set of shared parameters or latent variables. This type of model has been successfully applied in settings where the missingness mechanism is related to an underlying process that changes over time. These so-called joint models[4] combine information from a mixed model for a longitudinal outcome and a temporal event model for censoring events with a set of latent variables or random effects.

A common strategy for informative missingness is to directly model the relationship between the risk of a variable being missing and its unseen value [96–98]. This strategy is based on the Heckman selection model [95], and can

[4] In this context, 'joint' is used to describe models that share a parameter, and is not to be confused with joint models that fully describe a multivariate distribution.

be used to assess and correct potential non-random missingness of outcome data. Briefly, the selection model approach involves two equations to predict the missing value and their availability. Both equations are linked together through their residual error terms, which are modelled using a bivariate (e.g., normal) distribution. The correlation of this distribution is estimated from the available data and indicates to what extent the magnitude of the missing values affects their probability of missingness (i.e., presence of MNAR). A special situation arises when there is no correlation between the error terms, as the Heckman model then generates imputations under the MAR assumption. An important requirement for the implementation of Heckman-type imputation models is the availability of exclusion restriction variables. These variables are related to the probability of missingness, but not to the missing value itself. For example, if younger physicians are more motivated to routinely record data into EHR systems, the age of the treating healthcare professional could be treated as an exclusion restriction variable. Similarly, it is possible that CRP tests are ordered more frequently for patients with a certain healthcare insurance program or socioeconomic background. As discussed, information on missingness mechanisms could also be addressed using traditional imputation methods that adopt auxiliary variables, especially if their inclusion converts MNAR situations into MAR. Indeed, it has been demonstrated that Heckman-selection models perform comparably to traditional imputation methods when missing values do not depend on unobserved information [99]. However, Heckman-selection models do not require the MAR assumption and therefore appear more suitable when the missing data mechanisms are unclear. Several simulation studies have demonstrated that Heckman-selection models can greatly decrease bias, even when the proportion of missing data is substantial [96, 98, 99].

6.2 Longitudinal and Sequence Data

RWD are often collected over a period of time and may therefore contain multiple observations for one or more variables. Traditionally, these data are collected at frequent and regular time intervals. The recorded observations then describe a smooth trajectory that strongly resembles the underlying time process. In RWD, however, there are many challenges as compared to traditional longitudinal data. First, a large number of variables in the dataset are measured over time. For example, the MIMIC-III dataset contains patient medical records from 2001 to 2012 and includes thousands of variables with repeated measurements [100]. For standard longitudinal or sequence data, the number of variables is generally very small. Second, each variable generally has its own scheme of measurement times, and the measurement interval can be irregular and may even vary across individuals. As illustrated in Fig. 3, many clinical variables in the MIMIC-III dataset are affected by irregular measurement times. For standard longitudinal data, all variables typically follow the same scheme of measurement schedule, and for time series data, the measurement interval is fixed and remains the same for the entire series. Third, complex relationships can exist between measurements of different variables at different time points. Finally, missing data can be confounded with the irregularity of measurement schedule, and when missing data do exist, they tend to be informative and the missing rate can be very high for some variables. Due to these challenges, RWD are highly prone to MNAR mechanisms and intermittent patterns of missingness (Sect. 2.2). Traditional imputation methods are not capable of handling missing data in longitudinal datasets like EHR. In this section, we therefore discuss advanced imputation methods that are dedicated to longitudinal data. These methods can be used to reconstruct the entire trajectory of longitudinal variables for each distinct individual, but also to recover single observations at particular points in time (e.g., at the startpoint or endpoint of the study).

One approach to address the presence of missing values in longitudinal data is to recover each trajectory separately, using methods designed for time series (TS) reconstruction. Although TS methods were originally designed for the analysis of evenly spaced observations, some methods could also be used when measurement times are irregular [101]. It is, for instance, possible to replace the missing values by their respective mean or mode of the repeated measurements. These univariate algorithms are best suited for stationary series (i.e., when statistical properties of the data generation process do not change over time) and should generally be avoided because they tend to introduce bias for non-stationary series. More advanced univariate algorithms for TS imputation may account for trend (i.e., the long-term direction of the data), seasonality (i.e., systematic patterns that repeat periodically), or even certain irregularities (i.e., distribution of the residuals) of the repeated observations [102]. These algorithms often rely on moving averages or interpolation methods, and can be satisfactory when the stretches of missing data are short and if the TS is not much affected by noise [103]. Last observation carried forward (LOCF) is a special type of interpolation, where the last observed value replaces the next missing observations. Another common example is the use of autoregressive integrated moving average (ARIMA) models, which eliminate autoregressive parts from the TS and can also adjust for seasonality. However, because their implementation can distort the data distribution and their relation with other variables, univariate TS algorithms should be used with caution. Instead, multivariate TS algorithms could be used to create time lagged and lead data, and to include smooth basis functions over time in the imputation model [104]. Simulation studies found that this strategy tends to outperform simple univariate TS algorithms [103]. There are several R packages available for missing data imputation in time series. Due to space limitations, we will not list the packages individually, and refer the reader to https://CRAN.R-project.org/view=TimeSeries.

A different class of methods allows borrowing of information across individuals. When repeated measurements are structured in the wide format, time-related variables can be imputed using the methods discussed in Sect. 4 without the need for further adjustment. For instance, the Sequential Organ Failure Assessment (SOFA) score is widely employed in the daily monitoring of acute morbidity in critical care units [105]. It is calculated using information on the patient's respiratory, cardiovascular, hepatic, coagulation, renal and neurological systems, and prone to missing values when some test results are unavailable. For example, most predictors of the SOFA score were affected by missing values in MIMIC-III, with missingness rates ranging from 58.88–99.98% (Fig. 3). When repeated measurements of the SOFA score are formatted into separate columns with daily observations, corresponding variables can be imputed with joint modelling methods such as JM-MVN [30] or with conditional modelling methods such as FCS-fold [106]. Alternatively, recurrent neural networks can be used to capture long-term temporal dependencies without the need for distributional assumptions [29, 102, 107–109]. Also other machine learning methods have been customized to allow for imputation of longitudinal data, including matrix completion and nearest neighbor methods [102]. Unfortunately, these methods are not well suited to recover irregularly spaced observations (Figs. 8 and 9).

Because RWD are rarely collected at regular time intervals, it is often more helpful to structure sequential observations in the long format. Imputation methods then need to adjust for the time of measurement and the non-independence of observations. This requires to adopt hierarchical (also known as multilevel) models that group related observations, which can be achieved using joint modelling or conditional modelling imputation. A detailed overview of imputation methods for longitudinal data is provided by Huque et al. [110]. When adopting multilevel imputation methods, the longitudinal relation

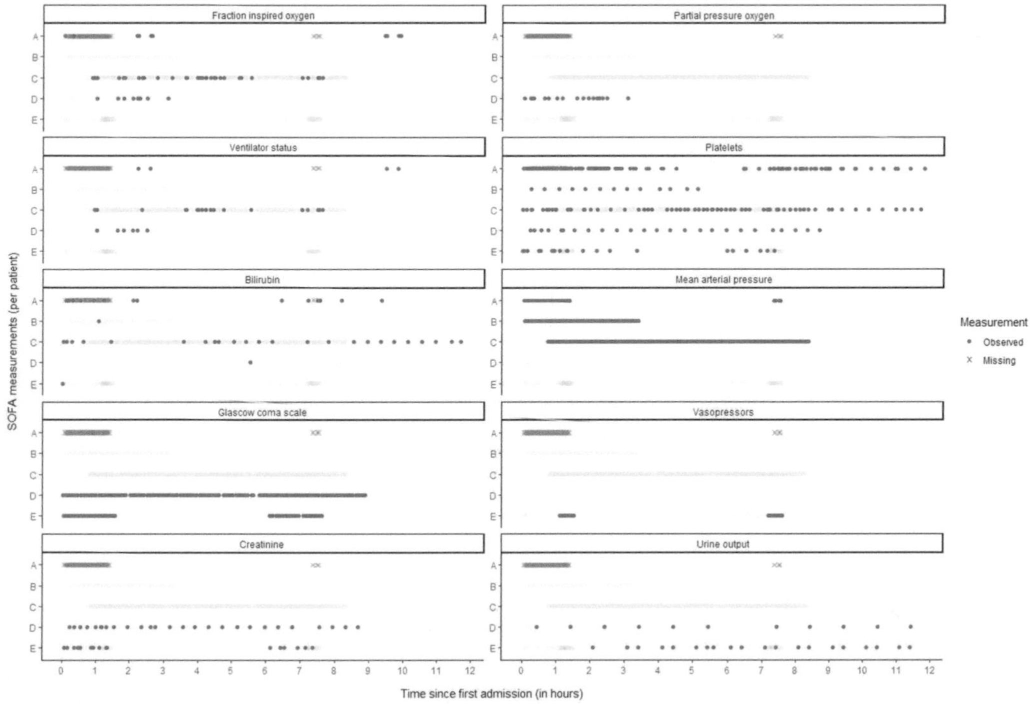

Fig. 8 Illustration of longitudinal data for five patients from MIMIC-III. Repeated measurements are presented for all predictors of the SOFA score. Each point represents a contact moment between the patient and healthcare provider

of repeated observations can be preserved by including measurement time as an explanatory (possibly random) variable. It is then common to assume a linear relationship for the effect of the time variable. Unfortunately, this approach may become problematic when there is no linear association between the incomplete variable and its predictors, when there is no compatibility between the joint distribution and the full conditional model, or when there is a lack of congeniality between the imputation model and the analysis model. Therefore, it has been proposed to adopt Bayesian substantive-model-compatible methods in which the joint distribution of the variables in the imputation model is specified by a substantive analysis model and an incomplete explanatory variable model [36, 111, 112]. Alternatively, van Buuren proposed the time raster imputation method [13] to convert irregular observations into a set of regular measurements using a piecewise linear mixed model. Initially, the user must specify an ordered set of *k* break times. Next, a B-spline model is used to represent each subject's time points with knots that are given by *k*. This approach then yields a k-column matrix *X*. Finally, the incomplete time-dependent variables are imputed using chained equations with a clustering method, using the reference variables, other time-dependent variables and *X* as predictors in the imputation method for each incomplete variable. More recently, Debray et al. developed conditional modelling imputation methods that adjust for clustering and autocorrelation. These methods were implemented using chained equations and can be used to recover missing observations at arbitrary time points [113]. Simulations showed that this approach substantially outperforms simpler imputation methods such as LOCF or rounding, and can also yield valid inferences when longitudinal data are MNAR.

It is also possible to impute longitudinal data using machine learning methods such as recurrent neural networks (RNNs). Although RNNs have been described since 1986 [114], they have rarely been used for longitudinal data analysis until the past decade. Standard RNNs bear many similarities to traditional feedforward neural networks, and can use the output from previous time steps as input for the next time step. In this manner, RNNs offer the ability to handle sequential or time series data. Traditional implementations of RNN cannot process information across many time steps and therefore have a short-term memory. This limitation can be addressed by adopting gated architectures that control the flow of information in the RNN [115]. The long short-term memory (LSTM) [116] and the Gated Recurrent Unit (GRU) are common examples of this architecture [117].

Traditional RNNs require that all variables have the same measurement schedule. For this reason, they are not well suited for the imputation and analysis of RWD. In the past few years, there have been tremendous research developments to facilitate the analysis of multivariate sequence data collected with irregular measurement schedules [102]. RNN methos can, for instance, be enhanced by adopting adversarial training, attention mechanisms, or multidirectional structures. We here distinguish between three common types of RNN for imputation of longitudinal data. A first type of RNN methods generate multiple imputed datasets, and include Bidirectional Recurrent Imputation for Time Series [118], multi-directional recurrent neural networks [119], and residual neural networks [120]. A second, similar type of RNN methods adopt generative adversarial networks to learn the overall distribution of a multivariate time series data and to generate imputed datasets [121]. Finally, a third type of RNN methods do not yield imputed datasets, but offer an integrated solution to the analysis of incomplete longitudinal data. To this purpose, they adopt missing indicators ("masks") and/or the time interval between the observed values as input values of the network [29, 122–124]. To increase the ability to capture long-term relations in the data, these non-imputation methods often adopt a GRU or LSTM architecture. Estimation of aforementioned RNNs is not straightforward and often requires dedicated software packages, which may not always be readily available or easy to use.

6.3 Choosing an Appropriate Imputation Method

The selection of an appropriate imputation method will often depend on the ultimate goal of the data analysis. If the goal is to make statistical inferences, such as estimating regression parameters or testing certain hypotheses, it is important that the imputation method provides not only unbiased estimates of parameters of interest, but also unbiased estimates of their associated (co)variance. On the other hand, if the goal of data analysis is to make predictions or classification, a suitable imputation method should be able to maintain the desired prediction or classification accuracy.

As discussed in this chapter, multiple imputation offers a generic solution to handle the presence of missing data. Multiple imputation can be used in both "inference-focused" and "prediction-focused" studies, and can also be used on a case-by-case basis (e.g., when calculating predictions in clinical practice). Multiple imputation methods that have widely been studied approximate the observed data using a well-known multivariate probability distribution (Sect. 4.1) or approximate this distribution through a series of conditional (often regression-based) models (Sect 4.2). Although these methods can greatly differ in operationalization and underlying assumptions, simulation studies have demonstrated that they generally achieve similar performance [19, 38, 125]. Overall, (semi-)parametric imputation methods can reliably be used for inference and prediction, and tend to perform well in datasets with a limited number of variables. Caution is, however, warranted when complex relations exist in the data (e.g., presence of treatment-covariate interactions), when observations are not independent (e.g., presence of repeated measurements) or when mechanisms of missingness are complex (e.g., presence of MNAR). In these situations, the required complexity of imputation methods drastically increases and manual configuration is often necessary to avoid bias (e.g., see Sects. 6.1 and 6.2) [36, 40]. In this regard, non-parametric methods offer several important advantages. First, there is no need to specify the functional form of the outcome relationship. Instead, non-linear effects and interactions are directly derived from the observed data. Second, there is no need to distinguish between different data types, as most machine learning methods can easily handle discrete, continuous and other data types. Third, because variable selection and dimensionality reduction are integrated into many machine learning procedures, they are well capable of dealing with high-dimensional datasets. Finally, because machine learning methods are extremely flexible, they are well suited to avoid incompatibilities between the imputation and substantive analysis model [40]. This is an important issue when pursuing statistical inference and is often overlooked. Machine learning methods are therefore particularly appealing when there is limited understanding about likely sources of variability in the data, as data-driven procedures are used to determine how the imputations should be generated.

Results from the literature review are summarized in Fig. 9. Each row in this figure represents

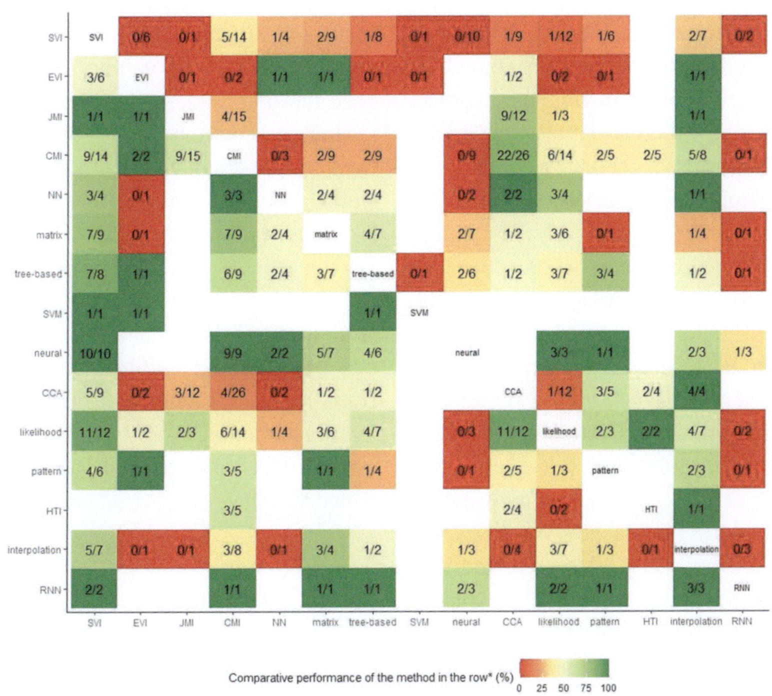

Fig. 9 Comparative performance of imputation methods as identified through a literature review. The color indicates the fraction of simulation studies in which the method in the row outperforms the method in the column. **Single imputation methods**: SVI = single value imputation; EVI = expected value imputation, **Multiple imputation methods**: JMI = joint modelling imputation, CMI = conditional modelling imputation, NN = nearest neighbor imputation, matrix = matrix factorization, tree-based = tree-based ensembles, SVM = support vector machine imputation, generative = neural network-based imputation, **Non-imputation methods**: CCA = complete case analysis, likelihood = likelihood-based approaches, pattern = missing data pattern methods, **Imputation of MNAR**: HTI = Heckman-type imputation, **Imputation of longitudinal data**: interpolation = interpolation methods (incl. last observation carried forward), RNN = recurrent neural networks

one method of accommodating missing data, in order of appearance in this chapter. In particular, we highlight single imputation (single value imputation, expected value imputation), joint modelling imputation, conditional modelling imputation, non-parametric imputation, non-imputation methods, and methods dedicated for informative missingness and longitudinal data. Each cell displays the total number of simulation studies in which the method in the row outperforms the method in the column. Methods that work comparatively well have a higher percentage of papers in which they outperform other methods, signified by rows with many green cells. Most studies evaluated performance by quantifying the mean squared error of imputed values.

Our literature review confirms that missing data is an important problem in RWD and requires dedicated methods. In particular, it is rarely justifiable to delete incomplete records, and to perform a so-called complete case analysis. Although missing values can accurately be recovered by adopting single imputation methods, simulation studies showed that their implementation usually leads to bias when estimating model parameters. For this reason, single imputation methods should be reserved for situations where imputations are needed on a case-by-case basis (e.g., when implementing a prediction model in clinical practice). Conversely, methods that perform consistently well are often based on multiple imputation using neural networks or other non-parametric approaches. As discussed, most of these methods can address mixed data types under various missingness mechanisms, and do not require user input to inform variable selection. Recurrent neural networks appear particularly useful because they can manage informative missingness and incomplete longitudinal data. However, when repeated measurements are relatively sparse, (semi-)parametric approaches that explicitly model their relatedness (e.g., through random effects) may be more suitable. Unfortunately, the implementation of multiple imputation methods can be very demanding w.r.t. available resources and may therefore not always be desirable. As discussed in Sect. 5, it is possible to avoid the need for imputation in some circumstances. For instance, when adopting statistical models for prediction, the presence of missing data can simply be addressed by estimating pattern submodels [92]. These models require fewer assumptions about the missing data mechanisms, and can perform well even when data are MNAR.

Finally, our review highlights several gaps in the published literature. Methods that appear promising but have not extensively been studied are based on SVM, or parametric models that estimate the joint distribution of the data and the missingness. Further, there is little consensus on appropriate strategies to evaluate missing data methods. For example, many simulation studies focus on situations where data are MCAR, or do not consider the validity of statistical inference that is based on imputed datasets. For this reason, it would be helpful to develop guidelines for the conduct and reporting of simulation studies focusing on missing data imputation, to facilitate fair comparisons between methods. For reasons of brevity, our review did not distinguish between different implementations of similar methods, such as the tree-based methods implemented within the chained equations framework. Uniting statistical and machine learning methods holds a promise to obtain imputations that are both accurate and confidence valid.

7 Summary

The analysis of RWD often requires extensive efforts to address data quality issues. In this chapter, we primarily focused on the presence of missing data and discussed several imputation methods. Although these methods are no panacea for poor quality RWD, their implementation may help address situations where RWD are incomplete or require recovery due to temporality or accuracy issues.

1. Assess whether missing data can be handled using non-imputation methods. For example, when the goal is to develop a prediction model, it is possible to avoid the need for imputation by adopting pattern submodels or built-in algorithms for dealing with missing values
2. When pursuing imputation strategies, multiple imputed values should be generated to preserve uncertainty (and thus allow for inference)
3. Include the covariates and outcome from the substantive (analysis) model [78]
4. Include as many variables as possible, especially (auxiliary) variables that are related to the variables of interest or the presence of missingness [24, 78]
5. Consider imputation methods that allow for informative missingness when missing data mechanisms cannot be ignored
6. Especially in very large data sets with many cases and variables (RWD): use flexible imputation models [24]. This can be achieved by adopting machine learning methods that have built-in procedures for variable selection and dimensionality reduction such as neural networks
7. Evaluate the quality of imputed data by inspecting trace plots and distribution of imputed values [125].

Acknowledgements

This project has received funding from the European Union's Horizon 2020 research and innovation programme under ReCoDID grant agreement No 825746.

References

1. Cave A, Kurz X, Arlett P. Real-world data for regulatory decision making: challenges and possible solutions for Europe. Clin Pharmacol Ther. 2019;106(1):36–9.
2. Makady A, de Boer A, Hillege H, Klungel O, Goettsch W. What is real-world data (RWD)? A review of definitions based on literature and stakeholder interviews. Value in Health [Internet]. 2017 May [cited 2017 Jun 12]; Available from: http://linkinghub.elsevier.com/retrieve/pii/S1098301517301717.
3. Cook JA, Collins GS. The rise of big clinical databases. Br J Surg. 2015;102(2):e93–101.
4. Michaels JA. Use of mortality rate after aortic surgery as a performance indicator. Br J Surg. 2003;90(7):827–31.
5. Black N, Payne M. Directory of clinical databases: improving and promoting their use. Qual Saf Health Care. 2003;12(5):348–52.
6. Aylin P, Lees T, Baker S, Prytherch D, Ashley S. Descriptive study comparing routine hospital administrative data with the Vascular Society of Great Britain and Ireland's National Vascular Database. Eur J Vasc Endovasc Surg. 2007;33(4):461–5; discussion 466.
7. Kelly M, Lamah M. Evaluating the accuracy of data entry in a regional colorectal cancer database: implications for national audit. Colorectal Dis. 2007;9(4):337–9.
8. Stey AM, Ko CY, Hall BL, Louie R, Lawson EH, Gibbons MM, et al. Are procedures codes in claims data a reliable indicator of intraoperative splenic injury compared with clinical registry data? J Am Coll Surg. 2014;219(2):237-244.e1.
9. Botsis T, Hartvigsen G, Chen F, Weng C. Secondary use of EHR: data quality issues and informatics opportunities. Summit on Translat Bioinforma. 2010;1(2010):1–5.
10. Peek N, Rodrigues PP. Three controversies in health data science. Int J Data Sci Anal [Internet]. 2018 [cited 2018 Mar 12]; Available from: https://doi.org/10.1007/s41060-018-0109-y.
11. Ehrenstein V, Kharrazi H, Lehmann H, Taylor CO. Obtaining data from electronic health records [Internet]. Tools and technologies for registry interoperability, registries for evaluating patient outcomes: A user's guide, 3rd ed., Addendum 2 [Internet]. Agency for Healthcare Research and Quality (US); 2019 [cited 2021 Aug 27]. Available from: https://www.ncbi.nlm.nih.gov/books/NBK551878/.
12. Feder SL. Data quality in electronic health records research: quality domains and assessment methods. West J Nurs Res. 2018;40(5):753–66.
13. van Buuren S. Longitudinal data. In: Flexible imputation of missing data, 2nd edn. Boca Raton: Chapman and Hall/CRC; 2018. (Chapman & Hall/CRC Interdisciplinary Statistics).
14. Diehl J. Preprocessing and visualization. Aachen, Germany: RWTH Aachen University; 2004 Jan. Report No.: 235087.
15. Rubin DB. Inference and missing data. Biometrika. 1976;63(3):581–92.
16. Carpenter JR, Kenward MG, White IR. Sensitivity analysis after multiple imputation under missing at random: a weighting approach. Stat Methods Med Res. 2007;16(3):259–75.
17. Little RJA, Rubin DB. Statistical analysis with missing data, 2nd edn. Hoboken, NJ: Wiley; 2002. 381 p. (Wiley series in probability and statistics).

18. van Buuren S. Flexible imputation of missing data [Internet], 2nd edn. Boca Raton: CRC Press, Taylor & Francis Group; 2018 [cited 2018 Nov 8]. 415 p. (Chapman & Hall/CRC Interdisciplinary Statistics). Available from: https://stefvanbuuren.name/fimd/.
19. Audigier V, White IR, Jolani S, Debray TPA, Quartagno M, Carpenter JR, et al. Multiple imputation for multilevel data with continuous and binary variables. Stat Sci. 2018;33(2):160–83.
20. Debray TPA, Snell KIE, Quartagno M, Jolani S, Moons KGM, Riley RD. Dealing with missing data in an IPD meta-analysis. In: Individual participant data meta-analysis: a handbook for healthcare research. Hoboken, NJ: Wiley; 2021. (Wiley series in statistics in practice).
21. Hunt NB, Gardarsdottir H, Bazelier MT, Klungel OH, Pajouheshnia R. A systematic review of how missing data are handled and reported in multi-database pharmacoepidemiologic studies. Pharmacoepidemiol Drug Saf. 2021;pds.5245.
22. Troyanskaya O, Cantor M, Sherlock G, Brown P, Hastie T, Tibshirani R, et al. Missing value estimation methods for DNA microarrays. Bioinformatics. 2001;17(6):520–5.
23. Murray JS. Multiple imputation: a review of practical and theoretical findings. Statist Sci [Internet]. 2018 [cited 2021 May 7];33(2). Available from: https://projecteuclid.org/journals/statistical-science/volume-33/issue-2/Multiple-Imputation-A-Review-of-Practical-and-Theoretical-Findings/10.1214/18-STS644.full.
24. Fernández-Delgado M, Cernadas E, Barro S, Amorim D. Do we need hundreds of classifiers to solve real world classification problems? J Mach Learn Res. 2014;15(90):3133–81.
25. van de Schoot R, de Bruin J, Schram R, Zahedi P, de Boer J, Weijdema F, et al. An open source machine learning framework for efficient and transparent systematic reviews. Nat Mach Intell. 2021;3(2):125–33.
26. Van de Schoot R, De Bruin J, Schram R, Zahedi P, De Boer J, Weijdema F, et al. ASReview: active learning for systematic reviews [Internet]. Zenodo; 2021 [cited 2021 Sep 8]. Available from: https://zenodo.org/record/5126631.
27. Johnson AEW, Pollard TJ, Shen L, Lehman LH, Feng M, Ghassemi M, et al. MIMIC-III, a freely accessible critical care database. Sci Data. 2016;24(3): 160035.
28. Johnson A, Pollard T, Mark R. MIMIC-III Clinical Database [Internet]. PhysioNet; 2019 [cited 2021 Sep 24]. Available from: https://physionet.org/content/mimiciii-demo.
29. Che Z, Purushotham S, Cho K, Sontag D, Liu Y. Recurrent neural networks for multivariate time series with missing values. Sci Rep. 2018;8(1):6085.
30. Schafer JL, Graham JW. Missing data: our view of the state of the art. Psychol Methods. 2002;7(2):147–77.
31. Nijman SWJ, Hoogland J, Groenhof TKJ, Brandjes M, Jacobs JJL, Bots ML, et al. Real-time imputation of missing predictor values in clinical practice. Eur Heart J Digital Health. 2020;2(1):154–64.
32. Nijman SWJ, Groenhof TKJ, Hoogland J, Bots ML, Brandjes M, Jacobs JJL, et al. Real-time imputation of missing predictor values improved the application of prediction models in daily practice. J Clin Epidemiol. 2021;19(134):22–34.
33. Rubin DB. Multiple imputation for nonresponse in surveys. New York: Wiley; 1987.
34. Harel O, Mitchell EM, Perkins NJ, Cole SR, Tchetgen Tchetgen EJ, Sun B, et al. Multiple Imputation for Incomplete Data in Epidemiologic Studies. Am J Epidemiol. 2018;187(3):576–84.
35. Carpenter JR, Kenward MG. Multiple imputation and its application [Internet]. 1st ed. John Wiley & Sons, Ltd; 2013 [cited 2014 Dec 18]. (Statistics in Practice). Available from: https://doi.org/10.1002/9781119942283.
36. Erler NS, Rizopoulos D, Jaddoe VW, Franco OH, Lesaffre EM. Bayesian imputation of time-varying covariates in linear mixed models. Stat Methods Med Res. 2019;28(2):555–68.
37. Erler NS, Rizopoulos D, Rosmalen J van, Jaddoe VWV, Franco OH, Lesaffre EMEH. Dealing with missing covariates in epidemiologic studies: a comparison between multiple imputation and a full Bayesian approach. Stat Med. (2016).
38. Hughes RA, White IR, Seaman SR, Carpenter JR, Tilling K, Sterne JAC. Joint modelling rationale for chained equations. BMC Med Res Methodol. 2014;14:28.
39. Buuren S, Groothuis-Oudshoorn K. mice: Multivariate imputation by chained equations in R. J Statistical Software [Internet]. 2011;45(3). Available from: http://doc.utwente.nl/78938/.
40. Meng X-L. Multiple-imputation inferences with uncongenial sources of input. Stat Sci. 1994;9(4):538–58.
41. Tutz G, Ramzan S. Improved methods for the imputation of missing data by nearest neighbor methods. Comput Stat Data Anal. 2015;1(90):84–99.
42. Bay SD. Combining nearest neighbor classifiers through multiple feature subsets. In: Proceedings of the fifteenth international conference on machine learning. San Francisco, CA, USA: Morgan Kaufmann Publishers Inc.; 1998. p. 37–45. (ICML '98).
43. Ding Y, Ross A. A comparison of imputation methods for handling missing scores in biometric fusion. Pattern Recogn. 2012;45(3):919–33.
44. Vink G, Frank LE, Pannekoek J, van Buuren S. Predictive mean matching imputation of semicontinuous variables: PMM imputation of semicontinuous variables. Stat Neerl. 2014;68(1):61–90.
45. Faisal S, Tutz G. Multiple imputation using nearest neighbor methods. Inf Sci. 2021;570:500–16.

46. Jadhav A, Pramod D, Ramanathan K. Comparison of performance of data imputation methods for numeric dataset. Appl Artif Intell. 2019;33(10):913–33.
47. Jerez JM, Molina I, García-Laencina PJ, Alba E, Ribelles N, Martín M, et al. Missing data imputation using statistical and machine learning methods in a real breast cancer problem. Artif Intell Med. 2010;50(2):105–15.
48. Thomas T, Rajabi E. A systematic review of machine learning-based missing value imputation techniques. Data Tech Appl. 2021;55(4):558–85.
49. Marimont RB, Shapiro MB. Nearest neighbour searches and the curse of dimensionality. IMA J Appl Math. 1979;24(1):59–70.
50. Davenport MA, Romberg J. An overview of low-rank matrix recovery from incomplete observations. IEEE J Sel Top Sig Proc. 2016;10(4):608–22.
51. Li XP, Huang L, So HC, Zhao B. A survey on matrix completion: Perspective of Signal Processing. arXiv:190110885 [eess] [Internet]. 2019 May 7 [cited 2021 Aug 20]; Available from: http://arxiv.org/abs/1901.10885.
52. Sportisse A, Boyer C, Josse J. Imputation and low-rank estimation with Missing Not At Random data. arXiv:181211409 [cs, stat] [Internet]. 2020 Jan 29 [cited 2021 Aug 20]; Available from: http://arxiv.org/abs/1812.11409.
53. Hernandez-Lobato JM, Houlsby N, Ghahramani Z. Probabilistic Matrix Factorization with non-random missing data. In: International conference on machine learning [Internet]. PMLR; 2014 [cited 2021 Aug 20]. p. 1512–20. Available from: https://proceedings.mlr.press/v32/hernandez-lobatob14.html.
54. Stekhoven DJ, Bühlmann P. MissForest—non-parametric missing value imputation for mixed-type data. Bioinformatics. 2012;28(1):112–8.
55. Shah AD, Bartlett JW, Carpenter J, Nicholas O, Hemingway H. Comparison of random forest and parametric imputation models for imputing missing data using MICE: a caliber study. Am J Epidemiol. 2014;179(6):764–74.
56. Ramosaj B, Pauly M. Who wins the miss contest for imputation methods? Our vote for miss BooPF. arXiv: 171111394 [stat] [Internet]. 2017 Nov 30 [cited 2021 Aug 24]; Available from: http://arxiv.org/abs/1711.11394.
57. Tang F, Ishwaran H. Random forest missing data algorithms. Stat Anal Data Min. 2017;10(6):363–77.
58. Breiman L. Manual for setting up, using, and understanding random forest V4.0 [Internet]. 2003. Available from: https://www.stat.berkeley.edu/~breiman/Using_random_forests_v4.0.pdf.
59. Ishwaran H, Kogalur UB, Blackstone EH, Lauer MS. Random survival forests. The Ann Appl Stat. 2008;2(3):841–60.
60. Burgette LF, Reiter JP. Multiple imputation for missing data via sequential regression trees. Am J Epidemiol. 2010;172(9):1070–6.
61. Hong S, Lynn HS. Accuracy of random-forest-based imputation of missing data in the presence of non-normality, non-linearity, and interaction. BMC Med Res Methodol. 2020;20(1):199.
62. Cortes C, Vapnik V. Support-vector networks. Mach Learn. 1995;20(3):273–97.
63. Vapnik V. The nature of statistical learning theory [Internet], 2nd edn. New York: Springer-Verlag; 2000 [cited 2021 Aug 24]. (Information Science and Statistics). Available from: https://www.springer.com/gp/book/9780387987804.
64. Pereira RC, Santos MS, Rodrigues PP, Abreu PH. Reviewing autoencoders for missing data imputation: technical trends, applications and outcomes. J Artif Intell Res. 2020;14(69):1255–85.
65. Beaulieu-Jones BK, Moore JH. Missing data imputation in the electronic health record using deeply learned autoencoders. Pac Symp Biocomput. 2017;22:207–18.
66. Vincent P, Larochelle H, Bengio Y, Manzagol P-A. Extracting and composing robust features with denoising autoencoders. In: Proceedings of the 25th international conference on machine learning [Internet]. New York, NY, USA: Association for Computing Machinery; 2008 [cited 2021 Aug 25]. p. 1096–103. (ICML '08). Available from: https://doi.org/10.1145/1390156.1390294.
67. Gondara L, Wang K. MIDA: multiple Imputation using denoising autoencoders. arXiv: 170502737 [cs, stat] [Internet]. 2018 Feb 17 [cited 2021 Aug 25]; Available from: http://arxiv.org/abs/1705.02737.
68. Lall R, Robinson T. The MIDAS touch: accurate and scalable missing-data imputation with deep learning. Polit Anal. 2021;26:1–18.
69. Kingma DP, Welling M. Auto-encoding variational bayes. arXiv:13126114 [cs, stat] [Internet]. 2014 May 1 [cited 2021 Aug 25]; Available from: http://arxiv.org/abs/1312.6114.
70. Rezende DJ, Mohamed S, Wierstra D. Stochastic backpropagation and approximate inference in deep generative models. In: Proceedings of the 31st international conference on international conference on machine learning, Vol. 32. Beijing, China: JMLR.org; 2014. p. II-1278-II–1286. (ICML'14).
71. Ma C, Tschiatschek S, Turner R, Hernández-Lobato JM, Zhang C. VAEM: a deep generative model for heterogeneous mixed type data. In: Advances in neural information processing systems [Internet]. Curran Associates, Inc.; 2020 [cited 2021 Aug 25]. p. 11237–47. Available from: https://papers.nips.cc/paper/2020/hash/8171ac2c5544a5cb54ac0f38bf477af4-Abstract.html.

72. Goodfellow IJ, Pouget-Abadie J, Mirza M, Xu B, Warde-Farley D, Ozair S, et al. Generative adversarial networks. arXiv:14062661 [cs, stat] [Internet]. 2014 Jun 10 [cited 2021 Aug 25]; Available from: http://arxiv.org/abs/1406.2661.
73. Li SC-X, Jiang B, Marlin B. MisGAN: learning from incomplete data with generative adversarial networks. arXiv:190209599 [cs, stat] [Internet]. 2019 Feb 25 [cited 2021 Aug 25]; Available from: http://arxiv.org/abs/1902.09599.
74. Shang C, Palmer A, Sun J, Chen K-S, Lu J, Bi J. VIGAN: missing view imputation with generative adversarial networks. arXiv:170806724 [cs, stat] [Internet]. 2017 Nov 1 [cited 2021 Aug 25]; Available from: http://arxiv.org/abs/1708.06724.
75. Yoon J, Jordon J, van der Schaar M. GAIN: missing data imputation using generative adversarial nets. arXiv:180602920 [cs, stat] [Internet]. 2018 Jun 7 [cited 2021 Aug 25]; Available from: http://arxiv.org/abs/1806.02920.
76. van Buuren S. Rubin's rules. In: Flexible imputation of missing data, 2nd edn. Boca Raton: CRC Press, Taylor & Francis Group; 2018. (Chapman & Hall/ CRC Interdisciplinary Statistics).
77. White IR, Royston P, Wood AM. Multiple imputation using chained equations: issues and guidance for practice. Stat Med. 2011;30(4):377–99.
78. Vink G, van Buuren S. Pooling multiple imputations when the sample happens to be the population. arXiv:14098542 [math, stat] [Internet]. 2014 Sep 30 [cited 2021 Aug 27]; Available from: http://arxiv.org/abs/1409.8542..
79. Wood AM, White IR, Royston P. How should variable selection be performed with multiply imputed data? Stat Med. 2008;27(17):3227–46.
80. Marshall A, Altman DG, Holder RL, Royston P. Combining estimates of interest in prognostic modelling studies after multiple imputation: current practice and guidelines. BMC Med Res Methodol. 2009;28(9):57.
81. Zhao Y, Long Q. Variable selection in the presence of missing data: imputation-based methods. Wiley Interdiscip Rev Comput Stat. 2017;9(5): e1402.
82. Little RJA. Regression with missing X's: a review. J Am Stat Assoc. 1992;87(420):1227–37.
83. Herring AH, Ibrahim JG. Likelihood-based methods for missing covariates in the cox proportional hazards model. J Am Stat Assoc. 2001;96(453):292–302.
84. Xie Y, Zhang B. Empirical Likelihood in Nonignorable covariate-missing data problems. Int J Biostat. [Internet]. 2017 [cited 2021 Sep 21];13(1). Available from: https://www.degruyter.com/document/doi/10.1515/ijb-2016-0053/html.
85. Fletcher Mercaldo S, Blume JD. Missing data and prediction: the pattern submodel. Biostatistics [Internet]. 2018 [cited 2018 Sep 27]; Available from: https://academic.oup.com/biostatistics/advance-article/doi/10.1093/biostatistics/kxy040/5092384.
86. Breiman L. Classification and regression trees. Wadsworth International Group; 1984. 376 p.
87. Chen T, Guestrin C. XGBoost: A scalable tree boosting system. Proceedings of the 22nd ACM SIGKDD international conference on knowledge discovery and data mining - KDD '16. 2016;785–94.
88. van Smeden M, Groenwold RHH, Moons KG. A cautionary note on the use of the missing indicator method for handling missing data in prediction research. J Clin Epidemiol. 2020.
89. Goldstein BA, Navar AM, Pencina MJ, Ioannidis JP. Opportunities and challenges in developing risk prediction models with electronic health records data: a systematic review. J Am Med Inform Assoc. 2016.
90. Haneuse S, Arterburn D, Daniels MJ. Assessing Missing Data Assumptions in EHR-Based Studies: A Complex and Underappreciated Task. JAMA Netw Open. 2021;4(2): e210184.
91. Hardt J, Herke M, Leonhart R. Auxiliary variables in multiple imputation in regression with missing X: a warning against including too many in small sample research. BMC Med Res Methodol. 2012;12:184.
92. Ibrahim JG, Molenberghs G. Missing data methods in longitudinal studies: a review. Test (Madr). 2009;18(1):1–43.
93. Michiels B, Molenberghs G, Bijnens L, Vangeneugden T, Thijs H. Selection models and pattern-mixture models to analyse longitudinal quality of life data subject to drop-out. Stat Med. 2002;21(8):1023–41.
94. Creemers A, Hens N, Aerts M, Molenberghs G, Verbeke G, Kenward MG. Generalized shared-parameter models and missingness at random. Stat Model. 2011;11(4):279–310.
95. Heckman JJ. The common structure of statistical models of truncation, sample selection and limited dependent variables and a simple estimator for such models. Ann Econ Soc Meas. 1976;5(4):475–92.
96. Koné S, Bonfoh B, Dao D, Koné I, Fink G. Heckman-type selection models to obtain unbiased estimates with missing measures outcome: theoretical considerations and an application to missing birth weight data. BMC Med Res Methodol. 2019;19(1):231.
97. Muñoz J, Hufstedler H, Gustafson P, Bärnighausen T, De Jong VMT, Debray TPA (2023) Dealing with missing data using the Heckman selection model: methods primer for epidemiologists. Int J Epidemiol 2(1):5–13
98. Galimard J-E, Chevret S, Curis E, Resche-Rigon M. Heckman imputation models for binary or continuous MNAR outcomes and MAR predictors. BMC Med Res Methodol. 2018;18(1):90.
99. Holmes FW. A comparison of the heckman selection model, ibrahim, and lipsitz methods for dealing with nonignorable missing data. J Psychiatry Behav Sci. 2021;4(1):1045.

100. Deasy J, Liò P, Ercole A. Dynamic survival prediction in intensive care units from heterogeneous time series without the need for variable selection or curation. Sci Rep. 2020;10(1):22129.
101. Eckner A. A Framework for the analysis of unevenly spaced time series data [Internet]. 2014 [cited 2021 Sep 24]. Available from: https://www.semanticscholar.org/paper/A-Framework-for-the-Analysis-of-Unevenly-Spaced-Eckner/bb307aa6671a5a65314d3a26fffa6c7ef48a3c86.
102. Fang C, Wang C. Time series data imputation: a survey on deep learning approaches. arXiv: 201111347 [cs] [Internet]. 2020 Nov 23 [cited 2021 Aug 25]; Available from: http://arxiv.org/abs/2011.11347.
103. Bauer J, Angelini O, Denev A. Imputation of multivariate time series data - performance benchmarks for multiple imputation and spectral techniques. SSRN J [Internet]. 2017 [cited 2021 Aug 27]; Available from: https://www.ssrn.com/abstract=2996611.
104. Zhang Z. Multiple imputation for time series data with Amelia package. Ann Transl Med. 2016;4(3):56.
105. Lambden S, Laterre PF, Levy MM, Francois B. The SOFA score—development, utility and challenges of accurate assessment in clinical trials. Crit Care. 2019;23(1):374.
106. Nevalainen J, Kenward MG, Virtanen SM. Missing values in longitudinal dietary data: a multiple imputation approach based on a fully conditional specification. Stat Med. 2009;28(29):3657–69.
107. Guo Y, Liu Z, Krishnswamy P, Ramasamy S. Bayesian recurrent framework for missing data imputation and prediction with clinical time series. arXiv: 191107572 [cs, stat] [Internet]. 2019 [cited 2021 May 7]; Available from: http://arxiv.org/abs/1911.07572..
108. Yu K, Zhang M, Cui T, Hauskrecht M. Monitoring ICU mortality risk with a long short-term memory recurrent neural network. Pac Symp Biocomput. 2020;25:103–14.
109. Li Q, Xu Y. VS-GRU: a variable sensitive gated recurrent neural network for multivariate time series with massive missing values. Appl Sci. 2019;9(15):3041.
110. Huque MH, Carlin JB, Simpson JA, Lee KJ. A comparison of multiple imputation methods for missing data in longitudinal studies. BMC Med Res Methodol. 2018;18(1):168.
111. Enders CK, Du H, Keller BT. A model-based imputation procedure for multilevel regression models with random coefficients, interaction effects, and nonlinear terms. Psychol Methods. 2020;25(1):88–112.
112. Goldstein H, Carpenter JR, Browne WJ. Fitting multilevel multivariate models with missing data in responses and covariates that may include interactions and non-linear terms. J R Stat Soc A Stat Soc. 2014;177(2):553–64.
113. Debray TP, Simoneau G, Copetti M, Platt RW, Shen C, Pellegrini F et al (2023) Methods for comparative effectiveness based on time to confirmed disability progression with irregular observations in multiple sclerosis. Stat Methods Med Res. https://doi.org/10.1177/09622802231172032
114. Rumelhart DE, Hinton GE, Williams RJ. Learning representations by back-propagating errors. Nature. 1986;323(6088):533–6.
115. Weerakody PB, Wong KW, Wang G, Ela W. A review of irregular time series data handling with gated recurrent neural networks. Neurocomputing. 2021;21(441):161–78.
116. Hochreiter S, Schmidhuber J. Long short-term memory. Neural Comput. 1997;9(8):1735–80.
117. Cho K, van Merriënboer B, Gulcehre C, Bahdanau D, Bougares F, Schwenk H, et al. Learning phrase representations using rnn encoder–decoder for statistical machine translation. In: Proceedings of the 2014 conference on empirical methods in natural language processing (EMNLP) [Internet]. Doha, Qatar: Association for Computational Linguistics; 2014 [cited 2021 Sep 22]. p. 1724–34. Available from: https://aclanthology.org/D14-1179.
118. Cao W, Wang D, Li J, Zhou H, Li L, Li Y. BRITS: Bidirectional recurrent imputation for time series. In: Advances in neural information processing systems [Internet]. Curran Associates, Inc.; 2018 [cited 2021 Sep 22]. Available from: https://proceedings.neurips.cc/paper/2018/hash/734e6bfcd358e25ac1db0a4241b95651-Abstract.html.
119. Yoon J, Zame WR, van der Schaar M. Estimating missing data in temporal data streams using multi-directional recurrent neural networks. IEEE Trans Biomed Eng. 2019;66(5):1477–90.
120. He K, Zhang X, Ren S, Sun J. Deep residual learning for image recognition. In: 2016 IEEE conference on computer vision and pattern recognition (CVPR). 2016. p. 770–8.
121. Luo Y, Cai X, ZHANG Y, Xu J, Xiaojie Y. Multivariate time series imputation with generative adversarial networks. In: Advances in neural information processing systems [Internet]. Curran Associates, Inc.; 2018 [cited 2021 Sep 22]. Available from: https://papers.nips.cc/paper/2018/hash/96b9bff013acedfb1d140579e2fbeb63-Abstract.html.
122. Lipton ZC, Kale DC, Wetzel R. Modeling Missing Data in Clinical time series with RNNs. Proc Mach Learn Healthc. 2016;2016:17.
123. Baytas IM, Xiao C, Zhang XS, Wang F, Jain AK, Zhou J. Patient subtyping via time-aware LSTM networks. KDD. 2017.

124. Choi E, Bahadori MT, Schuetz A, Stewart WF, Sun J. Doctor AI: Predicting clinical events via recurrent neural networks. In: Proceedings of the 1st machine learning for healthcare conference [Internet]. PMLR; 2016 [cited 2021 Sep 22]. p. 301–18. Available from: https://proceedings.mlr.press/v56/Choi16.html
125. Quartagno M, Carpenter JR. Multiple imputation for discrete data: Evaluation of the joint latent normal model. Biom J. 2019;61(4):1003–19.
126. Raghunathan T, Bondarenko I. Diagnostics for multiple imputations [Internet]. Rochester, NY: Social Science Research Network; 2007 Nov [cited 2021 Sep 24]. Report No.: ID 1031750. Available from: https://papers.ssrn.com/abstract=1031750.

Data Standards and Terminology Including Biomedical Ontologies

Spiros Denaxas and Christian Stoeckert

Abstract

Electronic health records are routinely collected as part of care and have variable data types, quality and structure. As a result, there is a need for standardization of clinical data from health records if these are to be used in software applications for data mining and/or machine learning and artificial intelligence approaches. Clinical terminologies and classification systems are available that can serve as standards to enable the harmonization of disparate data sources. In this chapter, we discuss different types of biomedical semantic standards including medically-relevant ontologies, their uses, and their limitations. We also discuss the application of semantic standards in order to provide features for use in machine learning particularly with respect to phenotypes. Finally, we discuss potential areas of improvement for the future such as covering genotypes and steps needed.

S. Denaxas (✉)
Institute of Health Informatics, University College London, London, UK
e-mail: s.denaxas@ucl.ac.uk

Data Science Centre, British Heart Foundation, London, UK

C. Stoeckert
University Of Pennsylvania, Philadelphia, USA
e-mail: stoeckrt@pennmedicine.upenn.edu

Keywords

EHR · Semantic standards · Ontologies · Clinical terminologies

1 Introduction

Medicine is inherently a data driven practice. The widespread adoption of electronic health record (EHR) systems in the US and Europe has rapidly increased the amounts of health related data that are electronically generated and captured during routine interactions of patients with the healthcare system [1]. Patient interactions with the healthcare system, for example an outpatient visit or a hospital admission, generate a substantial amount of data and metadata. These data are organized, recorded and curated using different healthcare standards and clinical terminologies. Healthcare standards enable the storage and exchange of health information across healthcare providers while clinical terminologies enable the systematic and standardized recording of healthcare information.

Before raw EHR data can be used as input features into analytical AI pipelines, a significant amount of preprocessing and harmonization must occur. For example, multiple EHR sources utilizing different clinical terminologies to record information need to be aligned to a common format. With unstructured data, such

F. W. Asselbergs et al. (eds.), *Clinical Applications of Artificial Intelligence in Real-World Data*,
https://doi.org/10.1007/978-3-031-36678-9_3

as information recorded in clinical text, Natural Language Processing (NLP) approaches can be deployed to extract clinically-meaningful markers and transform them into input features for the pipeline (this process is often referred as entity extraction). Finally, depending on the purpose of each dataset, different biases might exist in the data which need to be accounted for. For example, administrative hospitalization EHR might be influenced by local coding guidelines which in turn affect the observed data recording patterns and need to be accounted for prior to analyses.

The outcome of such a data preprocessing pipeline would be features extracted from complex, multidimensional EHR that can be used as input features to AI analytical approaches. Extracting clinically important markers from complex EHR (e.g. disease status, biomarkers, prescriptions, procedures, symptoms etc.) is often referred to as phenotyping [2]. The main objective therefore of this chapter is to provide a succinct overview of the main clinical terminologies used to record EHR data, their characteristics, and outline different approaches for creating and evaluating EHR-derived phenotypes. The methods outlined here will cover a set of phenotyping methodologies ranging from rule-based deterministic algorithms, to aggregated coding systems and finally to more complex learnt representations).

1.1 The Need for Standards and Their Application

Standards in the context of this chapter are defined as common representations of data. They may be approved by a governing body (e.g., ISO dates [3]) or they may simply represent established formats (Variant Call Format (VCF) files of genomic variants [4]). For clinical terminologies, standards may be mandated by the government, institution (e.g., National Institutes of Health [5]), or professional societies. Terminologies may be developed by communities adhering to common principles (e.g., OBO Foundry [6]).

Standards are needed in healthcare to effectively find, store and analyze data. If different representations are used for syntax and semantics, there is no guarantee that the data used for analysis is complete or can be correctly combined across sources. If data is not standardized, it can prevent information sharing and reuse of clinical data [7]. Often data can come from different systems even within the same institution and mappings to a common standard is needed. The challenge however is that there may be competing standards (PCORNet [8], FHIR [9], OMOP [10] and others).

To understand the need and application of standards consider the how, when and why data are generated during routine clinical interactions. Data can be generated by physicians and healthcare professionals entering data directly in the EHR for patient care. Data can also be generated through clinical coding for billing and reimbursement purposes can subsequently be used for research FInally, data may be processed and curated through clinical audits for registries, quality of care, and planning. Each of these may use different systems with different representations that need to be harmonized before analyses. Furthermore, different stakeholders and systems may attempt to record the same information but choose different levels of granularity. For example a healthcare professional might record detailed information on presenting signs, symptoms and diagnoses while a clinical coder might distill this information into a small number of terminology concepts. A coding system therefore should be able to account for these differences and enable their harmonization.

In this section, we will provide working definitions of key concepts in data standardization to guide understanding of the different options and complexity of choosing and applying a standard. An excellent review of different semantic representations is provided elsewhere [11]. Here we highlight commonly used and mentioned types of semantic standards and provide details of different levels of standardization and what they offer.

Semantic standards can be understood at three levels of abstraction of increasing complexity. The first is as entities (terms) that make up classes (general concepts) and instances (individual members) of those classes. For example, 'heart failure' is a class whereas 'the first heart failure diagnosis of a patient' is an instance of that class. Most usage of terminologies and ontologies is at this first level where terms are used as annotations. A second level is the organization of the entities into structures such as hierarchies or assertions and statements including axioms and logical definitions. Hierarchies can be simple taxonomies ('heart failure' is-a 'disorder of cardiac function') or can be poly-hierarchies to accommodate a term having more than one parent. The structure of assertions/statements can be in the form of triples: subject-predicate-object such as: 'heart failure' 'occurs in' 'heart structure'. These structures provide the ability to connect concepts in a defined manner. The third level is the representational model adhering to open versus closed worlds and languages such as Resource Description Framework (RDF) [12], Web Ontology Language (OWL), Simple Knowledge Organization System (SKOS) [13] and schema languages as part of the Semantic Web [14]. These can be employed in messaging systems such as FHIR and Common Data Models (CDM) like Observational Medical Outcomes Partnership (OMOP). The products of semantic standards can be browsed in repositories such as the NCBO BioPortal [15] or used in knowledge bases linking classes or terms (TBox) to instances or assertions (ABox) about data [16].

Clinical classification systems, medical ontologies, and clinical terminologies make use of these different levels of abstraction. In this context, ontologies are distinguished by formal relations between entities and use of logical definitions or axioms. The W3C provides approved standards such as OWL and a query language (SPARQL) which enables ontologies based on these standards to be programmatically accessed and searched [12]. Clinically relevant ontologies include the Disease Ontology [17], the Drug Ontology [18], and the Ontology for Biomedical Investigations [19] which can be used to link to diagnoses, medications, and lab tests respectively in EHR. Those ontologies, which are part of the OBO Foundry, not only provide hierarchies for capturing related data at different levels of granularity but also have formal links to other external ontologies (e.g., for chemicals in CHEBI [20]) that can be used to connect them and build more complex knowledge structures (e.g., classes of drugs containing chemicals that are used as an antineoplastic agent).

Multiple ontologies or terminologies may be needed to annotate or instantiate data. When this is done, care should be taken to avoid conflicts or redundancies, i.e. the chosen terminologies should be semantically interoperable. This however is not guaranteed if different sources of terms are used as they can have different contexts and thus different meanings. With the OBO Foundry, the objective is that adhering ontologies are semantically consistent with respect to meaning of terms and use of relations.

2 Controlled Clinical Terminologies and Clinical Classifications Systems

EHR provide the infrastructure for healthcare professionals to record information that is relevant for the care of a patient. This information can include symptoms, medical history information on the patient or their direct family, laboratory or anthropometric measurements, prescriptions, diagnoses, and surgical procedures. The data recorded within the EHR allow healthcare professionals to assess and treat a patient but are also widely used for a number of other purposes (often referred to as secondary uses) such as reimbursement, planning, billing, auditing and research. Although clinical terminologies and clinical classification systems are often used interchangeably, they serve two distinct purposes [21]. The former were created to enable healthcare professionals to record information that is pertinent to clinical care. The latter are a tool which enables the aggregation and statistical analyses of health information (Table 1).

Controlled clinical terminologies (also referred to as controlled clinical ontologies, controlled medical ontologies, controlled medical vocabularies) are the basic building blocks used by healthcare professionals to record information within an EHR system. The main purpose of clinical terminologies is to enable the consistent and systematic recording of clinical data and metadata which in turn are used for direct patient care. As a result, controlled clinical terminologies often encapsulate a wide and diverse set of domains and healthcare-related actions.

The US Bureau of Labor Statistics defines classification systems as "ways of grouping and organizing data so that they may be compared with other data" [22]. In the context of medicine, clinical classification systems enable the aggregation and analysis of data related to health can healthcare on a national or international level. One of the most commonly used classification systems worldwide is the ICD-10 which is maintained by the World Health Organization (WHO) [23]. Clinical classification systems are also used for other secondary purposes, one of the most common being reimbursement where clinical data get transformed and aggregated into a clinical classification system. The process by which raw data are transformed into ICD codes is defined as *coding*. The WHO defines coding as "the translation of diagnoses, procedures, comorbidities and complications that occur over the course of a patient's encounter from medical terminology to an internationally coded syntax" [24].

2.1 SNOMED-CT

SNOMED Clinical Terms (SNOMED-CT) is a controlled clinical terminology providing a set of hierarchically-organized, machine-readable codes, terms, synonyms and definitions used to record information related to health and healthcare within EHR information systems [25]. SNOMED-CT is maintained and distributed by the International Health Terminology Standards Development Organisation (IHTSDO). SNOMED-CT was created in 1965 as the Systematized Nomenclature of Pathology (SNOP) which in turn evolved in the SNOMED Reference Terminology (SNOMED-RT) and finally merged with the NHS Clinical Terms Version 3 (Read codes Version 3, CTV3) [26] to create SNOMED-CT in 2002. Similarly to ICD, different countries can maintain their own versions of SNOMED-CT that are tailored to their local healthcare system or needs; in the UK for example, the National Health Service (NHS) maintains a UK version of SNOMED-CT [27] that is used.

SNOMED-CT consists of three components [28] which are explained below (Tables 2 and 3):

Table 1 Comparison between ICD-10 (statistical classification system) and SNOMED (clinical terminology

	ICD-10	SNOMED-CT
Type	Clinical classification system	Controlled clinical terminology
N concepts	10^4	10^5
Relationships	A concept has a single parent	A concept can have multiple hierarchical relationships and multiple parents
Age related diagnoses	Information on age is encapsulated within the term	The term used is the same across all ages and the age of onset is derived by the date of diagnosis and the age of the patient
Fidelity	Information organized in mutually exclusive categories with generic "not otherwise specified" or "not elsewhere classified" terms used to record information if required	NOS/NEC are not used in SNOMED-CT

1. **Concept**: Every SNOMED-CT concept represents a unique clinical meaning and has a unique numerical identifier which is persistent across the ontology and can be used to reference the concept. The January 2021 version of SNOMED CT contains approximately 350,000 concepts.
2. **Description**: Each SNOMED-CT concept has a unique description, the Fully Specified Name (FSN), which offers an unambiguous description of the concept's meaning. Additionally, a concept can have one or more synonym terms (*Synonyms*) which are associated with the concept.
3. **Relationship**: SNOMED-CT offers several types of relationships between concepts in order to enable logical computable definitions of complex concepts. The terminology contains approx 1.4 million relationship entries defining these. All concepts are organized in an acyclic hierarchy using the "is-a" relationship and concepts can have multiple parents (as opposed to most statistical classification systems that only support a single parent child relationship). Additionally, SNOMED-CT offers more than 60 other relationship types for example finding site, causative agent and associate morphology.

Table 2 Example SNOMED-CT concept core components

Fully specified name	Heart failure (disorder)
SCTID	84,114,007
Synonyms	Heart failure Myocardial failure Weak heart Cardiac failure Heart failure (disorder) HF—Heart failure Cardiac insufficiency
Parents	Disorder of cardiac function (disorder)
Finding site (relationship)	Heart structure

Subsets of SNOMED-CT components (e.g. of concepts, their descriptions and relationships between concepts) can be represented using a standardized approach enabled by *Reference Sets*. Reference Sets are commonly used to provide a subset of the terminology that has been curated to serve a particular process and to enable the standardized recording of clinical data at the point of care (for example, in an emergency department [29]).

Precoordination and Postcoordination of Concepts

Complex clinical information can often be represented by combinations of multiple concepts or modifiers for example "chronic migraine", "major depression with psychotic symptoms", "recurrent deep vein thrombosis" or "accidental burning or scalding caused by boiling water". The concepts can contain information on the chronicity, morphology, severity or other aspect

Table 3 Selected top level SNOMED hierarchy concepts and examples (based on the SNOMED-CT UK hierarchy [30])

Name	Example
Body structure	83,419,000 Femoral vein structure (body structure)
Clinical finding	1,362,251,000,000,108 Recurrent bleeding from nose (finding)
Environment or geographical location	285,201,006 Hospital environment (environment)
Event	419,620,001 Death (event)
Procedure	414,089,002 Emergency percutaneous coronary intervention (procedure)
Qualifier value	90,734,009 Chronic (qualifier value)
Situation with explicit context	406,140,001 Discussion about care plan with family (situation)
Social concept	236,324,005 Factory worker (occupation)
Specimen	258,583,001 Bone marrow clot sample (specimen)
Staging and scales	1,077,341,000,000,105 Diagnosing Advanced Dementia Mandate Tool (assessment scale)
Substance	447,208,001 Alcaftadine (substance)

```
284196006 | burn of skin | :
  116676008 | associated morphology | = 80247002 | third degree burn injury |
, 272741003 | laterality | = 7771000 | left |
, 246075003 | causative agent | = 47448006 | hot water |
, 363698007 | finding site | = 83738005 | index finger structure
```

Fig. 1 Example of the SNOMED-CT compositional syntax used to create a postcoordinated concept which can be used to record a third degree burn caused by hot water of the left index finger (*Source* WIkipedia [33])

of the information being recorded. Clinical terminologies have traditionally tried to enable the recording of such information by creating and providing terms for them, a process often referred to as *precoordination*. The core SNOMED-CT ontology contains approx 350.000 precoordinated concepts as they are available upfront for use. The use of precoordinated concepts greatly improves the storage and manipulation of information as it effectively reduces the dimensionality of the data (i.e. the use of one concept versus the use of multiple concepts to record the same data point).

The approach of offering precoodinated concepts for any possible combination of clinically meaningful concepts however does not scale given the complex, highly heterogeneous, and multidisciplinary nature of health and healthcare. For example, it would be unreasonable to expect a precoordinated term for "third degree burn of left index finger caused by hot water". To enable the recording of complex concepts in a machine readable manner, SNOMED-CT offers a compositional grammar (Fig. 1) [31] that can be used to combine multiple concepts together into clinical expressions that are more accurate as opposed to only using a single concept. The created concepts are referred as "postcoordinated" as they are not available upfront in the ontology but have been created a posteriori. Postcoordination however introduces considerable challenges, both in terms of data recording by clinicians, storage and retrieval of information and significantly increases the complexity of the underlying data [32].

2.2 International Classification of Disease (ICD)

The 10th edition of the International Classification of Disease (ICD), commonly referred to as ICD-10, is maintained and published by the WHO and is the most commonly used statistical classification system worldwide. The 11th edition of ICD (ICD-11) officially came was adopted by the 72nd World Health Assembly in 2019 and came into effect on 1st January 2022 [34]. While the WHO maintains the core ICD system, individual countries often develop and deploy their own branches which are adapted to their own needs by often including additional terms or other changes. For example, secondary healthcare providers in the US make use of ICD-10 Clinical Modifications (ICD-10-CM) for discharge summaries and reimbursement purposes which is maintained by the US Centres for Disease Control and Prevention (CDC) [35] (Table 4).

ICD-10 is organized in 21 top level chapters which represent disease systems and are denoted by roman numerals e.g. chapter IX contains terms related to diseases of the circulatory system. Terms within each chapter are often organized in one or more blocks which define a range of codes e.g. block I20-I25 encapsulates terms related to ischaemic heart disease. Individual ICD-10 terms can have up to seven characters. All ICD-10 codes always begin with a letter that is associated with the chapter which they belong to e.g. codes related to circulatory diseases begin with the character "I". This is followed by one or two numbers which further specify the category of the diagnosis. The remaining characters indicate the disease aetiology, anatomic site, severity or other relevant clinical detail. The first three characters are separated by the remaining characters by a decimal character. Within individual codes, the 5th or 6th character length codes represent terms with the highest level of specificity. In certain disease chapters such as obstetrics, a 7th character can be used to denote the type of encounter (e.g. initial vs. subsequent). Within three and four character codes,

Table 4 Comparison of ICD-10 and ICD-10-CM terms used to record heart failure

ICD-10-CM	ICD-10
I50.1 Left ventricular failure, unspecified	I50.0 Congestive heart failure
I50.2 Systolic (congestive) heart failure	I50.1 Left ventricular failure
I50.20 Unspecified systolic (congestive) heart failure	I50.9 Heart failure, unspecified
I50.21 Acute systolic (congestive) heart failure	
I50.22 Chronic systolic (congestive) heart failure	
I50.23 Acute on chronic systolic (congestive) heart failure	
I50.3 Diastolic (congestive) heart failure	
I50.30 Unspecified diastolic (congestive) heart failure	
I50.31 Acute diastolic (congestive) heart failure	
I50.32 Chronic diastolic (congestive) heart failure	
I50.33 Acute on chronic diastolic (congestive) heart failure	
I50.4 Combined systolic (congestive) and diastolic (congestive) heart failure	
I50.40 Unspecified combined systolic (congestive) and diastolic (congestive) heart failure	
I50.41 Acute combined systolic (congestive) and diastolic (congestive) heart failure	
I50.42 Chronic combined systolic (congestive) and diastolic (congestive) heart failure	
I50.43 Acute on chronic combined systolic (congestive) and diastolic (congestive) heart failure	
I50.8 Other heart failure	
I50.81 Right heart failure	
I50.810 ...... unspecified	
I50.811 Acute right heart failure	
I50.812 Chronic right heart failure	
I50.813 Acute on chronic right heart failure	
I50.814 ...... due to left heart failure	
I50.82 Biventricular heart failure	
I50.83 High output heart failure	
I50.84 End stage heart failure	
I50.89 Other heart failure	
I50.9 Heart failure, unspecified	

a "rubric" often denotes a number of other diagnostic terms that are associated with that code such as other related syndromes, synonyms for the disease or common terms. Finally, when a conclusive diagnosis was not possible, for example when the presenting symptoms did not meet the diagnostic criteria for one of the existing defined codes in the hierarchy, generic, broader "Not Otherwise Specified" codes can be used e.g. "I50.9 Heart failure, unspecified".

Working Across ICD Versions

A key challenge of working with longitudinal data that has been recorded using ICD is dealing with different versions of the same coding system e.g. ICD-9 and ICD-10 [36]. Major new versions of an ontology will, by definition, contain a substantial amount of new entities that can be used to record information (e.g. ICD-9-CM contains 13,000 codes while ICD-10-CM contains 68,000 codes) which will often be organized differently. As a result, there are often many additional codes (and often in higher fidelity than before) that can be used to define clinical concepts.

To enable this translation of data between ICD versions, the Centers for Medicare & Medicaid Services (CMS) curates and provides a set of General Equivalent Maps (GEMs, these are often referred to as *crosswalks*) [37]. GEMs can provide forward maps (e.g. ICD-9-CM to ICD-10-CM) and backward maps (e.g. ICD-10-CM to ICD-9-CM). The use of GEMs however is not straightforward as newer concepts that exist in ICD-10-CM might not always exist in ICD-9-CM and some ICD-9-CM concepts might map to a combination of more than one ICD-10-CM codes. For example, the ICD-9-CM code "250.10 Diabetes with ketoacidosis, type II or unspecified type, not stated as uncontrolled" can potentially map to "E11.69 Type 2 diabetes mellitus with other specified complication" or "E13.10 Other specified diabetes mellitus with ketoacidosis without coma" ICD-10-CM codes. In their work, Fung et al. [38] show that the majority of ICD-10-CM codes are not represented in the forward map, and a significant portion of ICD-9-CM codes (25%) are not represented in the backward map e.g. the backward map provides 78,034 unique pairs of ICD-9-CM and ICD-10-CM codes (over three times more than the forward map), of which only 18,484 pairs (23.7%) are also found in the forward map.

Other Clinical Terminologies and Ontologies
A plethora of other clinical ontologies and terminologies exist that are used to record information related to health and healthcare. Information on drugs and medical devices is captured by RxNorm [39] in the US and the Dictionary of Medicines and Devices (DM+D) in the UK [40]. Similarly, surgical procedures and interventions in the US are recorded using the Current Procedural Terminology (CPT) [41] while in the UK using the Office of Population Censuses and Surveys Classification of Surgical Operations and Procedures, 4th revision (OPCS-4) classification which is maintained by the NHS [42]. Molecular pathology testing data and metadata can be standardized by using the LOINC (Logical Observation Identifier Names and Codes) ontology [43]. Semi-structured data, such as reports from investigative radiology procedures, can also contain clinically significant information that can benefit from harmonization and a bespoke ontology, RadLex, has been created to enable the standardized recording of entities [44].

3 Defining Diseases in Electronic Health Records

EHR data offer a rich source of information for research as they capture a diverse set of information on diagnoses, laboratory measurements, procedures, symptoms, medication prescriptions alongside metadata related to healthcare delivery such as referrals. The process of transforming raw EHR data and extracting clinical information for research is referred as *phenotyping* and involves the creation of algorithms (referred to as *phenotyping algorithms)* that can either be deterministic (rule based) or probabilistic [2]. Rule-based algorithms often combine multiple pieces of information, alongside logic rules, to identify patients with a given disease [42].

The use of EHR however for research is associated with significant challenges as the data are often fragmented, recorded using different controlled clinical terminologies and have variable data quality and completeness [45]. Importantly, the purpose and processes in which data are generated and captured varies significantly. For example, primary care EHR are generated by the clinician for direct patient care but are influenced by local clinical guidelines while secondary care claims data are recorded by clinical codes which in turn operate based on a predefined coding protocol. This in turn might influence how data are recorded within each source and how data should be merged across sources [46]. For example, a study comparing the recording of non-fatal myocardial infarctions (AMI) in linked data from primary care, hospitalization records and a myocardial ischaemia national audit observed that only a third of AMI events were recorded in all three sources [47]. As a result of these challenges, researchers must both study the underlying processes that generate the data and perform robust validation across multiple layers of evidence.

3.1 The Need for Aggregated Code Representations

One of the many challenges of working with coded data is that related concepts (e.g. all manifestations of a particular disease) can be fragmented across the terminology used to record information. For example, tuberculosis related diagnoses in ICD-10 occur in four different ICD chapters (e.g. infections, skin diseases, diseases of the genitourinary system and diseases of the musculoskeletal and connective tissue). Furthermore, when working with longitudinal data, researchers have to deal with changes within clinical terminologies and changes related to new major versions of ontologies such as the transition of ICD-9-CM to ICD-10-CM or SNOMED-CT concepts becoming inactive and replaced by newer alternative concepts. As a result, the creation of phenotyping algorithms to define diseases in complex EHR becomes significantly more challenging and requires a significant amount of resources.

To enable the scalable definition of diseases in EHR, using all available ICD diagnosis codes, a layer above source ICD codes has been developed by Bastarache et al. [48] that provides phenotype codes (*phecodes*) grouppings. Phecodes were originally developed in ICD-9-CM and derived partially from the Agency for Healthcare Research and Quality Clinical Classification Software for ICD-9-CM (CCS) [49]. Phecodes are manually curated, hierarchically organized groupings of ICD codes aiming to capture common adult diagnoses to facilitate phenome-wide genetic association studies (PheWAS) [50]. Phecodes version 1.2 condenses roughly 15,500 ICD-9-CM codes and 90,000 ICD-10-CM codes into 1867 phecodes. Subsequent research mapped phecodes to ICD-10 and ICD-10-CM codes [51] and phecodes have been shown to produce robust genotype–phenotype associations compared with other relevant approaches [52].

3.2 Bridging Molecules to Phenotypes

Phenotypes typically require aggregation of structured data fields in clinical records as described in the preceding section. Phenotypic inferences can be made based on an interpretation of lab test results, medications prescribed, diagnoses, and clinical notes. To make such inferences using a programmatic approach requires connecting phenotypes to structured representations of those clinical record elements. The OBO Foundry includes relevant ontologies for bridging molecules to phenotypes. The Chemical Entities of Biological Interest (ChEBI) ontology covers molecules and their roles while the Drug Ontology (DrON) captures the relationships between the molecules defined in ChEBI and the drugs where the molecules are active ingredients and also links to RxNorm terms (from the National Library of Medicine [39]). The human disease ontology (DO) has database-cross references to ICD-9 and ICD-10 codes as well as to SNOMED. The Monarch Disease Ontology (MonDO [53]) connects DO with additional disease resources (e.g., Orphanet [54], OMIM [55]). Genotyping results can be interpreted through the Gene Ontology (GO [56]) to identify the processes affected by mutations. The Ontology for Biomedical Investigations (OBI) [19] can be used to link lab test results with specimens and assays. Anatomy-based data can be interpreted through Uberon [57], a species neutral anatomy ontology, or the Foundational Model of Anatomy (FMA [58]) which is focused on human anatomy. The Human Phenotype Ontology [59] provides representation of phenotypes and connects to many of these listed OBO Foundry ontologies as well as clinical terminologies.

4 Application of Standards to Aid Machine Learning

Representing words as numerical vectors based on the contexts in which they appear has become the de facto method of natural language processing approaches. A survey of word embeddings for clinical text provides some good pointers on other approaches [60].

Learnt representations of controlled clinical terminologies can be used as the basis for features in machine learning. In order to utilize the information located in free text, it has to be converted to structured representation. This transformation however needs to take into consideration the structure of the clinical terminology itself as it provides essential contextual information. Artificial Intelligence approaches are increasingly being used to learn and predict phenotypes. An example of deep learning applied to EHR records is BEHRT [61], a deep neural sequence transduction model capable of simultaneously predicting the likelihood of 301 phenotypes (originally developed in the CALIBER resource [62]) in a patient's future visits. When trained and evaluated on the data from nearly 1.6 million individuals, BEHRT was able to show a striking improvement in terms of average precision scores for different tasks over the existing state-of-the-art deep EHR models. In addition to its scalability and improved accuracy, BEHRT enables personalized interpretation of its predictions. Its flexible architecture enables it to incorporate multiple heterogeneous concepts (e.g., diagnosis, medication, measurements, and more) to further improve the accuracy of its predictions; its (pre-)training results in disease and patient representations can be useful for future studies (i.e., transfer learning).

Tensor factorization methods such as Limestone and Granite have also provided phenotype predictions [63, 64]. EHR data do not always directly and reliably map to medical concepts that clinical researchers need or use. Some recent studies have focused on EHR-derived phenotyping, which aims at mapping the EHR data to specific medical concepts; however, most of these approaches require labor intensive supervision from experienced clinical professionals. Furthermore, existing approaches are often disease-centric and specialized to the idiosyncrasies of the information technology and/or business practices of a single healthcare organization. Limestone [64], a nonnegative tensor factorization method to derive phenotype candidates with virtually no human supervision. Limestone represents the data source interactions naturally using tensors (a generalization of matrices) and investigates the interaction of diagnoses and medications. The resulting tensor factors are reported as phenotype candidates that automatically reveal patient clusters on specific diagnoses and medications. Using the proposed method, multiple phenotypes can be identified simultaneously from data.

Standards in the form of biomedical ontologies can be used directly for analysis of annotated data. The most visible form of this approach is in the enrichment analysis of gene expression data using annotations of proteins and genes with the Gene Ontology. Those analyses while very successful do not take advantage of relationships encoded in the ontologies. Recent work has been done however using ontology-based network analysis and visualization for COVID-19 analysis [65]. In a similar vein, in the AI-driven cell ontology brain data standards project, ontologies are being used to capture results of analysis and learn more through reasoning [66].

Knowledge graphs provide the ability to connect clinical terminologies and encodings in EHR with biomedical ontologies and standards. For example, a knowledge graph framework has been developed for COVID-19 focused around molecular and chemical information, enabling users to conduct complex queries over relevant biological entities as well as machine learning analyses to generate graph embeddings for making predictions. This framework can also be applied to other problems in which siloed biomedical data must be quickly integrated for different research applications, including future pandemics [67].

5 Future directions

The proper use of standards is an active area of research. In a recent call for proposals, the issue of relating real-world data (RWD) (e.g., EHR, claims, and digital health technologies) between different sources was raised as not just an issue of mapping but also transforming the data and the underlying definition of its meaning as these can be similar but not identical. Even if standards are used, proper use of data from multiple sources will rely heavily on human interpretation and efforts are still needed for fully reliable computer-driven approaches. In this chapter, the emphasis has been on data for phenotyping. The same concerns and considerations about the choice and application of standards need to be applied for genotyping and genomics. Linkages of this type of data to clinical terminologies are either non-existent or in their infancy. There are standards for file formats and some relevant OBO Foundry ontologies exist (e.g., OBI, Sequence Ontology[68]) which should aid the ultimate goal of combining phenotyping and genotyping/genomics.

A fundamental difference between clinical terminologies/coding systems such as SNOMED-CT and ICD with OBO Foundry ontologies such as the Basic Formal Ontology (BFO) or the Disease Ontology (DO) is the modeling approach. SNOMED and ICD are representing information collected by a health care worker whereas BFO and DO are representing what happened or exists in the world. The former fits well with data models while the latter provides a common grounding in reality. It remains a challenge to leverage the benefits of both clinical standards like SNOMED-CT and OBO Foundry ontologies. SNOMED has greater adoption in the clinical area but lacks the semantic rigor and breadth (for example in genomic technologies) than OBO Foundry ontologies. The use of database cross-references in OBOF ontologies to SNOMED-CT does provide a bridge.

Resources for further reading:
We provide below several resources for further reading on topics covered in this chapter:

- Bodenreider and colleagues [69] provide an excellent overview and discussion of recent developments in SNOMED-CT, LOINC and RxNorm.
- Aspden and colleagues discuss the topic of healthcare data standards in depth and provide examples of their application in healthcare [7].
- Standards are by their nature about classes of concepts. However, when working with RWD, attention needs to be placed on their application to instances to establish when the diagnosis or even the patient being referred to is the same or different. This topic is covered in detail by Ceuster [70].
- Practical applications and theoretical background for applied ontology especially in the biomedical area can be found in Smith, Arp, and Spears Building Ontologies with Basic Formal Ontology [71].
- Hemingway and colleagues provide a detailed overview with examples on how electronic health records are utilized for early and late translational cardiovascular research [72].

References

1. The health information technology for economic and clinical health act (HITECH act). PsycEXTRA Dataset. American Psychological Association (APA); 2009. https://doi.org/10.1037/e500522017-001.
2. Shivade C, Raghavan P, Fosler-Lussier E, Embi PJ, Elhadad N, Johnson SB, et al. A review of approaches to identifying patient phenotype cohorts using electronic health records. J Am Med Inform Assoc. 2014;21:221–30.
3. ISO 8601-1:2019. In: ISO [Internet]. 2019 [cited 31 Jan 2022]. Available: https://www.iso.org/standard/70907.html.
4. Danecek P, Auton A, Abecasis G, Albers CA, Banks E, DePristo MA, et al. The variant call format and VCFtools. Bioinformatics. 2011;27:2156–8.
5. National Institutes of Health (NIH). In: National Institutes of Health (NIH) [Internet]. [cited 31 Jan 2022]. Available: https://www.nih.gov/.
6. Jackson R, Matentzoglu N, Overton JA, Vita R, Balhoff JP, Buttigieg PL, et al. OBO Foundry in 2021: operationalizing open data principles to evaluate ontologies. Database . 2021;2021. https://doi.org/10.1093/database/baab069.
7. Institute of Medicine (US) Committee on Data Standards for Patient Safety, Aspden P, Corrigan JM, Wolcott J, Erickson SM. Health Care Data Standards. National Academies Press (US); 2004.
8. McGlynn EA, Lieu TA, Durham ML, Bauck A, Laws R, Go AS, et al. Developing a data infrastructure for a learning health system: the portal network. J Am Med Inform Assoc. 2014;21:596–601.
9. Bender D, Sartipi K. HL7 FHIR: an agile and RESTful approach to healthcare information exchange. In: Proceedings of the 26th IEEE international symposium on computer-based medical systems. ieeexplore.ieee.org; 2013. p. 326–31.
10. OMOP Common Data Model. [cited 31 Jan 2022]. Available: https://www.ohdsi.org/data-standardization/the-common-data-model/.
11. Rector A, Schulz S, Rodrigues JM, Chute CG, Solbrig H. On beyond Gruber: "Ontologies" in today's biomedical information systems and the limits of OWL. J Biomed Inform. 2019;100S: 100002.
12. McGuinness DL, Van Harmelen F, Others. OWL web ontology language overview. W3C recommendation. 2004;10: 2004.

13. Miles A, Bechhofer S. SKOS simple knowledge organization system reference. W3C Recommendation. 2009 [cited 22 Feb 2022]. Available: https://www.escholar.manchester.ac.uk/uk-ac-man-scw:66505.
14. Semantic web - W3C. [cited 22 Feb 2022]. Available: https://www.w3.org/standards/semanticweb/.
15. Whetzel PL, Noy NF, Shah NH, Alexander PR, Nyulas C, Tudorache T, et al. BioPortal: enhanced functionality via new Web services from the national center for biomedical ontology to access and use ontologies in software applications. Nucleic Acids Res. 2011;39:W541–5.
16. Wikipedia contributors. Abox. In: Wikipedia, The Free Encyclopedia [Internet]. 19 Nov 2021. Available: https://en.wikipedia.org/w/index.php?title=Abox&oldid=1056049124.
17. Kibbe WA, Arze C, Felix V, Mitraka E, Bolton E, Fu G, et al. Disease Ontology 2015 update: an expanded and updated database of human diseases for linking biomedical knowledge through disease data. Nucleic Acids Res. 2015;43:D1071–8.
18. Hogan WR, Hanna J, Joseph E, Brochhausen M. Towards a consistent and scientifically accurate drug ontology. CEUR Workshop Proc. 2013;1060:68–73.
19. Bandrowski A, Brinkman R, Brochhausen M, Brush MH, Bug B, Chibucos MC, et al. The ontology for biomedical investigations. PLoS ONE. 2016;11: e0154556.
20. Hastings J, Owen G, Dekker A, Ennis M, Kale N, Muthukrishnan V, et al. ChEBI in 2016: improved services and an expanding collection of metabolites. Nucleic Acids Res. 2016;44:D1214–9.
21. Giannangelo K. Healthcare code sets, clinical terminologies, and classification systems, 3rd ed. American Health Information Management Association; 2014.
22. Classification Systems : U.S. Bureau of Labor Statistics. 30 Sep 2015 [cited 14 Jan 2022]. Available: https://www.bls.gov/opub/hom/topic/classification-systems.htm.
23. ICD-10 Version:2019. [cited 14 Jan 2022]. Available: https://icd.who.int/browse10/2019/en.
24. Nouraei SAR, Hudovsky A, Virk JS, Chatrath P, Sandhu GS. An audit of the nature and impact of clinical coding subjectivity variability and error in otolaryngology. Clin Otolaryngol. 2013;38:512–24.
25. Benson T. Principles of health interoperability HL7 and SNOMED. Springer London; 2010.
26. Read Codes—NHS Digital. [cited 5 Mar 2021]. Available: https://digital.nhs.uk/services/terminology-and-classifications/read-codes.
27. Lee D, Cornet R, Lau F, de Keizer N. A survey of SNOMED CT implementations. J Biomed Inform. 2013;46:87–96.
28. Kalet IJ. Chapter 4—Biomedical Information Access. In: Kalet IJ, editor. Principles of Biomedical Informatics. 2nd ed. San Diego: Academic Press; 2014. p. 397–478.
29. Hansen DP, Kemp ML, Mills SR, Mercer MA, Frosdick PA, Lawley MJ. Developing a national emergency department data reference set based on SNOMED CT. Med J Aust. 2011;194:S8-10.
30. NHS Digital. The NHS Digital SNOMED CT Browser. [cited 14 Jan 2022]. Available: https://termbrowser.nhs.uk/?.
31. Compositional Grammar—Specification and Guide—Compositional Grammar - SNOMED Confluence. [cited 14 Jan 2022]. Available: https://confluence.ihtsdotools.org/display/DOCSCG/Compositional+Grammar+-+Specification+and+Guide.
32. Karlsson D, Nyström M, Cornet R. Does SNOMED CT post-coordination scale? Stud Health Technol Inform. 2014;205:1048–52.
33. Wikipedia contributors. SNOMED CT. In: Wikipedia, The Free Encyclopedia [Internet]. 23 Dec 2021. Available: https://en.wikipedia.org/w/index.php?title=SNOMED_CT&oldid=1061690432.
34. ICD-11. [cited 22 Feb 2022]. Available: https://icd.who.int/en.
35. ICD-ICD-10-CM - International classification of diseases, tenth revision, clinical modification. 11 Feb 2022 [cited 22 Feb 2022]. Available: https://www.cdc.gov/nchs/icd/icd10cm.htm.
36. Cartwright DJ. ICD-9-CM to ICD-10-CM codes: what? why? how? Adv Wound Care. 2013;2:588–92.
37. ICD-10-CM and ICD-10 PCS and GEMs Archive. [cited 22 Feb 2022]. Available: https://www.cms.gov/Medicare/Coding/ICD10/Archive-ICD-10-CM-ICD-10-PCS-GEMs.
38. Fung KW, Richesson R, Smerek M, Pereira KC, Green BB, Patkar A, et al. Preparing for the ICD-10-CM transition: automated methods for translating ICD codes in clinical phenotype definitions. EGEMS (Wash DC). 2016;4:1211.
39. Liu S, Ma W, Moore R, Ganesan V, Nelson S. RxNorm: prescription for electronic drug information exchange. IT Prof. 2005;7:17–23.
40. Spiers I, Goulding J, Arrowsmith I. Clinical terminologies in the NHS: SNOMED CT and dm+ d. British J Pharmacy. 2017;2:80–7.
41. Association AM. Current procedural terminology: CPT. Am Med Ass. 2007.
42. Morley KI, Wallace J, Denaxas SC, Hunter RJ, Patel RS, Perel P, et al. Defining disease phenotypes using national linked electronic health records: a case study of atrial fibrillation. PLoS ONE. 2014;9: e110900.
43. Huff SM, Rocha RA, McDonald CJ, De Moor GJ, Fiers T, Bidgood WD Jr, et al. Development of the logical observation identifier names and codes (LOINC) vocabulary. J Am Med Inform Assoc. 1998;5:276–92.
44. Langlotz CP. RadLex: a new method for indexing online educational materials. Radiographics. 2006;26:1595–7.

45. Hripcsak G, Albers DJ. Next-generation phenotyping of electronic health records. J Am Med Inform Assoc. 2013;20:117–21.
46. Denaxas S, Gonzalez-Izquierdo A, Direk K, Fitzpatrick NK, Fatemifar G, Banerjee A, et al. UK phenomics platform for developing and validating electronic health record phenotypes: CALIBER. J Am Med Inform Assoc. 2019;26:1545–59.
47. Herrett E, Shah AD, Boggon R, Denaxas S, Smeeth L, van Staa T, et al. Completeness and diagnostic validity of recording acute myocardial infarction events in primary care, hospital care, disease registry, and national mortality records: cohort study. BMJ. 2013;346: f2350.
48. Bastarache L. Using phecodes for research with the electronic health record: from PheWAS to PheRS. Annu Rev Biomed Data Sci. 2021;4:1–19.
49. HCUP-US Tools & Software Page. [cited 22 Feb 2022]. Available: https://www.hcup-us.ahrq.gov/toolssoftware/ccs/ccsfactsheet.jsp.
50. Denny JC, Bastarache L, Ritchie MD, Carroll RJ, Zink R, Mosley JD, et al. Systematic comparison of phenome-wide association study of electronic medical record data and genome-wide association study data. Nat Biotechnol. 2013;31:1102–11.
51. Wu P, Gifford A, Meng X, Li X, Campbell H, Varley T, et al. Mapping ICD-10 and ICD-10-CM codes to phecodes: workflow development and initial evaluation. JMIR Med Inform. 2019;7: e14325.
52. Wei W-Q, Bastarache LA, Carroll RJ, Marlo JE, Osterman TJ, Gamazon ER, et al. Evaluating phecodes, clinical classification software, and ICD-9-CM codes for phenome-wide association studies in the electronic health record. PLoS ONE. 2017;12: e0175508.
53. Vasilevsky N, Essaid S, Matentzoglu N, Harris NL, Haendel M, Robinson P, et al. Mondo disease ontology: harmonizing disease concepts across the world. CEUR Workshop Proceedings. CEUR-WS; 2020. Available: http://ceur-ws.org/Vol-2807/abstractY.pdf.
54. Nguengang Wakap S, Lambert DM, Olry A, Rodwell C, Gueydan C, Lanneau V, et al. Estimating cumulative point prevalence of rare diseases: analysis of the Orphanet database. Eur J Hum Genet. 2020;28:165–73.
55. McKusick VA. Mendelian inheritance in man and its online version. OMIM Am J Hum Genet. 2007;80:588–604.
56. Gene Ontology Consortium. The gene ontology resource: enriching a GOld mine. Nucleic Acids Res. 2021;49:D325–34.
57. Mungall CJ, Torniai C, Gkoutos GV, Lewis SE, Haendel MA. Uberon, an integrative multi-species anatomy ontology. Genome Biol. 2012;13:R5.
58. Cook DL, Mejino JLV, Rosse C. The foundational model of anatomy: a template for the symbolic representation of multi-scale physiological functions. Conf Proc IEEE Eng Med Biol Soc. 2004;2004:5415–8.
59. Robinson PN, Köhler S, Bauer S, Seelow D, Horn D, Mundlos S. The human phenotype ontology: a tool for annotating and analyzing human hereditary disease. Am J Hum Genet. 2008;83:610–5.
60. Khattak FK, Jeblee S, Pou-Prom C, Abdalla M, Meaney C, Rudzicz F. A survey of word embeddings for clinical text. J Biomed Inform. 2019;100S: 100057.
61. Li Y, Rao S, Solares JRA, Hassaine A, Ramakrishnan R, Canoy D, et al. BEHRT: transformer for electronic health records. Sci Rep. 2020;10:7155.
62. Kuan V, Denaxas S, Gonzalez-Izquierdo A, Direk K, Bhatti O, Husain S, et al. A chronological map of 308 physical and mental health conditions from 4 million individuals in the English National Health Service. Lancet Digit Health. 2019;1:e63–77.
63. Henderson J, Ho JC, Kho AN, Denny JC, Malin BA, Sun J, et al. Granite: diversified, sparse tensor factorization for electronic health record-based phenotyping. In: 2017 IEEE international conference on healthcare informatics (ICHI); 2017. p. 214–23.
64. Ho JC, Ghosh J, Steinhubl SR, Stewart WF, Denny JC, Malin BA, et al. Limestone: high-throughput candidate phenotype generation via tensor factorization. J Biomed Inform. 2014;52:199–211.
65. Wang Z, He Y. Precision omics data integration and analysis with interoperable ontologies and their application for COVID-19 research. Brief Funct Genom. 2021;20:235–48.
66. Aevermann BD, Novotny M, Bakken T, Miller JA, Diehl AD, Osumi-Sutherland D, et al. Cell type discovery using single-cell transcriptomics: implications for ontological representation. Hum Mol Genet. 2018;27:R40–7.
67. Reese JT, Unni D, Callahan TJ, Cappelletti L, Ravanmehr V, Carbon S, et al. KG-COVID-19: a framework to produce customized knowledge graphs for COVID-19 response. Patterns (N Y). 2021;2: 100155.
68. Eilbeck K, Lewis SE, Mungall CJ, Yandell M, Stein L, Durbin R, et al. The sequence ontology: a tool for the unification of genome annotations. Genome Biol. 2005;6:R44.
69. Bodenreider O, Cornet R, Vreeman DJ. Recent developments in clinical terminologies—SNOMED CT, LOINC, and RxNorm. Yearb Med Inform. 2018;27:129–39.
70. Ceusters, W. The place of Referent Tracking in Biomedical Informatics. 2020. https://doi.org/10.31219/osf.io/q8hts.
71. Arp R, Smith B, Spear AD. Building ontologies with basic formal ontology. MIT Press; 2015.
72. Hemingway H, Asselbergs FW, Danesh J, Dobson R, Maniadakis N, Maggioni A, et al. Big data from electronic health records for early and late translational cardiovascular research: challenges and potential. Eur Heart J. 2018;39:1481–95.

Data Integration and Harmonisation

Maxim Moinat, Vaclav Papez and Spiros Denaxas

Abstract

Data harmonisation is an essential step for federated research, which often involves heterogeneous data sources. A standardised structure and terminology of the source allows application of standardised study protocol and analysis code. A Common Data Model (CDM) accompanied with standardised software supports standardised federated analytics. In this chapter we demonstrate the benefit of Common Data Models and the OMOP CDM in particular. We also introduce a general pipeline of an Extract Transform Load process to transform health data to the OMOP CDM and provide an overview of the supporting tooling that ensures a high-quality conversion. Finally, we discuss potential challenges of the harmonisation process and how to address them.

Keywords

Common data model · Electronic health records · Medical ontologies · OMOP · Mapping · Harmonisation

1 Introduction to Common Data Models

1.1 Introduction

The previous chapters, especially Chap. 3—*Data standards and terminology including Biomedical ontologies*, have introduced various standards used in healthcare and biomedical research. Each standard addresses a particular purpose and helps organising and interpreting data. Although many standards are global and used across domains, many data use local standards, like national drug coding or customised EHR systems built for a hospital.

For large-scale studies, fundamental for AI, it is essential to integrate data from various sources. For example to characterise treatment patterns at different healthcare settings [1] or predicting the risk of multiple outcomes after a

M. Moinat
The Hyve, Utrecht, Netherlands

Erasmus Medical Centre Rotterdam, Rotterdam, Netherlands

V. Papez (✉) · S. Denaxas
Institute of Health Informatics, University College London, London, UK
e-mail: v.papez@ucl.ac.uk

Health Data Research UK, London, UK

S. Denaxas
British Heart Foundation Data Science Centre, Health Data Research UK, London, UK

F. W. Asselbergs et al. (eds.), *Clinical Applications of Artificial Intelligence in Real-World Data*,
https://doi.org/10.1007/978-3-031-36678-9_4

COVID19 infection [2]. This enables interoperability and reusability of the collected information, which are two of the FAIR principles emphasising machine-actionability of data [3].

One way is to harmonise the data to a Common Data Model (CDM). Data harmonisation is not an easy task. Healthcare databases can consist of many tables from diverse systems, like inpatient, outpatient, lab, pharmacy. And the source model and the CDM might capture data at different granularities, leading either to loss of information or requiring to derive missing information. The choice of data model and terminology is important as is the support for the CDM of choice.

1.2 Common Data Models

An EMA workshop report from 2017 describes a CDM as: "a mechanism by which raw data are standardised to a common structure, format and terminology independently from any particular study in order to allow a combined analysis across several databases/datasets" [4]. In this report three CDMs (OMOP CDM, Sentinel, Pcornet) were compared for use for pan-European observational health studies to address regulatory questions in a timely manner. Specifically, to use a CDM for Post Authorisation Safety Studies, drug utilisation and drug effectiveness studies on a wide population.

This definition shows the main components of a CDM. The first is a common structure, where the elements of the model are defined. In traditional models this is the definition of the tables and fields, for graph databases these will be the attributes of nodes and edges. The second is a common format, the form in which the data is presented. This can be flat tables, preferably as a relational database, or nested documents, like JSON. The third is a common terminology, defining the semantics of the values in the model. For example, the target vocabulary used for diagnoses. Preferably the values are richly annotated with metadata about the terminology used.

All three elements are crucial for machines to process the data. Ideally the data is also richly annotated with interoperable metadata that describes the structure, format, and terminology of the data. This enables machines without any prior knowledge of the data to access it.

A CDM is not application specific. Therefore, in most cases the data is not stored natively in this model. Having data in a CDM requires extraction from the application specific system, applying transformations and loading it into the CDM.

1.3 Common Data Models in the Biomedical Domain

The notion of using a CDM for biomedical data is not new. For many years, data from different sources has been integrated at institutional, regional, and also global levels. Table 1 gives an overview of a selection of important open healthcare standards and their main purpose.

HL7 FHIR [5] and OpenEHR [6] are models that directly integrate with the systems of a clinical care site. Their aim is not so much on research, but on processing healthcare data for their primary purpose: patient care. These models are important, as they are important entry points for integrating with models aimed towards research.

The other models have their specific research purposes. The OMOP CDM, maintained by the global OHDSI open science collaborative [7], is the main topic of this section and will be addressed in detail later. The CDISC SDTM [8] is a well-established standard for submission of Clinical Trial data to regulatory bodies and is required by e.g., the FDA. The Sentinel CDM is at the basis of an FDA funded federated network of US claims data [4]. The i2b2 model is the only model that is aimed at translational medicine and can be used to combine real world data from healthcare and research data.

Table 1 Standards for biomedical data and their main purpose

Standard	Main purpose
HL7 FHIR	*Record Exchange*: Connecting digital resources like software and devices in order to improve healthcare delivery
OHDSI OMOP CDM	*Observational Research*: Representing clinical data to do reproducible large scale medical evidence generation
OpenEHR Archetypes	*Clinical Care*: Collecting and organising electronic health records (EHR) data at the source
CDISC SDTM	*Clinical Trial:* Submitting data from studies to regulatory bodies like the FDA
Sentinel CDM	*Regulatory Observational Analysis:* Studies on a FDA network of US claims data
i2b2 model	*Translational Medicine:* Integrating data from healthcare and research

HL7 FHIR: Health Level Seven Fast Healthcare Interoperability Resource, OHDSI: Observational Health Data Sciences and Informatics, OMOP CDM: Observational Medical Outcomes Partnership Common Data Model, CDISC SDTM: Clinical Data Interchange Standards Consortium Standard Data Tabulation Model, i2b2: Informatics for Integrating Biology and the Bedside

1.4 Benefits of Harmonisation to a CDM

One of the benefits of a CDM is to enable large scale evidence generation across a federated network of data sources [9]. We assume here that federation means that the analysis is run locally and only the study results are shared back with the central study coordinator. The analysis, or study code, consists of two main pieces: phenotype algorithms for the target, comparator and outcome cohorts, and a statistical program e.g., written in R, SAS, or SPSS.

Let us assume we want to execute a study protocol across a set of similar, but structurally and semantically different, datasets. The protocol can be as simple as characterising a population of interest or as complex as building and (externally) validating a predictive model. The study protocol describes in text all the definitions and analytical procedures needed to execute the study. This includes among other the inclusion/exclusion criteria, the medical codes used for each, statistical methods, and outcome measures.

Without a CDM, the protocol has to be translated into four separate pieces of study code (Fig. 1, top left). This can be implemented in any programming language or statistical framework.

The re-implementation of the study protocol is not only labour intensive but will also result in other issues. Different interpretations of the protocol can result in analysis code being implemented differently. If the analysis procedure is not identical across sources, it is difficult to determine if any differences observed are due to the data or due to the analysis. And variations in the output format of the study results make aggregation of the final results harder.

With a CDM, the protocol has to be translated to study code only once (Fig. 1, top-right) and the code is shared between sites. This ensures each site executes exactly the study definition and outputs results in the same format. However, there is a high upfront cost to harmonise each data source to a CDM. Regardless of the choice of CDM, this is a big amount of effort and also variations can occur between data sources on the conventions used to populate the CDM. A common data quality assessment is key to spot any issues early on, which we will elaborate in the section.

It might be clear that a CDM will make cross-institutional network studies more reliable. However, an observant reader might have noticed that with a CDM a total of five 'translations' are necessary (four CDM, one study

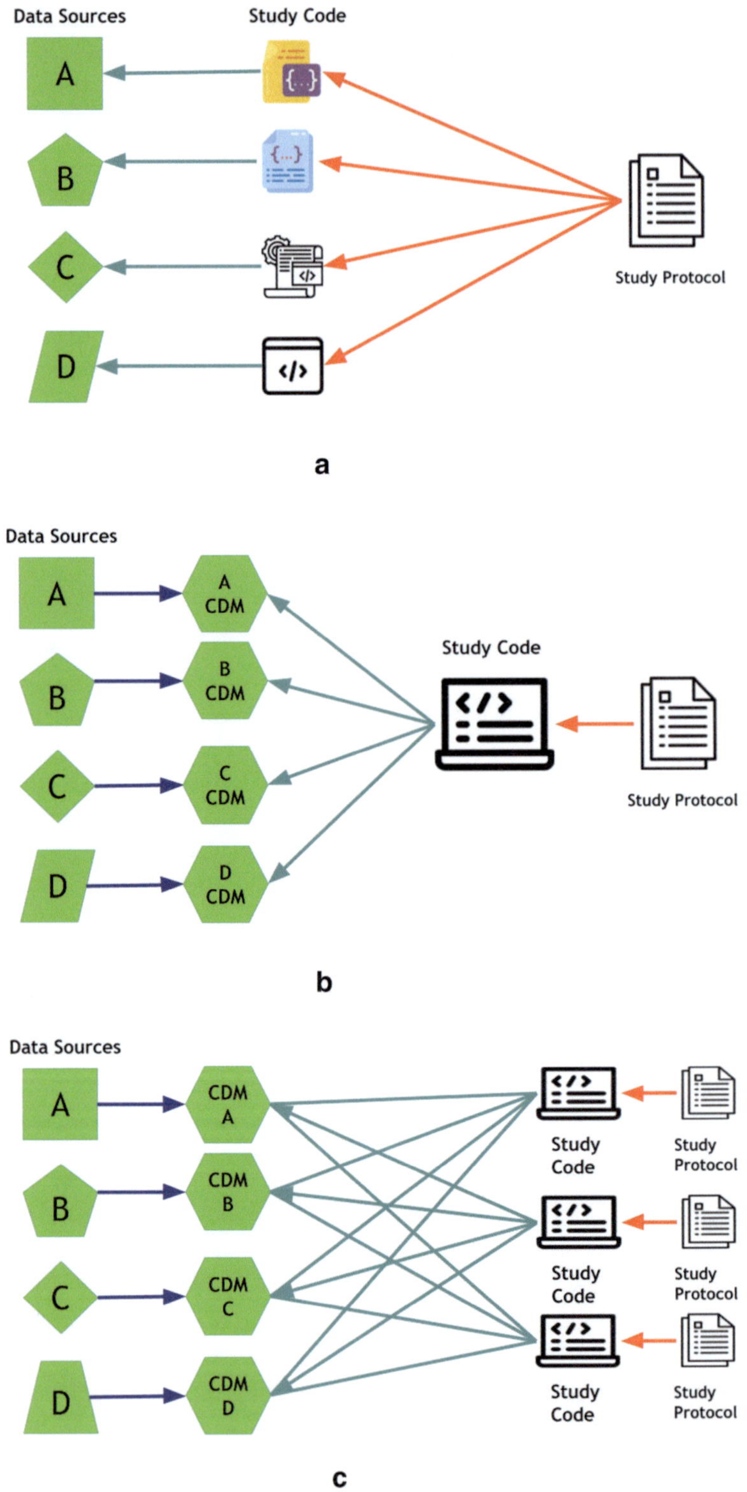

Fig. 1 Cross-institutional study of four structurally and semantically different databases (A, B, C, D). In the diagram on the top-left without a common data model. The protocol has to be 'translated' to study code for each of the data sources. In the diagram on the top-right each data source is harmonised to a CDM after which the protocol is 'translated' to one piece of study code that is executed against each CDM. In both scenarios the analysis is run locally and only study results are shared back with the central study coordinator. In the diagram on the bottom, performing multiple cross-institutional studies with a common data model is shown. After an initial harmonisation to a CDM, multiple studies are executed. Each requires translation to study code once

code) where without a CDM just four 'translations' are necessary (all study code). Also, harmonising a full data source to a CDM is often more work than creating a piece of study code focussed on a specific subset of variables. Thus, for one particular study using a CDM might not be worthwhile.

The real benefit of a CDM comes when executing a series of studies on the same network of data sources (Fig. 1, bottom). Without a CDM the number of code translations needed grows by multiplying the number of databases and studies. Executing one study across four databases requires 4 interfaces, executing ten studies across ten databases requires 100 interfaces. Instead of having to translate each protocol four times to code (resulting in twelve separate translations), this only has to be done three times in total (plus four CDM conversions). The number of databases is a constant for translations needed. And this scales of course when executing more studies across the network [10].

Furthermore, this goes beyond studies. A CDM enables the reuse of standard tooling for data quality assessment, visualisations, reporting and analysis. The OHDSI open science collaborative is a good example of a community that has produced a large library of standard tools and analytical methods around a CDM.

Standard research may be more costly for a single researcher compared with a bespoke study. But standardised research scales and benefits a community as a whole by enabling reuse. Akin 'Tragedy of Commons' where adding one cow to a field benefits a farmer, but degrades the field and negatively impacts the community as a whole [11].

Another benefit is that the conversion splits the path to evidence (i.e., study results) into two parts; the data harmonisation and the analysis execution. The harmonisation can be developed and evaluated separately from the analysis design.

2 The OMOP CDM

In this section we will dive deeper into one particular CDM, the OMOP CDM, which is used for research on real world healthcare data.

2.1 History

The OMOP CDM was born out of the Observational Medical Outcomes Partnership (OMOP), a public–private partnership chaired by the US FDA. This collaboration focussed on active medical product safety surveillance using observational healthcare data. In order to run studies across a heterogeneous set of databases, the OMOP Common Data Model was designed. This included standardised vocabularies for semantic interoperability. The OMOP studies showed successfully that it was possible to facilitate cross-institutional collaboration on safety studies [12].

After the lifetime of the OMOP project, the journey was continued as the currently well-known open science collaborative named OHDSI (Observational Health Data Sciences and Informatics, pronounced 'odyssey'). Under this collaboration, the use of the OMOP CDM was expanded to support a wide set of analytical use cases, like general comparative effectiveness of medical interventions, database characteristics and prediction models. All work is done collaboratively and published in the open domain. This includes data standards, ETL (Extract Transform Load) conventions, methodological research, and development of clinical applications.

2.2 The OMOP CDM

The OMOP CDM [13] is a relational database model consisting of 39 tables (Fig. 2), designed to store longitudinal health records

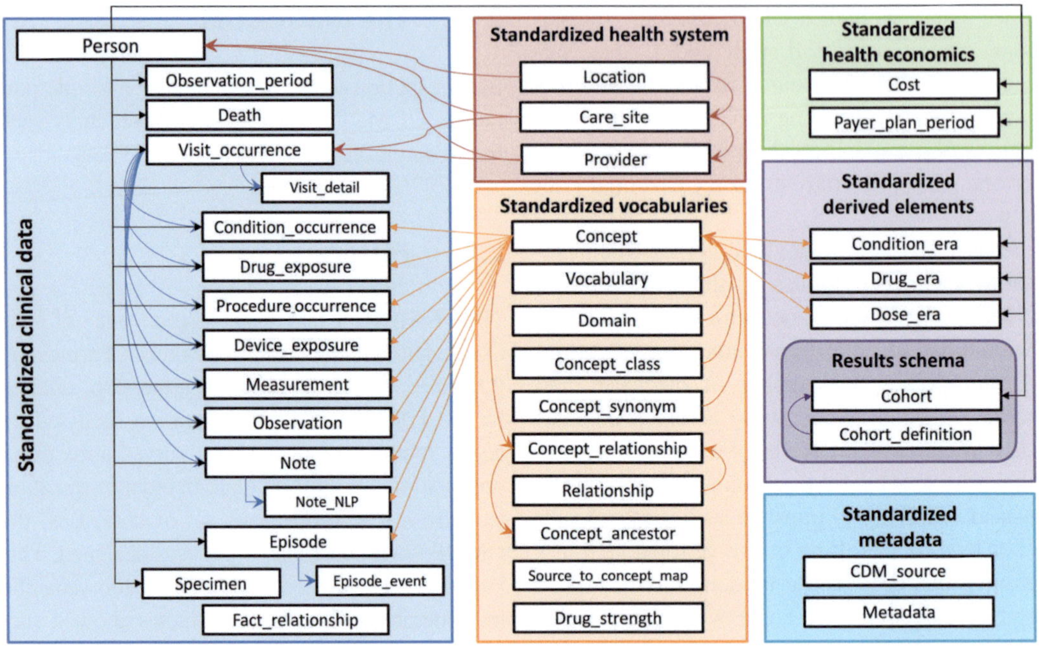

Fig. 2 The OMOP CDM overview of tables and relations between them [13]. The Person and Observation_period tables are the only ones required to be populated. The coloured boxes show the logical groupings of tables

collected from routine care. These are divided into seven logical groups. The tables from the 'Standardized clinical data' contain the main variables. Only the Person and Observation_period tables are required to be populated. The 'Standardized health system' tables provide additional context about who gave the care. The 'Standardized health economics' can contain associated costs of procedures and drugs and who pays these costs. Both the health system and economics data is often not made available by the source. The 'Standardized derived elements' are derived from the populated clinical data. The 'Standardized metadata' can provide information about the name of the data source, date of extraction and vocabulary version.

Every clinical event is captured in one of the eight domains, which each are stored in a separate table (Table 2). All clinical events, regardless of the domain, require at least a person_id (who), a fully specified date (when) and a concept_id (what). The concept_id has to refer to a standard concept from the OMOP Standardized vocabularies, explained in the next section.

Table 2 The eight domains of the OMOP CDM

Domain	Type of data
Condition occurrence	Diagnoses and symptoms
Drug exposure	Medications
Procedure occurrence	Diagnostic or surgical operations
Measurement	Lab results
Observation	Other clinical facts
Specimen	Sample, biopt
Device exposure	Medical equipment, Implantations, supplies
Note	Free text

Here we provide a short description of the most important tables in the OMOP CDM:

- Person contains demographic information. At least a year of birth and gender are required.
- Observation Period contains the periods of time for which we expect clinical events to be recorded for each person. This is important to determine 'healthy' time.

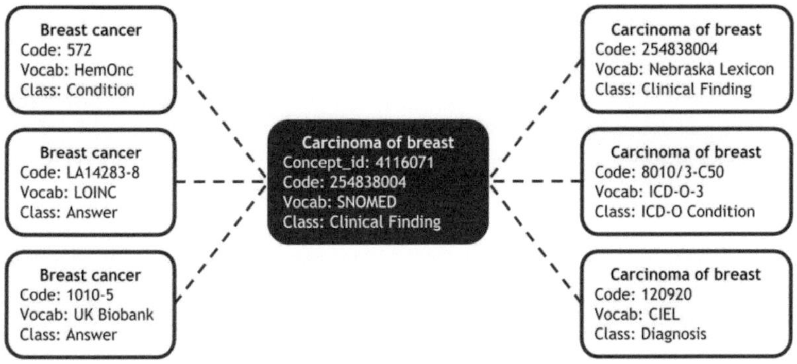

Fig. 3 The concept 'Carcinoma of breast' (SNOMED: 254838004) is the standard concept. Terms from other vocabularies with the same clinical meaning are mapped to this standard concept

- Death. At least the date is required, optionally the cause of death.
- Visit Occurrence contains the healthcare encounter, which can be anything between a short outpatient consult to a long hospitalisation.
- Drug Era is derived by combining single Drug Occurrences into longer periods of use of a particular ingredient.
- CDM Source. Contains the name of the dataset, date of extraction, link to ETL documentation, date of ETL process and vocabulary version.

2.3 The OMOP Standardised Vocabularies

"*The Standard Vocabulary is a foundational tool initially developed by some of us at OMOP that enables transparent and consistent content across disparate observational databases, and serves to support the OHDSI research community in conducting efficient and reproducible observational research.*" [14]

The OMOP Standardised Vocabularies provide semantic interoperability. It combines over 140 existing medical vocabularies, like ICD10, OPCS, SNOMED-CT, READ and RxNorm, into one vocabulary. See Chap. 3 for a more in-depth description of clinical terminologies. This is enriched with the mappings between the terms from these different vocabularies. Specifically, for each clinical idea (e.g. Type 2 Diabetes) one term is assigned as a **standard concept** and all similar terms are mapped to this standard concept (Fig. 3).

The latest release of the OMOP Standardised Vocabulary can be downloaded from Athena [15].

Not all medical ontologies are included in the OMOP Standardised Vocabularies. Especially local ontologies might be missing, for example a national medication vocabulary. In these cases for the mapping to the OMOP CDM, a manual conversion has to be created. This is explained in the sections below.

2.4 Use Cases from the OHDSI Community

The OHDSI community has created a wide range of tooling based on the OMOP CDM. We can roughly divide these tools into three categories: tools to help convert your data to the OMOP CDM, tools to design studies and tools to execute studies.

Using the study tooling, the OHDSI community has executed a quickly growing number of epidemiological studies. These studies can be separated into three pillars: characterization studies, comparative effectiveness/safety studies and prediction studies. Below we have selected three exemplary studies from the OHDSI community for each of these pillars. The focus is on reproducible studies, each paper building new open-source standardised analytics or improving on existing analytics. All studies below are designed using Atlas [16]: a common analysis tool on a common data model.

3 General Pipeline of the Data Source Transformation to OMOP CDM Process

The ETL pipeline represents a series of steps which leads to a conversion of a source data model into a harmonised one. Whilst the desired goal is to automatize most steps in the pipeline, a manual intervention, mainly in source data preparation and terminology mappings, is often necessary.

A typical ETL pipeline consists of source preparation, environment setup, source data profiling, syntactic mapping, semantic mapping and finally validation and quality assessment of the target dataset. Some steps are usually realised iteratively, like going back to the syntactic mapping after quality assessment (Fig. 4, [17]).

Each of the ETL pipeline steps involve participation in one of more of the four typical roles. These groups are not necessarily disjunctive, and one person could fulfil multiple roles.

- Source data expert
- OMOP expert
- Technical ETL expert
- Clinical expert.

3.1 Source Preparation

By the source data we will assume a large dataset of structured (typically tabular) electronic health records (EHRs). This data needs to be analysed and prepared to be compatible with the ETL input interface. Patient level EHRs usually have restricted access and therefore a data governance process for corresponding roles is fundamental. For instance, source data experts and clinicians will typically have full access to the (pseudonymised) data, but OMOP or technical ETL experts might need only access to a subset or only a generated dataset.

Structured EHRs are usually stored in relational databases or plain text files like Comma Separated Values (CSV) files. In case of a plain text file, we need to know some basic file metadata: the coding set in which the files are saved, size of the files, container type if any (.zip archive,.tar.gz, etc.), presence of a table header row, separators between the table columns used (tabs, commas, semi-colons, etc.), quotation marks of character strings used (single or double quotation), end of the line characters used (linux based or windows based) and beginning of the line character used. In some cases this is well documented, in other cases this requires some investigation to get this information.

An upfront analysis of source data could help to estimate required computation power, storage, and free memory. Such information could help with setting up the environment to be supporting the ETL process.

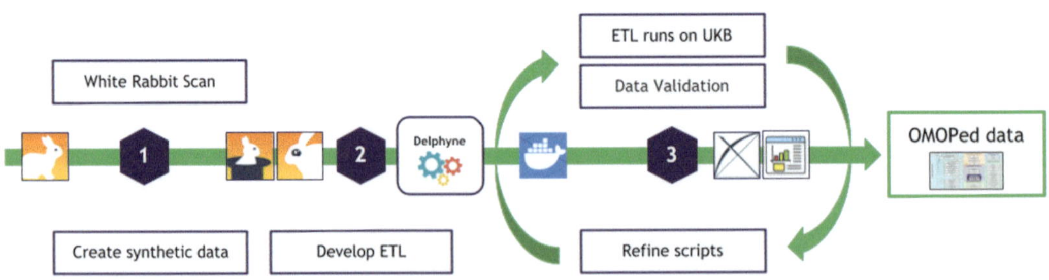

Fig. 4 ETL Pipeline—Transformation of UK Biobank into OMOP CDM use-case [17]

3.2 Environment Setup

The ETL environment consists of a database and an environment to run data transformation scripts. This runtime environment could be dedicated to the ETL or an existing shared environment could be used. Having a dedicated environment (both physical or virtual) means that all software requirements can be installed in isolation and hardware resources would not be shared with other processes. That decreases a risk of negative impact on a shared source data server as well as the ETL stability in case of a potential hardware overload or software incompatibility between the source server requirements and ETL requirements. A drawback of a fully dedicated environment could be a necessity of source data duplication. Also, a dedicated physical environment usually requires extra hardware, which adds overhead cost.

A specification of the ETL runtime environment requirements should contain hardware resources, hosting OS, required target DB system, required input form of source data, list of preinstalled tools, compilers, interpreters, and system and language specific libraries and packages. Main environmental dependency for OMOP CDM ETL is compatible DBMS. OMOP CDM v6 supports multiple DBMS including Oracle DB, PostgreSQL, and MS SQL Server. Other typical environmental requirements are Python 3 and R.

The minimal requirements for setting up an OMOP CDM and analysis environment are listed below:

- Server with about 3× the size of the source data (for raw source, OMOPed data, vocabulary data and Data Quality results)
- Relational database (Oracle DB, PostgreSQL, MS SQL Server)
- The OMOP vocabulary
- Java (White Rabbit, Usagi)
- R+OHDSI R packages for DQ (Achilles, DataQualityDashboard)
- Python (optional, being used as a workflow wrapper)
- OHDSI HADES R packages (analysis)
- OHDSI WebApi+Atlas (analysis)
- Bespoke mapping tools (optional, for example delphyne [17] or Perseus [18])

3.3 Data Profiling

A source data profile provides essential information required for ETL design, synthetic data generation (if necessary), data extraction code and validation test design. The data profile could be created using a dedicated tool like OHDSI WhiteRabbit [19] or by a direct query to all source data tables. Dedicated tools can be connected to the source data, and these will provide the report automatically. In both cases the analysis report ideally contains the following information for all tables:

- Table name with a description
- Field or attribute names
- Number of rows per table
- Number and/or percentage of values in each field—total, unique and empty
- Field data types
- List of most occurring values (e.g., diagnostic codes, measurement values, etc.) for each domain including their frequencies.

With a data profile, a data extraction and two types of transformation—syntactic and semantic—need to be performed. With syntactic mapping we describe a transformation of source attributes onto those of OMOP CDM tables and source values formatting. The semantic mapping covers a translation of source coding systems into systems supported by OMOP CDM.

3.4 Syntactic Mapping

In syntactic, or structural, mapping we define which source table fields/attributes map to which fields of the target model. This step could also include changes in source values structure, e.g., year taken from the date. An example of

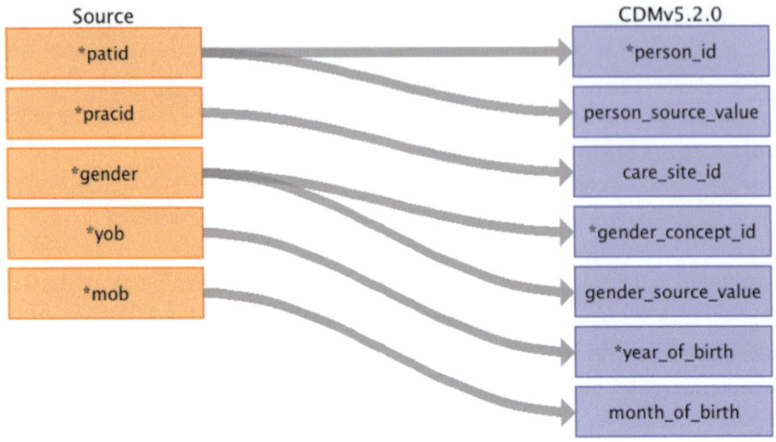

Fig. 5 A Syntax mapping between the CPRD patient table and Person table of OMOP CDM. Graphical representation was generated by the Rabbit-in-a-hat tool

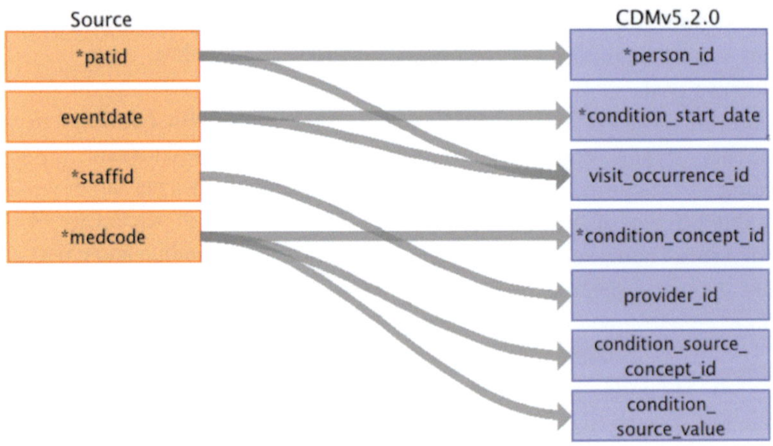

Fig. 6 A Syntax mapping between the CPRD clinical table and Condition Occurrence table of OMOP CDM. Graphical representation was generated by the Rabbit-in-a-hat tool

syntax mapping of a CPRD patient table onto OMOP CDM person table and CPRD clinical table onto OMOP CDM Condition Occurrence table can be seen in Figs. 5 and 6 respectively. The figures were generated by a Rabbit in a Hat tool [20]. Rabbit in a Hat is a syntax mapping assistant for OMOP CDM ETL development. Its graphical user interface (GUI) allows users to visualise syntax mapping between source data structure imported via WhiteRabbit scan report and target version of OMOP CDM. The tool helps with the manual mapping design via graphical representation and mapping document generation, however, the transformation code itself has to be implemented manually.

Two main issues for syntactic mapping could occur.

- the source data is missing for the required field in the target model
- source data elements do not have any equivalents in the target structure.

The first situation can be handled by a logic populating the missing and required target fields, e.g., a fixed value. The second situation may represent a challenge. A main question in that case should be if the data without the equivalent fields in the target structure are necessary or if these could be omitted, e.g., administrative data may not be of interest for population research. If the data is necessary, then the solution depends on the flexibility and robustness of the target data model and potential workarounds. OMOP CDM provides categorised, yet generic, elements/fields suitable for most health-related data to minimise a potential data loss.

3.5 Semantic Mapping

The semantic mapping is often done in the first stages of the ETL development and applied at the same time as the syntactic mapping. i.e., when transforming a local source code field to a standard concept field, we apply the prepared semantic to translate one coding system into the other.

Electronic health data is captured using a variety of medical terminologies (see Chap. 3). These terminologies, or coding systems, allow us to structurally capture things like diagnosis codes, drug codes, measurement units, ethnicity, etc. Often data sites use a mix of local and global terminologies. For network research, we need to harmonise the local coding systems to an agreed upon global standard. For OMOP specifically, we need to map source codes to the standard OMOP vocabulary concepts (see Sect. 2 The OMOP CDM).

Whilst syntactic mapping is mainly manual work, semantic mapping could be effectively automated when a machine-readable validated dictionary lookup between source and target vocabularies exists. Within an OMOP vocabulary, such a lookup is called *concept mapping*. In general, a concept mapping between the source and target terminology could have four existential forms:

1. Direct concept mapping between the source and the target vocabulary exists
2. Direct concept mapping between the source and the target vocabulary does not exist, however an intermediate mapping exists and could be used
3. The concept mapping does not exist
4. Source and target use the same vocabulary (e.g., SNOMED CT).

In the first situation, the concept mapping could be implemented directly into the ETL scripts. A large repository of OMOP CDM compatible dictionaries could be found in the OHDSI Athena Repository [15]. An example of such a scenario could be a mapping between ICD10 terminology and SNOMED CT.

In the second situation, a chain of existing suitable concatenated mappings could substitute a missing direct trustworthy concept mapping. Such a solution is challenging and data loss risk increases with each additional mapping involved (see Sect. 4 Challenges). Figure 7 provides an example observed within a transformation of the CALIBER data source [21, 22].

Thirdly, when no direct or indirect mapping dictionary between the source and target vocabulary exists a new concept mapping needs to be created and reviewed by domain experts thoroughly. Tools designed to ease the new mapping development exist, like OHDSI Usagi [23]. Usagi provides a graphical user interface comparing the uploaded source terminology with selected standard terminologies supported by OMOP CDM. Within the comparison, Usagi calculates a match score based on a similarity between the source and target terms and automatically matches the most likely terms. Each suggestion has to be reviewed by a clinical expert to create a validated concept mapping. There can be thousands of codes that need to be reviewed, which is a considerable amount of work. We can prioritise this work by using the term frequency (Fig. 8).

Finally, when the source data uses a coding system that is already used as standard concepts in OMOP, only a simple lookup of the OMOP concept id is needed. For example, part of the UK data is coded at the source with SNOMED codes. This code is present in the OMOP vocabularies and can be retrieved with a simple SQL query. One consideration is to check whether the

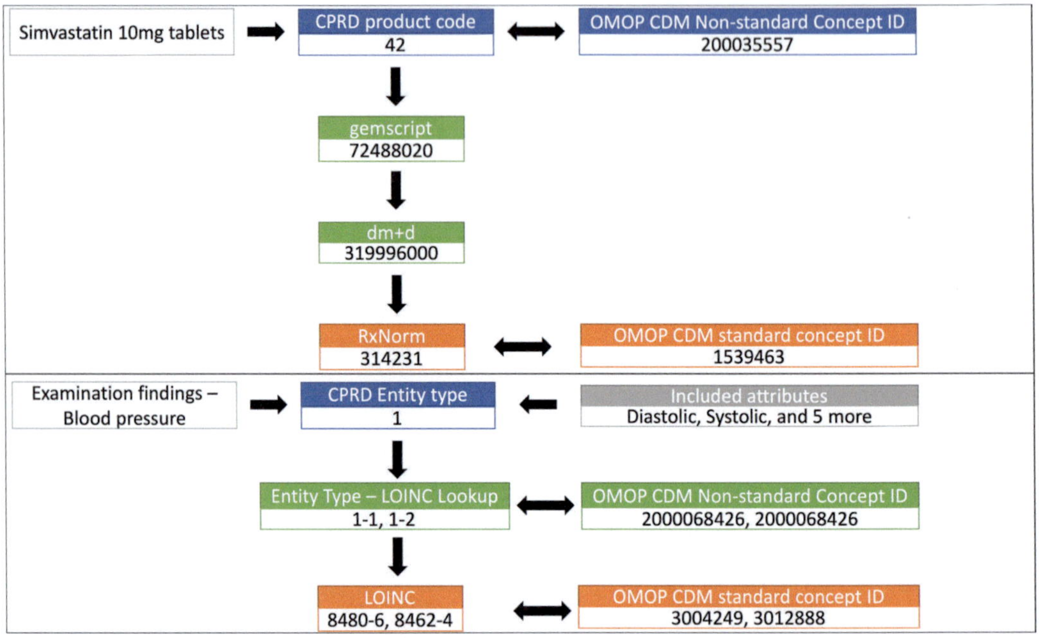

Fig. 7 Two examples where additional mappings were used. In the first case, CPRD product codes were translated into a gemscript terminology, then to dm+d terminology and finally to a target RxNorm terminology. In the second example, CPRD Entity types were firstly translated via a manual mapping file

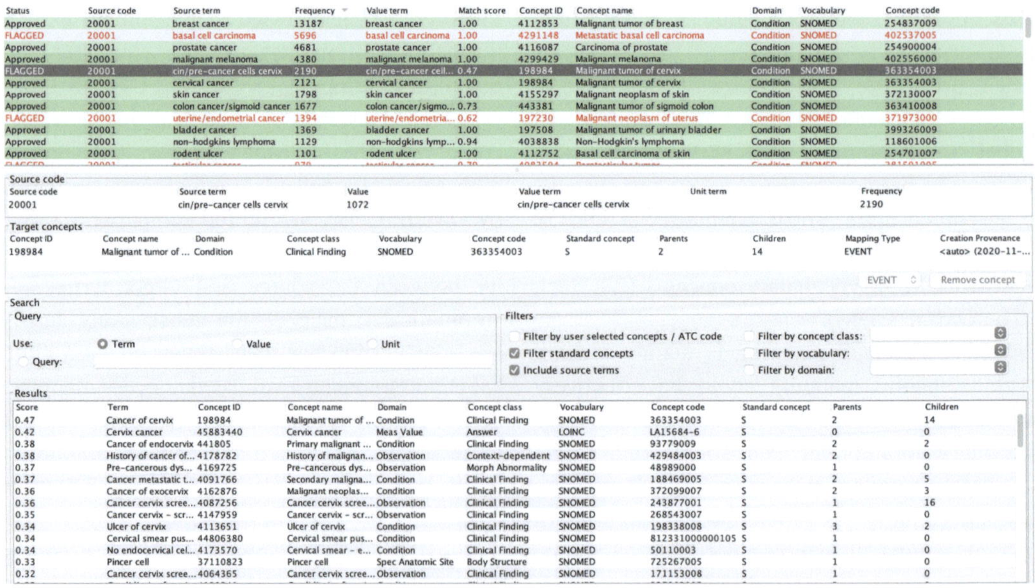

Fig. 8 OHDSI USAGI mapping tool comparing source participant self-reported cancer-illness UK Biobank vocabulary and target SNOMED vocabulary. Codes are ordered by the frequency of used terms

code in the OMOP vocabulary is still valid. If not, the OMOP vocabulary provides a mapping to the equivalent valid concept.

3.6 Validation

Validation starts during the ETL development by implementing a set of unit and/or end-to-end tests. Unit tests are for validating particular data manipulation functions and end-to-end tests allow validation of the whole pipeline by providing a known input and the expected output. The latter is especially important for validating the complete ETL pipeline. It makes it possible to detect any unwanted effects of code changes before running the ETL on actual data. We should note that it takes considerable effort to get a high coverage of tests, covering the most occurring scenarios.

Once the ETL is finished, a comprehensive validation of the target database including correctness of both semantic and syntactic mappings needs to be performed.

A first check on the ETL completeness is given by a comparison of general counts representing the dataset between the source and target databases. These counts typically include the number of patients, ratio between sex/ethnicity, average patient age, the number of events/prescriptions or median follow-up. Analytic tools like Achilles [24], Data Quality Dashboard (DQD) [25] and CDM Inspection [26] help to easily retrieve these overall counts from the OMOP CDM. The DQD provides a series of checks resulting in a data quality score. This score makes heterogeneous source datasets comparable on the same data quality metrics.

Another tool developed by OHDSI, the CDM Inspection report, contains a list of most used mapped and unmapped terms. Thus, the unmapped terms could be investigated individually based on their significance.

For use-case based (non-systematic) ETL evaluation miscellaneous codelists/cohort definitions to identify specific patient cohorts covering diverse fields of health care can be used. In previous research we have shown the validation process, comparing results on the source data and OMOP-transformed data for lifestyle data (smoking status, deprivation index), clinical measures (BMI, Blood pressure, haemoglobin concentration), clinical diagnosis (diabetes, cancer) or drug prescriptions (Beta blockers, loop diuretics) [22]. As the thorough test of all the used codes is time consuming, we should prioritise tests on the most frequently used codes and most needed codes according to the use case.

The OHDSI community has developed a tool, Cohort Diagnostics, that does something similar. Based on a set of phenotypes it will make suggestions on what other concepts are relevant and produce aggregate statistics to manually inspect [27].

4 Challenges of Harmonisation

Harmonisation of diverse data models into a common one in the health/bioinformatics domain is accompanied by several inevitable challenges.

4.1 Data and Information Loss

One of the most crucial challenges is to prevent the harmonisation from relevant data and/or information loss. Relevance of data depends on the purpose of the harmonised dataset, e.g., administrative details or internal hospital information would not be relevant for population-level studies and thus could be lost with no harm.

While data loss is mainly (not exclusively) caused by the structural mapping when part of the source data is not transformed into a target model, an information loss could be given also by the incorrect or imprecise interpretation and translation of the transformed data during the semantic mapping.

4.1.1 Data Loss

Data could get lost in the ETL process and/or due to issues/inconsistencies in the original datasets. Source data providers may use diverse recording practices (table structures, used coding systems), documentation practices, management of missing data, technicalities of data distribution, data cleaning processes before the distribution, etc. Combination of these factors within the same source dataset could lead to scenarios predisposed to data losses, e.g.:

- A source record does not include a data field which is mandatory from the perspective of CDM. This can be handled in two ways—making an assumption for this field or removing the patient during the ETL, e.g., a registration date may be inferred from other fields, however, records belonging to patients with missing mandatory demographic details like gender or year of birth would be removed during the ETL. These patients are deemed to be of too low quality for population research.
- Unexpected value in a domain for a specific data field, e.g., values are expected to be positive only, however a negative value appears
- Diagnostic events happen outside the patient's observation period which starts with a patient's registration date at GP and ends with the last event or the patient's death.
- A broken follow up when a patient changes GP; the scenario could lead to a situation when one patient is being considered as two different ones.
- Same data field is using multiple different coding systems (e.g., ICD10 and SNOMED CT) and these are not explicitly distinguished.
- Source record contains a clinical code unrecognised in a mapping dictionary / target vocabulary used.
- Inconsistent records for unvarying data fields, e.g., a same patient would have a different sex during different visits.

Some of these scenarios can be fixed during the ETL (e.g., handling unexpected values), but others are inherent to incompatibilities between source and target data model. Therefore, a potential risk of data loss is inevitable.

4.1.2 Information Loss

Despite the correct and complete syntactic transformation, the information derived from the source records may not be fully reflected in the target CDM. Such information loss is often caused by an imprecise semantic translation from the source to the target coding system.

A source and target terminology could have a different level of granularity. This gives problems if the source terminology contains terms with more detail than the target terminology. Generalisation of the source term solves the problem at a cost of losing details. Incompleteness could be also found in a translation relation itself. Figure 9 shows the loss of information on a fragment of Chronic Obstructive Pulmonary Disease (COPD) phenotype. The loss of information of this type causes another secondary issue which is an incompatibility of source clinically approved phenotyping codelists with transformed CDM as these codelists cannot be precisely translated into the target terminology.

In the OMOP CDM, the granularity is preserved in the 'source concepts'. Locally, we can still define phenotypes based on the original codes. However, definitions based on source concepts instead of standard concepts are not executable at other data sites as these will not, very likely, share same local source concepts.

We can distinguish between several levels of equivalence of code translation (Table 3) [28]. The two top-levels without information loss are equal (exactly the same term) and equivalent (similar definition). Information loss occurs when a translation is wider (target term is more general), narrower (target term is more specific) or inexact (both source and target have meaning not covered in the other). The latter three levels still capture a part of the information but can lead to issues as described in Fig. 7. Most information loss occurs when a source code is unmatched in the target coding system (or 'unmapped'). Unfortunately, this is often unavoidable, and the percentage of unmapped codes is an important quality metric. In all cases this is

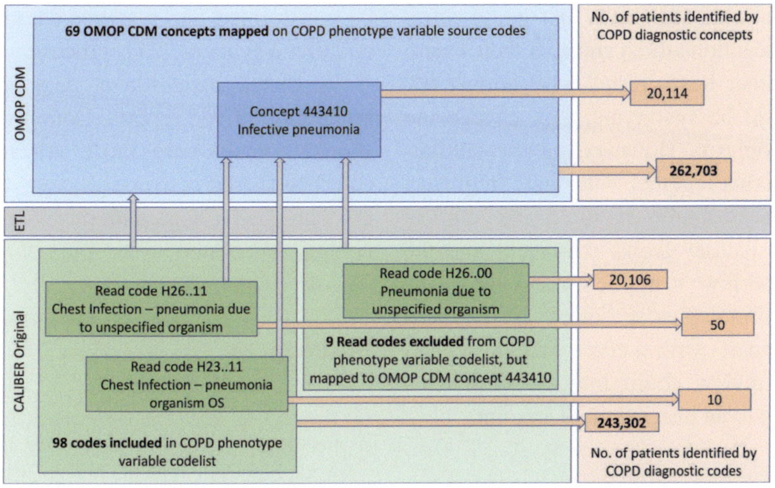

Fig. 9 Papez et al. [22] Example of inconsistency between original and converted records demonstrated with codelist from the Chronic Obstructive Pulmonary Disease (COPD) phenotype. Multiple source terminology terms codes (Read codes in green boxes) are mapped onto the same OMOP CDM target concept (blue box). The mapped concept however includes a broader set of clinical diagnoses which are not part of the original COPD phenotype. As a result, the number of patients retrieved (orange boxes) in the raw data using the original phenotype terms (243,302) is significantly lower than the number of patients retrieved using the OMOP CDM phenotype (262,703). Main result difference is caused by the Read code H26.0.00 Pneumonia due to unspecified organism used in more that 20,106 patients, which is excluded from COPD phenotype, but mapped to the same concept of Infective pneumonia as other Read codes from the phenotype

Table 3 Examples of equivalence levels

Equivalence level	Description	Example
Equivalent	Source and target contain the same information	Source—Depression Assessment Test Target—Assessment of depressed mood
Wider	The target is a more general concept than the source. In the mapping some information is lost, but the general information is captured	Source—Release of the median nerve at the carpal tunnel, by video surgery Target—Transposition of median nerve at carpal tunnel
Narrower	The target is a more specific concept than the source. In the mapping some information is added	Source—Corneal pachymetry Target—Ophthalmic ultrasound, diagnostic; corneal pachymetry, unilateral or bilateral (determination of corneal thickness)
Inexact	The target and source contain information that is not present in the other. In the mapping information is both lost and added	Source—Screening tests for deafness before the age of 3 years old Target—Ear disorder screening

a subject worthy of investigation whether it can be improved.

A key resource when fixing above mentioned issues is time. While the source and target terms with similar descriptions could be handled automatically, the others must be manually mapped or at least reviewed. Tools like Usagi provide a great help in sorting the terms by their frequency in the source dataset and calculation of text similarity weight between source and mostly probable target term. This speeds up the review process of mostly used terms rapidly. It is still good to be aware that even highly similar terms are not necessarily synonyms diverse in a punctuation or case sensitivity but could differ in presented negation which changes their meaning; on the other hand, terms with almost 0% similarity could be synonyms, e.g., cancer and malignant neoplasm. However, as the similarity between terms together with their frequency decrease, time resource required per clinical record in the dataset grows massively and the rule of the vital few[1] is applied. A review of the controlled terminologies and mappings is a task for domain experts with a corresponding expertise. Such a review could increase demanded time resources to an unacceptable amount.

4.2 Data Privacy and Sensitivity

Working with personal-level health data is usually accompanied with a strict policy regarding data privacy and sensitivity. Usually, only a selected subset of people involved in the ETL development has an approval to access the health data that the ETL is being developed for. Also, a common practice is that the health data must not leave the datacenter the data is stored in, which in some cases differs from the centre where the ETL code is being developed, tested or even performed in case of the dedicated ETL environment. Therefore, the ETL development might have to be realised using synthetic data only. Despite the identical structure the synthetic data could have with the real data, unexpected differences in the value domains could appear (see Sect. 4.1.1 Data loss).

Usually, synthetic data are generated by bespoke tools designed for one specific purpose like the tool Tofu [29] for UK Biobank data or by a generic tool for synthetic EHRs like Synthea [30]. A usage of a generic synthetic data could lead to an additional challenge when the structure of the synthetic data needs to be transformed into a source data structure, i.e., additional syntactic ETL process.

Restricted patient-level data access is also related to derived reports. Data profiling reports should contain only those information which could be shared between all developers and testers who need it, e.g., data profiling report would contain aggregated information only.

[1] The Pareto Principle, also 80/20 principle; applied on the mapping problem the principle says that by covering 20% of most frequently used terms, an 80% of all records will be mapped correctly. In the opposite way, to cover/map the last 20% of source terms will take approx. 80% of time.

References

1. Hripcsak G, Ryan PB, Duke JD, et al. Characterizing treatment pathways at scale using the OHDSI network. Proc Natl Acad Sci U S A. 2016;113:7329–36. https://doi.org/10.1073/pnas.1510502113.
2. Williams RD, Markus AF, Yang C, et al. Seek COVER: development and validation of a personalized risk calculator for COVID-19 outcomes in an international network. bioRxiv. 2020. https://doi.org/10.1101/2020.05.26.20112649.
3. FAIR principles. GO FAIR. 2017. https://www.go-fair.org/fair-principles/ (Accessed 29 Jun 2022).
4. EMA. A common data model in Europe? – Why? Which? How? European Medicines Agency. 2018. https://www.ema.europa.eu/events/common-data-model-europe-why-which-how (Accessed 29 Jun 2022).
5. FHIR v4.3.0. http://hl7.org/fhir/R4B (Accessed 29 Jun 2022).
6. Kalra D, Beale T, Heard S. The openEHR Foundation. Stud Health Technol Inform 2005;115:153–73. https://www.ncbi.nlm.nih.gov/pubmed/16160223.
7. OHDSI—observational health data sciences and informatics. http://ohdsi.org (Accessed 29 Jun 2022).
8. SDTM. https://www.cdisc.org/standards/foundational/sdtm (Accessed 29 Jun 2022).
9. Schuemie MJ, Ryan PB, Pratt N, et al. Large-scale evidence generation and evaluation across a network of databases (LEGEND): assessing validity using hypertension as a case study. J Am Med Inform Assoc. 2020;27:1268–77. https://doi.org/10.1093/jamia/ocaa124.
10. Overhage JM, Ryan PB, Reich CG, et al. Validation of a common data model for active safety surveillance research. J Am Med Inform Assoc. 2012;19:54–60. https://doi.org/10.1136/amiajnl-2011-000376.
11. Benson T, Grieve G. Principles of health interoperability: FHIR, HL7 and SNOMED CT. Springer Nature 2020. https://play.google.com/store/books/details?id=TiwEEAAAQBAJ.
12. Observational Health Data Sciences, Informatics. Chapter 1 the OHDSI community. 2021.https://ohdsi.github.io/TheBookOfOhdsi/OhdsiCommunity.html (Accessed 29 Jun 2022).

13. index.knit. https://ohdsi.github.io/CommonDataModel/index.html (Accessed 29 Jun 2022).
14. Data standardization. https://ohdsi.org/data-standardization/ (Accessed 29 Jun 2022).
15. Liu J, Li D, Gioiosa R, et al. Athena. In: Proceedings of the ACM international conference on supercomputing. New York, NY, USA: ACM 2021. https://doi.org/10.1145/3447818.3460355.
16. Kernighan BW, Plauger PJ. Software tools. SIGSOFT Softw Eng Notes. 1976;1:15–20. https://doi.org/10.1145/1010726.1010728.
17. Digital Natives. Mapping UK Biobank to the OMOP CDM using the flexible ETL framework Delphyne. the-hyve. https://www.thehyve.nl/cases/mapping-uk-biobank-to-omop-using-delphyne (Accessed 19 Jul 2022).
18. 'Perseus': Design and run your own ETL to CDM. https://ohdsi.org/2021-global-symposium-showcase-79/ (Accessed 19 Jul 2022).
19. *OHDSI WhiteRabbit tool.* Github https://github.com/OHDSI/WhiteRabbit (Accessed 25 May 2022).
20. Rabbit in a Hat. http://ohdsi.github.io/WhiteRabbit/RabbitInAHat.html (Accessed 29 Jun 2022).
21. Denaxas SC, George J, Herrett E, et al. Data resource profile: cardiovascular disease research using linked bespoke studies and electronic health records (CALIBER). Int J Epidemiol. 2012;41:1625–38. https://doi.org/10.1093/ije/dys188.
22. Papez V, Moinat M, Payralbe S, et al. Transforming and evaluating electronic health record disease phenotyping algorithms using the OMOP common data model: a case study in heart failure. JAMIA Open 2021;4:ooab001. https://doi.org/10.1093/jamiaopen/ooab001.
23. USAGI for vocabulary mapping. https://www.ohdsi.org/analytic-tools/usagi/ (Accessed 29 Jun 2022).
24. ACHILLES for data characterization. https://www.ohdsi.org/analytic-tools/achilles-for-data-characterization/ (Accessed 29 Jun 2022).
25. DataQualityDashboard: A tool to help improve data quality standards in observational data science. Github https://github.com/OHDSI/DataQualityDashboard (Accessed 29 Jun 2022).
26. CdmInspection: R Package to support quality control inspection of an OMOP-CDM instance. Github https://github.com/EHDEN/CdmInspection (Accessed 29 Jun 2022).
27. Diagnostics for OHDSI cohorts. https://ohdsi.github.io/CohortDiagnostics/ (Accessed 29 Jun 2022).
28. Valueset-concept-map-equivalence - FHIR v4.3.0. https://www.hl7.org/fhir/valueset-concept-map-equivalence.html (Accessed 29 Jun 2022).
29. Denaxas S. spiros/tofu: Updated release for DOI. 2020. https://doi.org/10.5281/zenodo.3634604.
30. synthetichealth. Github https://github.com/synthetichealth (Accessed 29 Jun 2022).

Natural Language Processing and Text Mining (Turning Unstructured Data into Structured)

Ayoub Bagheri, Anastasia Giachanou, Pablo Mosteiro and Suzan Verberne

Abstract

The integration of natural language processing (NLP) and text mining techniques has emerged as a key approach to harnessing the potential of unstructured clinical text data. This chapter discusses the challenges posed by clinical narratives and explores the need to transform them into structured formats for improved data accessibility and analysis. The chapter navigates through key concepts, including text pre-processing, text classification, text clustering, topic modeling, and advances in language models and transformers. It highlights the dynamic interplay between these techniques and their applications in tasks ranging from disease classification to extraction of side effects. In addition, the chapter acknowledges the importance of addressing bias and ensuring model explainability in the context of clinical prediction systems. By providing a comprehensive overview, the chapter offers insights into the synergy of NLP and text mining techniques in shaping the future of biomedical AI, ultimately leading to safer, more efficient, and more informed healthcare decisions.

Keywords

Natural language processing · Text mining · Clinical text · Text pre-processing · Language models · Text classification · Text clustering · Topic modeling · Explainability · Bias detection · Clinical NLP

1 Introduction

The field of biomedical artificial intelligence (AI) is undergoing a revolution. The widespread use of biomedical data sources next to electronic health records (EHR) systems provides a large amount of data in healthcare, leading to new areas for clinical research. These resources are rich in data with the potential to leverage applications that provide safer care, reduce medical errors, reduce healthcare expenditure, and enable providers to improve their productivity, quality and efficiency [1, 2]. A major portion of this data is inside free text in the form of physicians' notes, discharge summaries, and radiology reports among many other types of clinical narratives such as patient experiences. This clinical text follows the patient through the care procedures and documents the patient's complaints and symptoms, physical exam, diagnostic

A. Bagheri (✉) · A. Giachanou · P. Mosteiro
University Utrecht, Utrecht, Netherlands
e-mail: a.bagheri@uu.nl

S. Verberne
Leiden University, Leiden, Netherlands

F. W. Asselbergs et al. (eds.), *Clinical Applications of Artificial Intelligence in Real-World Data*,
https://doi.org/10.1007/978-3-031-36678-9_5

tests, conclusions, treatments, and outcomes of the treatment.

Free text in the clinical domain is unstructured information, which is difficult to process automatically. Despite many attempts to encode text in the form of structured data [3], free text continues to be used in EHRs. Additionally, clinical texts are packed with substantial amounts of abbreviations, special characters, stop words, and spelling errors. Therefore, natural language processing (NLP) and text mining techniques can be applied to create a more structured representation of a text, making its content more accessible for data science, machine learning and statistics, and for medical prediction models.

A widely accepted definition of text mining has been provided by Hearst [4], as "the discovery by computer of new, previously unknown information, by automatically extracting information from different written resources". Text mining is about looking for patterns in text, in a similar way that data mining can be loosely described as looking for patterns in data. According to [5], NLP is one of the most widely used big data analytical techniques in healthcare, and is defined as "any computer-based algorithm that handles, augments, and transforms natural language so that it can be represented for computation" [6]. There is therefore often an overlap of the tasks, methods, and goals for text mining and NLP, and the concepts are sometimes used interchangeably. Fleuren and Alkema [7] describe clinical text mining as automated processing and analysis of text in relevant textual biources. Text mining typically involves a number of distinct phases including information retrieval, named entity recognition, information extraction and knowledge discovery. The first step concerns collecting and filtering relevant documents. After information retrieval, the resulting document collection can be analyzed by classification or clustering algorithms. As a last step, information extraction is performed to generate structured data from unstructured text.

Text mining and NLP techniques have been applied to numerous health applications involving text de-identification tools [8], clinical decision support systems [2], patient identification [9–12], disease classification [13–15], disease history [16], ICD10 classification [17], hospital readmission prediction [18], and chronic disease prediction [19].

Although those systems can now achieve high performance in various clinical prediction tasks, they come with some limitations. A common issue is related to whether there is any bias introduced in any step involved in learning process. This is important because we know that systems are trained on data which contain societal stereotypes, and can therefore learn to reproduce them in their predictions. Another limitation is that clinicians are reluctant to widely use those systems because, among other reasons, they do not understand the complicated processes on which the predictions are made. Those limitations have led to the necessity of systems that can produce explanations regarding their learning mechanism and decisions.

The successive sections of this chapter are organised as follows: Sect. 2 provides a gentle introduction on NLP and the common techniques when conducting biomedical and clinical text analysis. Subsequently, we discuss state-of-the-art pre-trained language models in Sect. 3, and NLP tasks and their challenges in healthcare in Sect. 4. Finally, we overview bias and explainability of NLP-based models for biomedical and clinical text in Sects. 5 and 6, respectively. We conclude the chapter with a summary and recommendations.

2 What Is Natural Language Processing

Natural language processing is an area of artificial intelligence concerned with the interactions between computers and human languages. There are many applications of NLP in specific domains, such as machine translation of legal documents, mental disease detection, news summarization, patent information retrieval, and so on.

2.1 Text Preprocessing

With the advancements of NLP, it is possible to develop methodologies and automate different natural language tasks. NLP tasks can be divided in document-level tasks (Sects. 2.2 and 2.3), sequence labelling tasks (Sect. 2.4), and sequence-to-sequence processing (not discussed in this chapter). There are two types of document-level tasks: *text classification* and *text clustering*. The former refers to tasks of adding labels from a pre-defined label set to a text. In other words, we are interested in classifying texts into pre-defined categories. Annotating a piece of text as expressing positive or negative sentiment or classifying an EHR regarding the patient's risk of disease are two text classification examples. Text clustering refers to automatically group textual documents into clusters based on their content similarity. In this case, there are no pre-defined categories. Topic clustering of textual documents is one example of such a task. In sequence labelling tasks, one label is added to each word in a text, to identify and extract specific relevant information such as named entities. Finally, in sequence-to-sequence tasks, both the input and the output is text, like in translation or summarization.

Text from natural language is often noisy and unstructured and needs to be pre-processed before it can be used in one of these tasks. Pre-processing transforms text into a consistent form that is readable from the machines. The most common steps are sentence segmentation, word tokenization, lowercasing, stemming or lemmatization, stop word removal, and spelling correction.

Here, we should note that an NLP system can involve some or all of those steps. The steps and the techniques that will be used depends on the data, the task and the method used. For example, social media posts contain special characters and emoticons and the NLP researcher can decide how to handle them, whereas domain specific stop words may be necessary when EHRs are analyzed. In addition, for sequence labelling it is important to keep capitalisation, punctuation and word order, while these aspects can be disregarded in text classification or clustering. Below we will briefly describe the most common steps, which are the sentence segmentation, tokenization and stemming/lemmatization.

Segmentation The NLP pipeline usually starts with the sentence segmentation that refers to divide the text into sentences. Although this looks like a trivial task, there are some challenges. For example, in social media texts users tend to use emoticons that are a combination of symbols including a period (.), question mark (?) or exclamation mark (!). Additionally, a period is used in many abbreviations (e.g., Mr.) that makes the sentence segmentation more challenging. Packages such as NLTK and Spacy can perform sentence segmentation for a range of languages.

Tokenization Tokenization is one of the core steps in pre-processing and refers to converting a sentence into tokens. Traditionally, tokens are words, punctuation marks, or numbers, but in some contexts subwords can be used as tokens (see Sect. 3.3). In some tasks, we can also add tokens that capture other type of information such as word order or part-of-speech tags (i.e., information that refers to the type such as noun, verb etc.).

Stemming and Lemmatization Both stemming and lemmatization aim to normalize the tokens that refer to the same base but appear in a different form in the text (e.g., disease and diseases). Stemming is based on a more heuristic process and cuts the ends of the words, whereas lemmatization is based on the morphological analysis of words, and aims to return the base of a word (known as the lemma). For example, stemming of the verb *saw* can result to no changes while lemmatization will return the base form of the word which is *see*.

2.2 Text Classification

Text classification is the task of assigning one or more predefined categories to documents based on their contents. Given a document d and a set of n_C class labels $C_L \in \{1, \ldots, n_C\}$, text classification tries to learn a classification function $f : D \rightarrow C_L$ that maps a set of documents to labels. Text classification can be implemented as an automated process involving none or a small amount of interaction with expert users [20]. A general pipeline for a text classification system is illustrated in Fig. 1.

In binary text classification each document is assigned to either a specific predefined label or to the complement of that label (e.g. relevant or non-relevant). On the other hand, multi-class classification refers to the situation where each document is assigned a label from a set of n classes (where $n > 2$). Multi-label text classification refers to the case in which a document can be associated with more than one label. Text classification contains four different levels of scope that can be applied: (1) Document level, (2) Paragraph level, (3) Sentence level, and (4) Phrase level.

2.3 Text Clustering and Topic Modeling

With unsupervised learning such as clustering, there are no labeled examples to learn from, instead the goal is to find some structure or patterns in the input data [21]. Text clustering is an example of unsupervised learning, which aims to group texts or words according to some measure of similarity [22]. The goal of clustering is to identify the underlying structure of the observed data, such that there are a few clusters of points, each of which is internally coherent. Clustering algorithms assign each data point to a discrete cluster $c_i \in 1, 2, \ldots, K$.

Broadly speaking, clustering can be divided into subgroups; hard and soft clustering. Hard clustering groups the data in such a way that each item is assigned to one cluster, whereas in soft clustering one item can belong to multiple clusters. Topic modeling is a type of soft clustering [23, 24]. Topic modeling provides a convenient unsupervised way to analyze high-dimensional data such as text. It is a form of text analysis in which a collection is assumed to cover a set of topics; a topic is defined as a probability distribution over all words in the collection (some words being very prominent for the topic and other words not related to the topic) and each document is represented by a probability distribution over all topics (some topics being very prominent in the document, and other topics not covered).

There have been a number of topic modeling algorithms proposed in the literature. The most popular topic model is the Latent Dirichlet Allocation (LDA) that is a powerful generative latent topic model [23]. It applies unsupervised learning on texts to induce sets of associated words. LDA defines every topic as a distribution over the words of the vocabulary, and every document as a distribution over the topics.

LDA specifies a probabilistic procedure by which documents can be generated. Figure 2 shows a text generation process by a topic model. Topic 1 and topic 2 shown in the figure have different word distributions so that they can constitute documents by choosing the words which have different importance degree to the topic. Document 1 and document 3 are generated by the respective random sampling of topic 1 and topic 2. But, topic 1 and topic 2 generate document 2 according to the mixture of their different topic distributions. Here, the numbers at the right side of a word are its belonging topic numbers and, the word is obtained by the random sampling of the numbered topic.

LDA uses a K-dimensional latent random variable which obeys the Dirichlet distribution to represent the topic mixture ratio of the document, which simulates the generation process of the document. Let K be the multinomial topic distributions for the dataset containing V elements each, where V is the number of terms in the dataset. Let β_i represent the multinomial for the i-th topic, where the size of β_i is V. Given these distributions, the LDA generative process is as follows:

Algorithm 1: Generative process in LDA

for *each document* **do**
  (a) Randomly choose a K-dimensional multinomial distribution over topics
  for *each word in the document* **do**
    (i) Probabilistically draw β_j from the distribution over topics obtained in (a)
    (ii) Probabilistically draw one of the V words from β_j
  end
end

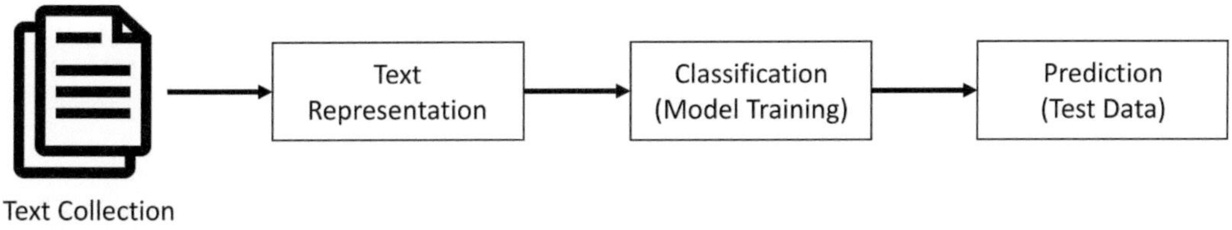

Fig. 1 The general pipeline of a text classification system

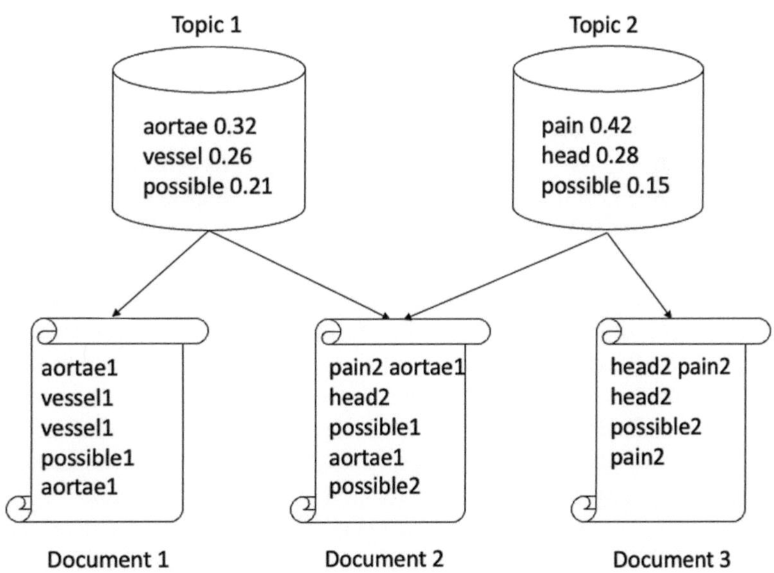

Fig. 2 The generative process of topic modeling

LDA emphasizes that documents contain multiple topics. For instance, a discharge letter might have words drawn from the topic related to the patient's symptoms and words drawn from the topic related to the patient's treatment. LDA uses sampling from the Dirichlet distribution to generate a text with the specific topic multinomial distribution, where the text is usually composed of some latent topics. And then, these topics are sampled repeatedly to generate each word for the document. Thus, the latent topics can be seen as the probability distribution of the words in the LDA model. And, each document is expressed as the random mixture of these latent topics according to the specific proportion.

The goal of LDA is to automatically discover the topics from a collection of documents. Standard statistical techniques can be used to invert the generative process of LDA, thus inferring the set of topics that were responsible for generating a collection of documents. The exact inference in LDA is generally intractable, therefore approximate inference algorithms are needed for posterior estimation. The most common approaches that are used for approximate inference are expectation-maximization, Gibbs sampling and variational method [25].

LDA has been applied in the health domain as well. Duarte et al. [26] applied LDA on a collection of electronic health records and showed that some topics occur more often in the deceased patients, like renal diseases, and others (e.g., diabetes) appear more often in the discharge collection. Li et al. [27] used LDA to cluster patient diagnostics groups from Rochester Epidemiology Projects (REP) that contains medical records. In their study, they identified 20 topics that could almost be connected with some group of diseases. However, they also observed that the same diagnosis code group might fall into different topics. LDA has not only been used to extract topics, but also as an alternative way to represent the documents [28].

LDA is accessible to work with, thanks to the implementation of the model in packages such as gensim.[1] There are a few challenges for the user though: First, the topics are unlabeled so a human has to assign labels to the topics to make them quickly interpretable. Second, LDA is not deterministic; in multiple runs it will give multiple different outputs. Third, the number of topics needs to be determined beforehand, e.g. through optimizing the model for topic coherence [29].

2.4 Information Extraction

As discussed in Sect. 2.2, in text classification tasks, labels are assigned to a text as a whole (a whole document, paragraph, or sentence). In information extraction tasks on the other hand, labels are assigned to each token in the text. The token labels identify tokens as being part of a relevant term, typically an entity such as a name. The task of identifying entities in text is called *Named Entity Recognition*. Machine learning tasks that learn to assign a label to each token are called *sequence labelling* tasks.

In sequence labelling, word order is important, because subsequent words might together form an entity (e.g. 'New York', 'breast cancer'), and words in the context of the entity words can give information about the presence of an entity. Take for example the sentence "Since taking Gleevec, the patient has peripheral edema". Even without ever having seen the word Gleevec, you can deduce from its context that it is a medication name. Apart from word order and context, capitalisation and punctuation are relevant in sequence labelling tasks: names are often capitalised, and punctuation such as bracketing sometimes provides information about the presence of an entity or the relation between two entities. These characteristics set information extraction tasks apart from text classification tasks, despite both being supervised learning tasks.

When creating labelled data for sequence labelling, words and word groups are marked in

[1] https://radimrehurek.com/gensim/.

Table 1 Example of IOB labelling with one medication name and one adverse drug reaction (ADR)

Since	Taking	Gleevec	,	The	Patient	Has	Peripheral	Edema
O	O	B-MED	O	O	O	O	B-ADR	I-ADR

annotation tools such as doccano[2] and inception.[3] These annotations are then converted to a file format with one label per token. The common token labelling scheme for named entity recognition is *IOB labelling*, in which each token gets one of three labels: 'I' if the token is inside an entity; 'O' if it is outside an entity; 'B' if it is the first token of an entity. The B and I labels have a suffix, indicating their type. Table 1 gives an example of IOB labelling for one sentence. Here, B-MED indicates the first word of the medication name, B-ADR the beginning of the adverse drug reaction (ADR), and I-ADR the subsequent word of a the ADR entity.

Based on token-level labelled data, sequence labelling models can be trained that take a vector representation for each token as input and learn the output label. For sequence labelling, we need machine learning models that take the context of tokens into account. The most commonly used feature-based sequence labelling model is Conditional Random Fields (CRF).[4] Since around 2016, CRF was typically used on top of a neural sequence model, Bi-LSTM [30]. LSTMs (Long Short-Term Memory models) are recurrent neural networks. These are neural network models that, instead of classifying each token independently, use the learned representations of the previous words for learning the label of the current token. Bi-LSTM-CRFs were the state of the art for named entity recognition for some years, before they were superseded by transformer-based models (see Sect. 3.1).

In addition to named entity recognition, *relation extraction* is often relevant: we not only want to identify medications and ADRs, but also which ADR is related to which medication. Another prominent relation extraction task in the biomedical domain is the relation between genes, proteins and diseases. Information extraction methods rely on co-occurrence of entities, both for unsupervised or supervised labelling. In supervised labelling, co-occurrence is combined with representations of the entities and their context to decide for a pair of entities whether or not there is a relation between them. An overview of methods is provided by Nasar et al. [31].

2.5 Text Representations

As introduced in Sect. 2.1, the first step of the NLP pipeline is to prepare the raw text into a representation that can be used for further processing. We have introduced classification, clustering and extraction tasks. In this subsection we will explain commonly used text representations: how to represent texts in a form that can be used as input to machine learning models.

2.5.1 Bag-of-Word Models

To perform text classification and after the text pre-processing, the question is how to represent each text document [22, 32]. A document can be seen as an observation in the dataset, e.g. a patient discharge letter in a collection of discharge summaries, or a chest x-ray report. A common approach is to use vector models of a co-occurrence matrix. A co-occurrence matrix is a way of representing how often words co-occur. An example of such co-occurrence matrices is a document-term matrix, in which each row represents a document from the dataset and each matrix column represents a word in the vocabulary of the dataset. Table 2 shows a small selection from a document-term matrix of radiology reports showing the occurrence of seven words in five documents.

[2] https://doccano.github.io/doccano/.

[3] https://inception-project.github.io/.

[4] A tutorial with a description of features for named entity recognition can be found on https://sklearn-crfsuite.readthedocs.io/en/latest/tutorial.html.

Table 2 Document-term matrix

Document	Abnormalities	Aortae	Possible	Nicotine	Pain	Thoracic
1	1	0	1	0	0	0
2	1	1	1	1	0	0
3	1	0	0	0	1	0
4	1	0	0	0	0	0
5	1	0	0	1	0	1

In Table 2, each document is represented as a vector of word counts. This representation is often called a *bag-of-words*, because it includes only information about the count of each word, and not the order in which the words appear. With the bag-of-words representation, we are ignoring grammar and order of the words. Yet the bag-of-words model is surprisingly effective for text classification [22].

There are three commonly used bag-of-words representations of text data, corresponding to the *binary*, the TF, and the $TFiDF$ model. A binary representation model corresponds to whether or not a word is present in the document. In some applications, such as finding frequently co-occurring groups of k words, it is sufficient to use a binary representation. However, it may lead to the loss of information because it does not contain the frequencies of the words [32].

The most basic form of frequency-based text feature extraction is TF. TF stands for the term frequency. In this method, each word is mapped to its number of occurrences in the text. However, this approach is limited by the fact that particular words (e.g., patient in a health application) that are commonly used in the language may dominate such representations. Most representations of text use normalized frequencies of the words. One approach is the $TFiDF$, where iDF stands for the inverse document frequency. The mathematical representation of the weight of the term t in the document d by TFiDF is given in:

$$TFiDF(d,t) = TF(d,t)log\left(\frac{N}{DF(t)}\right) \quad (1)$$

where $TF(d,t)$ is the frequency of the term t in document d, N is the number of documents and $DF(t)$ is the number of documents containing the term t. Although TFiDF tries to overcome the problem of common words in the document, it still suffers from the fact that it cannot account for the order of the words and the similarity between them in the document since each word is independently presented. Another issue with TFiDF is that even though it removes common words, it might decrease the performance by increasing the frequencies of misspellings that were not properly handled at the pre-processing step [20, 22].

2.5.2 Word Embeddings

There is a quote by Firth [33], denoting that "words occurring in similar contexts tend to have similar meanings". It outlines the idea in NLP that a statistical approach, that considers how words and phrases are used in text documents, might replicate the human notions of semantic similarity. This idea is known as the distributional hypothesis.

Word embeddings are dense vector representations of words. The embeddings vector space has much lower dimensionality than the sparse bag-of-words vector space (100–400 as opposed to tens of thousands). In the embeddings space, words that are more similar (semantically and syntactically) are closer to each other than non-similar words. In other words, embeddings are a distributional semantics representation of words. Embeddings can be learning with several algorithms. The most common algorithm is called word2vec and is a neural network-based model. Word2vec [34, 35] includes two main algorithms: continuous bag-of-words (CBOW) and skip-gram.

1. CBOW: Predicting target word from contexts. This model tries to predict the tth word, w_t, in a sentence using a window of width C around the word. Therefore, the context words $w_{t-C}, w_{t-C+1}, \ldots, w_{t-1}, w_{t+1}, \ldots,$

w_{t+C-1}, w_{t+C} are at the input layer of the neural network model to predict the target word w_t.
2. Skip-gram: Predicting contexts from target word.
This model is the opposite of the CBOW model. The target word is at the input layer, and the context words are on the output layer.

Continuous Bag-of-Words The CBOW model is similar to a feed-forward neural network, where the hidden layer is removed and the projection layer is shared for all words. The model architecture is shown in Fig. 3.

The model receives as input context words and seeks to predict the target word w_t by minimizing the CBOW loss function:

$$L_{\text{CBOW}} = -\frac{1}{|C|}\sum_{t=1}^{|C|} \log P(w_t|w_{t-C},\ldots,w_{t-1},w_{t+1},\ldots,w_{t+C})$$

$P(w_t|w_{t-C},\ldots,w_{t-1},w_{t+1},\ldots,w_{t+C})$ is computed using the softmax function:

$$P(w_t|w_{t-C},\ldots,w_{t-1},w_{t+1},\ldots,w_{t+C}) = \frac{\exp(\hat{x}_t^{\mathrm{T}} x_s)}{\sum_{i=1}^{|V|}\exp(\hat{x}_i^{\mathrm{T}} x_s)}$$

where x_i and $\hat{x}_i$ are the word and context word embeddings of word w_i respectively. x_s is the sum of the word embeddings of the words $w_{t-C},\ldots,w_{t-1},w_{t+1},\ldots,w_{t+C}$, and V is the vocabulary of the text dataset.

Mikolov et al. [34] called the CBOW model a bag-of-words because the order of the context words does not influence the projection. It is also called continuous, because rather than conditioning on the words themselves, we condition on a continuous vector constructed from the word embeddings.

Skip-Gram The skip-gram model is similar to CBOW, but instead of predicting a word based on the context, the context is predicted from the word. More precisely, the skip-gram architecture can be seen as a neural network without a hidden layer. It uses each word as input to the network to predict words within a certain range before and after that word (context size). This yields to the loss function:

$$L_{\text{Skip-Gram}} = -\frac{1}{|C|}\sum_{t=1}^{|C|}\sum_{-C\le j\le C, j\ne 0} \log P(w_{t+j}|w_t)$$

$P(w_{t+j}|w_t)$ is computed using the softmax function:

$$P(w_{t+j}|w_t) = \frac{\exp(\hat{x}_{t+j}^{\mathrm{T}} x_t)}{\sum_{i=1}^{|V|}\exp(\hat{x}_i^{\mathrm{T}} x_t)}$$

The skip-gram architecture is shown in Fig. 3. In this architecture, each word is generated multiple times; each time it is conditioned only on a single word. Increasing the context size in the skip-gram model increases the computational complexity, but it also improves quality of the resulting word vectors.

By training the word2vec model on this language modelling task (predicting words in context), the weights on the nodes in the neural network are continuously adapted in such a way that more similar words have more similar vector representations than less similar words. After training, the hidden layer of the network is stored as a dense vector representation for each word in the vocabulary. In the resulting vector space, closeness of words represents their similarity.

3 Pre-trained Language Models

As explained in the previous section, word embeddings are rich language representations: a dense vector for each term in the vocabulary. They are useful for word similarity applications, but if we want to use word embeddings models for the purpose of document representation instead, we need to go from word representations to document representations. One option is to combine the embeddings of all words in the document (e.g. by averaging), or to use a model such as doc2vec [36], which adds a document indicator to an embedding vector to learn document embeddings. Either way, these

Fig. 3 Model architectures for the CBOW and the skip-gram model [34]

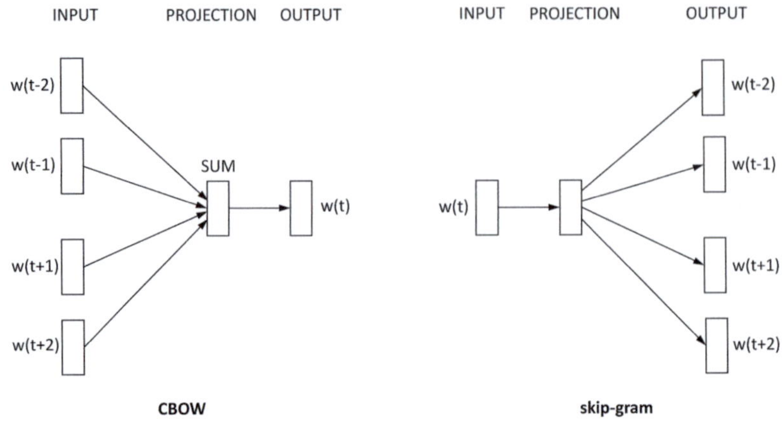

embeddings models are *static* in nature; they can be used as the input to a predictive model but are not updated during training.

A big leap forward in text representations for NLP was made by the introduction of pre-trained language models in the form of *dynamic* embeddings. These embeddings models can be directly used in supervised learning tasks by adding a classification layer on top of the embeddings architecture. During the supervised learning, the full network—including the input embeddings—is updated. This gave rise to the potential of *transfer learning* for text data [37]. Transfer learning is the principle of training a model on a large dataset and then transferring the learned parameters and finetuning them to a more specific, smaller dataset. Until 2018 transfer learning was possible for image data [38], not for text. Transfer learning is further described in Sect. 3.2. First, the next subsection will introduce BERT (Bidirectional Encoder Representations from Transformers), the most popular type of embeddings model in recent NLP.

3.1 Transformers and BERT

In 2017, a research team from Google introduced a new, powerful architecture for sequence-to-sequence learning: the transformer [39]. A transformer is an encoder-decoder architecture: in the encoder part it creates embeddings from input text; in the decoder part it generates text from the stored embeddings.

The core of the transformer architecture is the *self-attention mechanism* [40]. Prior architectures for sequential data (recurrent neural networks such as LSTMs) process text as a sequence: left-to-right and right-to-left. This makes them inefficient because parallellization of the process on a computer cluster is not possible. The self-attention mechanism computes the relation between each pair of input words, thus processing the whole input in parallel. As a result, the context that is taken into account by a transformer is much larger (i.e. the complete input) than in an LSTM (see Sect. 2.4), which has to be trained strictly sequentially (token by token). The longer context in transformer models makes long-distance linguistic relationships possible. This is necessary for language understanding tasks. For example, in the sentence "My lectures, taught in lecture hall 1 to computer science master students on Wednesday mornings at 9 a.m., are about Text Mining", the verb *are* has *my lectures* as subject. With long-distance attention, transformer models can process this correctly—evidenced by the correct translation of the sentence by Google Translate. A disadvantage of self-attention is that it is memory-heavy: since it computes the relation (dot-product) between the embeddings vectors of each pair of words in the input, the computational complexity is quadratic to the number of tokens in the input.

The consequence is that training transformer models required high-memory GPUs.

A year after the introduction of the transformer, BERT was introduced: Bidirectional Encoder Representations from Transformers [41].[5] BERT is a transformer model with only an encoder part. This means that it serves to convert text to embeddings.[6] BERT was designed for transfer learning, which is further explained in the next subsection.

3.2 Transfer Learning: Pre-training and Fine-Tuning

BERT models are trained in two stages: the model is pre-trained on a large—huge[7]—unlabeled text collection and then fine-tuned with a much smaller amount of labelled data to any supervised NLP task. BERT uses almost the same architecture for pre-training and fine-tuning: the dynamic embeddings vectors learned during pre-training are updated during fine-tuning.

The pre-training stage is *self-supervised*, following the same language modelling principles as static word embeddings without any labelled data. In BERT, two language modelling tasks are used during pre-training: Masked Language Modelling and Sentence Prediction. Masked Language Modelling is the task of predicting words based on their context. A proportion (typically 15%) of all tokens is replaced by the token [MASK] and while processing the text collection the model tries to predict what the word in place of the [MASK] token is. The second pre-training task, Sentence Prediction, takes place in parallel with Masked Language Modelling: based on the current sentence, the model tries to predict which of two alternatives is the next sentence. The goal is to learn relations between sentences, which is valuable for tasks such as question answering. Huge amounts of text data are needed to pre-train a BERT model, but thanks to the developers and the research community, pre-trained BERT models are shared for re-use by others. The largest repository of transformers, Hugging Face, contains almost 100,000 models, of which almost 10,000 BERT models for over 150 languages at the time of writing.[8]

Once pre-trained, the embeddings can be fine-tuned using labelled data to a supervised learning task. This can be a classification task (e.g. clinical code prediction, sentiment classification) or a sequence labelling task (e.g. named entity recognition). The last layer of the model defines the loss function and the labels that the model learns to predict.[9]

3.3 BERT Models in the Health Domain

BERT proved to be highly effective for many NLP tasks, outperforming state-of-the-art models. BBecause of its popularity and effectiveness, researchers have trained and released BERT models for specific domains. Generally speaking, there are three strategies for creating a domain-specific model: (1) pre-training a model from scratch on domain-specific data; (2) further pre-training an existing, generic, BERT model by adding domain-specific data to it; (3) no domain-specific pre-training, but only fine-tuning a generic model to a domain-specific task. The first strategy requires a huge amount of data and advanced computational resources (high-memory GPU cores) and is not a realistic choice for most researchers. The second strategy is therefore more common. In both the second and third strategy, the vocabulary of the original model is kept, as a result of which some of the domain-specific terms are not in the model's vocabulary and will be split in sub-words by the tokenizer.

BERT and other transformer models use a tailored tokenization method, called WordPiece [42]. The principle is that the vocabulary size (number of terms) is pre-given and fixed,

[5] The preprint was released in 2018; the paper published in a conference in 2019.

[6] A text generation transformer such as GPT-2 is decoder-only, generating text from embeddings.

[7] Typically, the whole wikipedia and a large book corpus.

[8] https://huggingface.co/models?search=bert.

[9] Hugging Face has example code available for fine-tuning: https://huggingface.co/docs/transformers/training.

typically at 30,000. While pre-training, WordPiece optimizes the coverage of the vocabulary of the collection using 30,000 terms. Words that are relatively frequent will become a term on their own, while words that are infrequent are split into more frequent subtokens. This splitting is not necessarily linguistically motivated. The authors of the BioBERT paper [43] give the example of *Immunoglobulin* that is tokenized by WordPiece as `I ##mm ##uno ##g ##lo ##bul ##in`, the hashes indicating that the tokens are subwords.

BioBERT was the first BERT model in the biomedical domain. BioBERT was pre-trained on PubMed Abstracts and PMC Full-text articles together with the English Wikipedia and BooksCorpus. In the paper it was shown to be successful on biomedical NLP tasks in 15 datasets for three types of tasks: named entity recognition (e.g. extracting disease names), relation extraction (e.g. extracting the relation between genes and diseases), and question answering [43]. Later, more biomedical models followed, specifically Clinical BERT [44], pretrained on the MIMIC-III data.

It became common in the past years to not only release pre-trained models on Huggingface, but also models that have been fine-tuned to a specific task, for example named entity recognition[10] or sentiment classification[11] [45]. This is valuable for users who don't have the computational resources or labelled data to fine-tune a model themselves. In addition, these models can also serve as a starting point for more specific fine-tuning tasks. For example, one could re-use a BioBERT model that was fine-tuned for named entity recognition of diseases, and use it either as-is ('zero-shot use') to label an unlabelled collection with disease names, or fine-tune it further to another set of labelled data for disease recognition.[12]

[10]e.g. https://huggingface.co/raynardj/ner-disease-ncbi-bionlp-bc5cdr-pubmed.

[11]e.g. https://huggingface.co/raynardj/ner-disease-ncbi-bionlp-bc5cdr-pubmed.

[12]It is good to be aware of the distinction between *cased* and *uncased* models. Cased models have been pre-trained with capitalisation preferred, while uncased models have all capitals removed.

A challenge when extracting biomedical entities in text (e.g. diseases, medications, side effects), is that the extracted entities need to be normalized for spelling errors and other variations: there are multiple ways to refer to the same entity, e.g. because of the difference between specialist and layman language. The common approach to entity normalization is *ontology linking*: connecting a mention in a text (e.g. "cannot sleep") to a concept in a medical term base (e.g. *insomnia*). Medical terminologies, of which the most commonly used in the clinical domain is SNOMED CT, can be huge, with tens of thousands different labels. A model linking entities from the text to the SNOMED terminology needs to be able to connect terms it has not seen during training time to labels from this huge label space. A BERT model fine-tuned for this particular task is SapBERT [46].

4 NLP Tasks and Challenges in Healthcare

Text data are abundant in the health and biomedical domain. There exist a large variety of text data types from which information extraction could be valuable, ranging from scientific literature to health social media. In this section we will discuss issues related to data privacy, existing datasets and applications of NLP in the health and biomedical domain.

4.1 Data Privacy

Healthcare information exchange can benefit both healthcare providers and patients. Healthcare data are universally considered sensitive data and are subject to particularly strict rules to be protected from unauthorized access. Because of privacy concerns, healthcare organizations have been extremely reluctant to allow access to care data for researchers from outside the associated institutions. Such restricted access to data has hindered collaboration and information exchange among research groups. Because of the recent introduction of technologies such as differential privacy [47, 48], federated learning [49], synthetic data generation [50] and text de-identification (text anonymization) [51], we expect the increase in data sharing, facilitating collaboration, and external validity of analysis using integrated data of multiple healthcare organizations. The extent of data sharing required for widespread adoption of data science and specifically natural language processing technologies across health systems will require extensive collaborative efforts.

Clinical **text de-identification** is one of the easiest methods enables collaborative research while protecting patient privacy and confidentiality; however, concerns persist about the reduction in the utility of the de-identified text for information extraction and natural language processing tasks. On the other hand, growing interest in **synthetic data** has stimulated development and advancement of a large variety of deep learning-based models for a wide range of applications including healthcare.

Federated learning enables collaborative model training, while training data remains distributed over many clients, minimizing data exposure. On the contrary, **differential privacy** is a system for publicly sharing information about a dataset by describing the patterns of groups within the dataset while withholding information about individuals in the dataset.

4.2 Biomedical Data Sources and Their Challenges

Scientific papers and patents. In their 2015 paper, Fleuren and Alkema [7] show the strong increase of the number of scientific publications between 1994, 2004 and 2014. We can only imagine how much this increase has progressed since then. Scientific papers are challenging for NLP techniques because they are long, often stored as PDF with headers, footers, captions, mid-sentence line endings, potential encoding issues, containing figures and tables, and technical language. Similarly challenging to process are patent documents; the amount of biomedical and biotechnical patents is large. Patents are a rich source of information, but also long, multilingual, and with technical and legal language [52].

Electronic Health Records (EHRs).EHRs receive a substantial amount of research in biomedical NLP [53]. The text data in EHRs, consisting of doctor notes and letters, provide rich information in addition to the structured data in the records, and therefore are promising sources for mining biomedical knowledge (see Sect. 4.3 for some key examples). The use of patient health records brings challenges related to pre-processing: doctor notes are written under time pressure, and contain typos and doctor-specific abbreviations. For example, the word *patient* is abbreviated by one doctor to 'pnt', by the second doctor to 'pt' and by the third even to 'p'. Another challenge for the use EHRs is data privacy: the anonymization of text data is challenging [8]. Recently, some work has addressed the potential of generating artificial EHR text for use in benchmarking contexts [54]. This direction is promising, and can be expanded upon in the near future with the fast improving quality of large generative language models such as Generative Pre-trained Transformers (GPT) [55].

Health social media. A more freely available source of patient experiences is health social media [56]: information shared on general platforms such as Twitter, and Reddit, but also disease-specific discussion forums in patient support groups. These data are direct personal accounts of experiences, without filtering through a questionnaire or interview. This makes the data potentially rich, but also noisy—not all information in the patient accounts is necessarily correct and of high-quality. Like with EHRs, the use of health social media data poses challenges with pre-processing and normalization, such as spelling errors and the use of medical language by laymen [57], and with data privacy. Under the GDPR, medical information shared online, also on a public channel, is considered personal information and should be handled with care.

An anonymous alternative source of patient experiences are the patient surveys conducted by hospitals. These surveys are not asking for specific medical and personal information, but for customer satisfaction aspects: how did patients experience their stay and what can be improved [58]. These data are less privacy sensitive and therefore easier to use, but also less rich in content and can only be used to analyze general trends of patient satisfaction [59].

4.3 Tasks and Applications

NLP tasks in the biomedical domain directly relate to the data sources that are available. We will discuss tasks related to the three types of data sources described in the previous subsection.

Scientific papers and patents. For the purpose of biomedical scientific research, mining knowledge from large bodies of biomedical papers is relevant, because individual papers only address one topic at the time, and the amount of papers published is large. Fleuren and Alkema [7] describe biomedical text mining task for scientific publications: starting with information retrieval to select the topically relevant papers from a large collection, followed by named entity recognition, relation extraction, knowledge discovery, and visualization. The most commonly addressed named entity recognition task is the extraction of diseases, genes and protein names from scientific tasks. Fleuren and Alkema [7] list benchmark tasks that have helped advancing the methods development for named entity recognition. The task of gene, protein, disease extraction can be expanded from scientific papers to patents, thereby also expanding from English-only to multiple languages [60].

NLP technology can also support the task of systematic reviewing of scientific publications, typically performed by clinical librarians or medical scholars [61]. Systematic reviewing is a challenging task, even for trained users, who compose long Boolean queries to select relevant papers to the topic of their review [62]. Text classification models can help the process of paper selection, but since the task is high-recall—the user cannot miss any relevant paper—should always be conducted in interaction with the human expert. Techniques such as Continuous Active Learning [63] allow for this interaction.

Electronic Health Records (EHRs). In the past two decades, biomedical NLP research has largely aimed at development of predictive models for EHRs [64]. Predictive models are classification tasks for the purpose of predicting future events. Past records are used as training data. Examples of such tasks are the prediction of clinical risks [65], the prediction of diagnosis codes based on free-text notes [66], the prediction of a patient's time to death for general practitioners [67], the prediction of hospital admissions in emergency departments [68], and the prediction of re-admissions after discharge [69].

Challenges in some clinical prediction tasks are huge label spaces: the ICD-10 coding system, used to code a patient's diagnosis, has tens of thousands of codes.[13] When training a machine learning model, the codes that are frequent in the training data will be well represented by the model and easy to predict, while the rare diseases have not sufficient training data to be correctly predicted in the test data. A second challenge is bringing the developed models to the clinical practice. Before a hospital takes the step to involve machine learning and NLP in the clinical workflow, the developed applications need to be evaluated in an end-to-end setting with user involvement. The models are typically aimed to not replace the human expert (the doctor or the clinical information specialist), but to assist them in making the right decisions. One example application in the hospital context is to discover misclassifications or inconsistencies in previously coded data [70, 71]. Another application is to use the machine learning model to make suggestions in an interactive task context, e.g. suggest the most likely diagnosis code based on the text typed by the doctor or coder [72].

Health social media. Health social media data can be used for the extraction of structured information, such as side effects for medications [73, 74], but also for more social-emotional aspects of patients' well-being, such as patient empower-

[13] https://www.cdc.gov/nchs/icd/icd10.htm.

ment [75]. The most commonly addressed health-related task with social media is the extraction of adverse drug reactions (ADRs), for which high-quality benchmarks have been developed [76]. The extraction of ADRs is defined as an information extraction task consisting of three steps: (1) named entity recognition to identify medications and ADRs; (2) ontology linking to normalize the extracted ADR string (e.g. "cannot fall asleep") to the correct term in a medical database (e.g. *insomnia*); (3) relation extraction to identify that the mentioned ADR is indeed connected to the mentioned medication.

5 Bias and Fairness

In this chapter we have seen how we can apply artificial intelligence algorithms to extract information and insights from real-world clinical text data. These AI algorithms draw their insights and information by generalizing observations from their training data to new samples. Sometimes this generalization can be grounded on an incorrectly assessed correlation between an input feature and an effect. This is known as *bias* [77]. As an example, consider an image classifier that is trained to distinguish wolves from dogs. If the classifier decides something is a wolf (rather than a dog) based on the snow in the background [78], then it is biased because it is not the snow that makes a wolf a wolf. This classifier will struggle to distinguish dogs from wolves in scenarios where the background is not visible, or if a dog happens to be surrounded by snow.

A related but somewhat distinct concept is *fairness*: how well people who are similar to each other are treated similarly by an AI system [79]. To see how fairness relates to bias, consider the following example [80]. An AI system is trained to determine whether benzodiazepines should be prescribed to a psychiatric patient, on the basis of certain information about the patient. The training data would be annotated with real prescriptions from past data. Suppose that one of the pieces of information available to the AI system is the biological gender of the patient, and suppose further that there is a high correlation between biological gender and past prescriptions [81]. The AI system might use the correlation between gender and past prescriptions to inform future predictions. This is biased, because biological gender is not expected to have any impact on whether a patient should be prescribed benzodiazepines [82, 83]. It is also unfair, because by discriminating on biological gender, the system might be treating otherwise equal patients differently. For a real-world example, Singh et al [84] found that a predictive model for mortality risk failed to generalize from one hospital to another, and that this resulted in disparate impact for different races.

Bias and fairness in AI have garnered attention for several years [85, 86]. We will use the terms bias and unfairness interchangeably to describe a situation in which an AI system uses certain *protected attributes* [79] implicitly or explicitly for a purpose that is unrelated to the value of the protected attribute. Protected attributes vary by country and by domain, but they typically include gender, nationality, race, and age, among others [87]. The challenge can sometimes arise from the fact that these attributes can be correlated with other features in the dataset, so that removing the protected attribute from the features used in the AI system does not remove the bias [88].

In this section we will outline some of the causes of bias in AI applications for clinical text analyses, as well as how to measure and mitigate those biases. We will also highlight some of the challenges associated with the study of bias given the limitations imposed by real-world clinical data.

5.1 Bias in Clinical NLP

Bias can be introduced at multiple points in the AI pipeline for clinical applications. We will introduce four common ways in which bias can occur. First, *selection bias* can be present in the dataset used for training an algorithm due to a sampling problem [89]. A notable example is *healthcare access bias* [77]: patients admitted to an institution do not necessarily represent the whole population they are drawn from. Therefore, using data from a single institution to draw insights about a population might be biased.

Second, bias can be intrinsically incorporated in the population, as in the case where more members of a protected group have a certain characteristic than non-members for historical reasons. Take the classical example of loan approvals presented in the introduction to this section. The correlation between ethnicity and postal code is due to social or historical reasons, and is not related to loan approval.

Third, bias can be caused by design choices in the AI system. For example, a clinician might decide to work on implementing a classifier to detect a sickness that only affects a subset of the population, while ignoring other sickness that affect another segment of the population [90].

Fourth, bias can also happen when systems trained on language varieties that are considered "standard" work less well on texts written by certain sociodemographic groups [91]. In the clinical practice, this could have a significant impact when designing models trained on texts written by patients from a given institution [92], as the application of these models on other institutions might lead to bias.

Bias can be dangerous for clinical NLP and text mining applications, but before we can do something about it, we must be able to identify bias. This can be complicated because it is not always clear whether bias should be removed. As an extreme example, consider an AI system trained to predict the probability of a (biologically) female patient becoming pregnant in the next three months based on reports written by doctors during general screenings. Suppose that the doctors are instructed to never write the age of the patient in the reports. They might, however, write other information that correlates with age. The AI system could then associate this information with the pregnancy status and use it to predict pregnancy. As a result, the AI system would "bias" its predictions against older women. As age can be considered a protected attribute, this could be considered unfair bias. In this case, however, there might be a medical reason why the prediction should be different for different ages.

Nevertheless, there are cases in which it is clear that bias should be mitigated if possible. As an example, consider an NLP system designed to predict a diagnosis from a written report. Suppose this NLP system is biased against a protected group, and that the illness the system tries to diagnose is potentially fatal. As a result, members of the protected group go undetected and die more often as a result of the sickness. This means that fewer patients come back for further treatment, and as a result there are fewer written reports about patients from the protected group to use as training data for newer models. This creates a feedback loop that results in the bias becoming even larger [93].

5.2 Bias Measurement

Bias can be measured using multiple metrics, depending on the specific details of the case. The very definition of bias is highly contested, with a recent review citing more than ten of them [93]. Listing all possible definitions is beyond the scope of this chapter, but we can sketch out two of them to give an idea of where differences in definitions come from. For illustrative purposes, consider a dataset containing patient records for white and black patients.[14] Suppose this dataset is annotated with *gold labels* representing whether the patient is diagnosed with a particular sickness or not. We want to train a binary classifier to predict this diagnosis in new non-annotated data: given a new patient record, the *predicted label* is *positive* if the model thinks the patient has the sickness, or *negative* if not. The *equal opportunity* definition of fairness requires that datapoints with a positive gold label have the same probability of being assigned a positive predicted label by the model; in other words: if we knew that a given patient has the sickness, the model should have the same probability of predicting *true positives* regardless of the race of the patients. The *equalized odds* definition requires exactly the same, and additionally

[14]In other words, we remove all records for patients who identify as belonging to any other race from the dataset for this example.

that all protected groups having a *negative* gold label should have the same probability of being (incorrectly) predicted as positive [94]; in other words: the model should have the same probability of predicting true positives *and false positives* regardless of the patient race.

Additionally, another question to be considered is whether we want *individual* fairness or *group* fairness. Individual fairness means that similar individuals get treated similarly. In the example above, this would mean that two patients with similar age, socioeconomic status, health status, etc., but of different races, should receive the same treatment by the model. Group fairness requires that each group gets treated similarly, so that the performance of the model is similar for each group. In the example above, this could mean that the accuracy of the model is the same for black and white patients. Individual fairness is very hard to implement, given that some kind of similarity metric needs to be defined.

Guidelines for selecting an appropriate bias measure depend on the specific use case [95]. As an example, suppose you are developing a system to help clinicians diagnose a disease. We assume that receiving a diagnosis is desirable, as it helps speed up treatment. As such, the designer of the system will prioritize minimizing the false negatives, to ensure no sick people go undetected. In that case, equal opportunity might be a better bias measure than equalized odds, as we are not so concerned with bias occurring in false positives. In a concrete example from the literature [96], a model trained to predict depression from clinical notes found a bias against patients of a given gender. They quantified the bias using the False Negative Rate Ratio (FNRR), i.e., the false negative rate for members of that gender divided by the false negative rate for other patients. The false negative rate is the fraction of patients with depression that were diagnosed by the model as not having the condition. They found the FNRR to be different from 1, which is the value expected if the classifier were fair. In practice, it's often not possible to satisfy multiple fairness metrics at the same time, therefore making it even more important to select one based on the domain.

An important remark to be made when it comes to measuring bias in clinical NLP applications is that clinical datasets are often heavily imbalanced. Often clinical NLP systems aim at extracting rare symptoms, detecting rare diseases, or predicting rare events. This should be taken into consideration when choosing a bias measure. For example, metrics emphasizing differences in the True Negative Rate are often inappropriate, as the True Negative Rate is usually very large due to the imbalanced nature of the dataset.

5.3 Bias Mitigation

Multiple bias mitigation techniques have been proposed [87] for machine learning applications. These can be classified as pre-processing, in-processing, or post-processing techniques. Pre-processing mitigation techniques attempt to debias by making modifications to the training dataset, such as applying different weights to sample from different protected groups. In-processing mitigation techniques attempt to debias by modifying the NLP and text mining algorithms; a popular example is the *prejudice remover* [97]. Finally, post-processing techniques attempt to debias by modifying the way predictions from the model are interpreted. As in the case of measuring bias, mitigating bias is also context-dependent, and the right tool should be chosen based on the domain and the task.

In recent literature, one study uses data augmentation to mitigate bias: they create new datapoints by swapping gender pronouns in the input documents, and find a difference in the fairness measures [96]. A recent survey outlines several more studies that used bias mitigation techniques [98]. As a complementary strategy, some argue that every dataset should be accompanied by a *data statements* providing enough information so that users can understand what biases might be present in the dataset [99].

6 Explainability

The advancements in AI and NLP with the emergence of deep learning approaches have led to systems with high predictive accuracy, which however, are based on very complex learning processes that are very difficult for users and researchers to understand. The difficulty to understand the internal logic and how those systems are reaching predictions is known as the *Black Box problem* and has led to an increasing interest of researchers to explainable AI (XAI) and interpretable AI.

Although the term XAI is mentioned already in a study published in 2004 [100], there is still no standarized technical definition. In literature, many times *transparency*, *explainability* and *interpretability* are used interchangeably [101]. Many researchers have already attempted to give formal definitions. Gilpin et al. [102] stated that both interpretability and fidelity are required to achieve explainability. According to Gilpin et al. *interpretability* refers to whether the explanation is understandable by humans, whereas *fidelity* refers to whether the explanation describes the method accurately. Based on that, Markus et al. [103] defined *explainability* as follows: *An AI system is explainable if the task model is intrinsically interpretable or if the non-interpretable task model is complemented with an interpretable and faithful explanation.* On the other hand, *transparency* has been defined as providing stakeholders with relevant information about how the model works that can include documentation of the training procedure and code releases [104].

From the above definitions, it is evident that XAI and transparency are very important for AI and NLP systems developed for the clinical domain. XAI models in healthcare should align with clinicians' expectations and acquire their trust, increase the transparency of the system, assure results quality, and allow addressing fairness, and ethical concerns [105].

In this section we will outline some of the main methodologies that have been used for explainability of AI applications for clinical text analyses, and how they were evaluated. We will also highlight some of the challenges and limitations associated with the explainability in AI and NLP in clinical applications.

6.1 Methods for Explainability

One of the aims of a XAI model is to produce explanations regarding the system's process and outcome predictions. Those explanations can be categorized in two groups: local and global [106]. The *local* explanations refer to providing explanation on an individual prediction, whereas the global refers to the model's prediction process as a whole. The *global* explanations can either emerge from the prediction process (self-explaining) or after post-processing (post-hoc).

There are several well known techniques that can have been proposed to generate explanations. One of the most well known models is LIME (Local Interpretable Model-Agnostic Explanations) that focuses on local explanations [78]. LIME is based on surrogate models which are trained to approximate the predictions of the initial non-explainable model. Surrogate models can also be learned for global explanations [107]. Although XAI methods based on surrogate models became very popular, they have a main drawback which is that the original model and the learned surrogate models may have completely different ways to reach the predictions.

SHapley Additive exPlanation (SHAP) is another popular Explainable AI (XAI) model that can provide model-agnostic local explainability for different types of data [108]. SHAP is based on Shapley values, which is a concept popularly used in Game Theory and is applies additive feature importance.

Many researchers also tried to derive explanations using the importance scores of different features on the output predictions. This can be applied on manual features derived from traditional feature engineering [109], lexical features [66] or gradient-based methods such as DeepLIFT [110] or Grad-CAM [111]. In particular, DeepLIFT is designed to compute feature importance in feed-forward neural networks, whereas Grad-CAM uses the gradients of a target concept flowing into the final convolutional layer and produces a coarse localization map highlighting the important regions for predicting the concept.

The extraction of weights from the attention mechanism is also a very popular way to enable feature-based explanations. Attention layers that can be added to most neural network architectures, indicate the parts that the network focuses. The package BERTviz[15] uses this premise to visualize the attention between input tokens, in particular between the [CLS] token—which has information for the prediction itself—to each of the input tokens. However, they have become a topic of debate on whether they can be used as a means of explanation or not. Jain and Wallace [112] claimed that there is no correlation between attention scores and other feature-important measures concluding that attention is not explanation. However, Wiegreffe and Pinter [113] proposed diagnostic tests to allow for meaningful interpretation of attention, but also showed that adversarial attention distributions could not achieve the performance of real model attention.

6.2 Evaluation of Explainability

One of the current challenges in XAI refers to their proper evaluation. It is important that the explainable models to be evaluated not only on their performance but also on the quality of the explanations. Taking into account that explainability is a relatively new field, there is still no agreement regarding a standarized evaluation of the XAI models.

One approach that has been applied, is to present an informal evaluation of the explanations and high level discussions of how some of the generated explanations agree with human intuition. In some cases explanations are even compared to other reference approaches [114] such as LIME.

[15]https://github.com/jessevig/bertviz.

A more formal way to evaluate an XAI approach is to use human evaluations that can quantify a system's performance [115]. The collected ground truth can be then compared with the generated explanations and state-of-the-art performance metrics such as Precision/Recall/F1 and BLUE scores can be calculated. Instead of collecting ground truth beforehand, an alternative evaluation approach is to ask humans to evaluate the explanations generated by the XAI system [66]. Although collecting human labels is a way to quantify the performance of those systems, they are not always of high quality. Also, humans have many biases that can be also reflected in the collected ground truth. Multiple annotators of diverse backgrounds and high inter-annotator agreement is a way to ensure the quality of the labels.

Attention based explanations have been also evaluated by more specific approaches. For example, Serrano and Smith [116] performed experiments in which they repeatedly set the maximal entry generated by the attention layer to zero. The idea behind this mechanism is that turning off those weights should lead to different explanations in the case that they actually explain the predictions.

One limitation of the current studies is the limited or even absent elaboration on what is being actually evaluated. Explanations can be evaluated from different angles such as fidelity and comprehensibility [117]. One exception is the study by Lertvittayakumjorn and Toni [118] who proposed human evaluation experiments targeting the following three goals: model behavior, model predictions and assist humans in investigating uncertain predictions.

6.3 Explainability in Clinical NLP Tasks

The widespread use of AI and NLP models into clinical practice have made transparency and explainability of critical importance, especially if we consider not only that practitioners usually work with complex sources of data [119] but also that incorrect predictions can lead to severe consequences [120]. In order to build trust between clinicians and AI models, clinicians should be able to understand the logic of the system and detect cases in which the model gave incorrect or unexpected predictions.

There have been several attempts for XAI models for different prediction tasks in the medical domain ranging in the type of data they use [119, 121]. Some of those works focus on XAI models for text prediction tasks in the medical domain. The easiest and most straightforward way is to apply well known models such as LIME, SHAP and DeepLIFT to generate explanations. For example, Uddin et al. [122] proposed an RNN system for depression detection from text and applied LIME to generate explanations of the predictions. Caicedo-Torres and Gutierrez [123] applied SHAP to generate explanations of their proposed deep learning system that was trained to predict patient mortality inside the ICU based on free-medical notes. DeepLIFT that is designed to compute feature importance in feed-forward neural networks was used by Caicedo-Torres and Gutierrez [123] to find word embeddings that deemed as most important for survival and death prediction.

Combing convolution with attention has been proved efficient in different NLP tasks. To this end, Mullenbach et al. [66] applied attentional convolution to highlight the most relevant parts of the clinical text of each ICD code. Hu et al. [124] focused also on ICD classification and proposed SWAM which established the correspondences between the informative snippet and convolution filter. Blanco et al. [125] proposed a bidirectional Gated Recurrent Units (GRU) with attention mechanism that allowed to understand which fragment contributed the most in the cause of death prediction.

7 Summary and Recommendations

7.1 Clinical Natural Language Processing

As the amount of unstructured text narratives that biomedical and healthcare systems produce grows, so does the need to intelligently process it and extract different types of knowledge from it. In the future, with an active role of the health community, more clinical NLP-based expert systems will be deployed in practice to accurately recognize the knowledge within clinical text, and feed this knowledge automatically into patient daily care.

7.2 Transfer Learning in Health

In NLP as well as in many areas of machine learning, the standard way to train a model is to annotate a number of examples that are then provided to the model. Recent deep learning-based transfer learning methods and pre-trained language models have achieved remarkable successes on a wide range of NLP tasks. Given the lack of annotated datasets for training and benchmarking in clinical text mining, in the future, it is expected that the knowledge from related tasks or domains are combined. We also expect, for the NLP tasks in healthcare, more effective approaches that combine semi-supervised learning with transfer learning.

7.3 Bias and Fairness

Bias in NLP occurs when an algorithm or model exploits certain properties of texts to solve a task that is unrelated to those properties. *Fairness* is a requirement that machine learning models treat members of different *protected groups* equally. For our purpose, we consider an NLP or text mining model to be biased or unfair if it uses certain protected attributes implicitly or explicitly to solve a problem unrelated to those attributes. There are multiple definitions of bias, as well as multiple bias metrics, such as *equal opportunity* and *equalized odds*. There are also several *mitigation* strategies that can be adopted to reduce the bias. The choice of a bias definition, a bias measure, and a bias mitigation strategy is dependent on the domain and the task, as different measures cannot be optimized simultaneously, and different tasks require different measures. Some work on bias measurement and mitigation has been done on the clinical NLP domain, but it is very much a nascent field, and no measure or mitigation strategy should be adopted without careful evaluation.

7.4 Explainability

In Sect. 6 we discussed what is XAI and the main methodologies that exist. In medical domain, XAI models aim to increase the trust of the practitioners and patients by providing transparent systems that are understandable by humans. Developing automated systems that could potentially take decisions for diagnosis and treatment is a multidisciplinary process. Models should be developed in collaboration with experts input from the appropriate areas. That will allow to understand domain-specific needs such as the purpose of the system, the need and level of required transparency and explainability. Additionally, the type of explanations should be decided considering not only the aspects of ethics and fairness, but also the limitations of the audience [126].

Another remaining challenge is related to the evaluation, a topic of a great discussion in the area. The majority of studies are using subjective measurements, such as user satisfaction, and researchers' intuition on the explanations [126]. From the previous studies, it is evident that there is an overall lack of validated and reliable evaluation metrics on which more work is needed. Zhou et al. [127] gave a summary of quantitative metrics for the evaluation of explainability aspects (i.e., clarity, broadness, parsimony, completeness, and soundness). In their study, they conclude that *the evaluation of ML explanations is a multidisciplinary research topic.* and that *It is also not possible to define an implementation of evaluation metrics, which can be applied to all explanation methods.*

References

1. Bagheri A. Text mining in healthcare: bringing structure to electronic health records. PhD thesis, Utrecht University; 2021.
2. Sutton RT, Pincock D, Baumgart DC, Sadowski DC, Fedorak RN, Kroeker KI. An overview of clinical decision support systems: Benefits, risks, and strategies for success. NPJ Digital Med. 2020;3(1):1–10.
3. Spasic I, Nenadic G, et al. Clinical text data in machine learning: systematic review. JMIR Med Inform. 2020;8(3): e17984.
4. Hearst MA. Untangling text data mining. In: Proceedings of the 37th annual meeting of the association for computational linguistics; 1999. p. 3–10.
5. Mehta N, Pandit A. Concurrence of big data analytics and healthcare: a systematic review. Int J Med Informa. 2018;114:57–65.
6. Yim W-W, Yetisgen M, Harris WP, Kwan SW. Natural language processing in oncology: a review. JAMA Oncol. 2016;2(6):797–804.
7. Fleuren WW, Alkema W. Application of text mining in the biomedical domain. Methods. 2015;74:97–106.
8. Menger V, Scheepers F, van Wijk L, Spruit M. DEDUCE: a pattern matching method for automatic de-identification of Dutch medical text. Telematics Inform. 2018;35(4):727–36.
9. Byrd R, Steinhubl S, Sun J, Ebadollahi S, Stewart W. Automatic identification of heart failure diagnostic criteria, using text analysis of clinical notes from electronic health records. Int J Med Inform. 2014;83(12):983–92.
10. Jamian L, Wheless L, Crofford LJ, Barnado A. Rule-based and machine learning algorithms identify patients with systemic sclerosis accurately in the electronic health record. Arthritis Res Ther. 2019;21(1):305.
11. Jonnalagadda S, Adupa A, Garg R, Corona-Cox J, Shah S. Text mining of the electronic health record: an information extraction approach for automated identification and subphenotyping of HFPEF patients for clinical trials. J Cardiovasc Transl Res. 2017;10(3):313–21.
12. Wu X, Zhao Y, Radev D, Malhotra A. Identification of patients with carotid stenosis using natural language processing. Eur Radiol. 2020;1–9.
13. Kocbek S, Cavedon L, Martinez D, Bain C, Mac Manus C, Haffari G, Zukerman I, Verspoor K. Text mining electronic hospital records to automatically classify admissions against disease: measuring the impact of linking data sources. J Biomed Inform. 2016;64:158–67.
14. Koopman B, Karimi S, Nguyen A, McGuire R, Muscatello D, Kemp M, Truran D, Zhang M, Thackway S. Automatic classification of diseases from free-text death certificates for real-time surveillance. BMC Med Inform Dec Making. 2015;15(1):53.

15. Torii M, Fan J, Yang W, Lee T, Wiley M, Zisook D, Huang Y. Risk factor detection for heart disease by applying text analytics in electronic medical records. J Biomed Inform. 2015;58:S164-70.
16. Bagheri A, Sammani A, van der Heijden PG, Asselbergs FW, Oberski DL. Etm: Enrichment by topic modeling for automated clinical sentence classification to detect patients' disease history. J Intell Inform Syst. 2020;55(2):329–49.
17. Sammani A, Bagheri A, van der Heijden PG, Te Riele AS, Baas AF, Oosters C, Oberski D, Asselbergs FW. Automatic multilabel detection of icd10 codes in dutch cardiology discharge letters using neural networks. NPJ Dig Med. 2021;4(1):1–10.
18. Huang K, Altosaar J, Ranganath R. ClinicalBERT: modeling clinical notes and predicting hospital readmission; 2019. ArXiv preprint arXiv:1904.05342
19. Jonnagaddala J, Liaw S, Ray P, Kumar M, Chang N, Dai H. Coronary artery disease risk assessment from unstructured electronic health records using text mining. J Biomed Inf. 2015;58:S203-10.
20. Kowsari K, Jafari Meimandi K, Heidarysafa M, Mendu S, Barnes L, Brown D. Text classification algorithms: a survey. Information. 2019;10(4):150.
21. Murphy KP. Machine learning: a probabilistic perspective. MIT Press; 2012.
22. Aggarwal C. Machine learning for text. Springer; 2018.
23. Blei D, Ng A, Jordan M. Latent Dirichlet allocation. J Mach Learn Res. 2003;3(1):993–1022.
24. Reed C. Latent dirichlet allocation: towards a deeper understanding. Available at obphio.us; 2012:1–13
25. Bagheri A, Saraee M, De Jong F. ADM-LDA: an aspect detection model based on topic modelling using the structure of review sentences. J Inform Sci. 2014;40(5):621–36.
26. Duarte D, Puerari I, Dal Bianco G, Lima JF. Exploratory analysis of electronic health records using topic modeling. J Inform Data Manage. 2020;11(2).
27. Li DC, Thermeau T, Chute C, Liu H. Discovering associations among diagnosis groups using topic modeling. AMIA Summits Transl Sci Proceed. 2014;2014:43.
28. Mosteiro P, Rijcken E, Zervanou K, Kaymak U, Scheepers F, Spruit M. Making sense of violence risk predictions using clinical notes. In: Huang Z, Siuly S, Wang H, Zhou R, Zhang Y, editors. Health information science. Cham: Springer International Publishing; 2020. p. 3–14.
29. Stevens K, Kegelmeyer P, Andrzejewski D, Buttler D. Exploring topic coherence over many models and many topics. In Proceedings of the 2012 joint conference on empirical methods in natural language processing and computational natural language learning; 2012. p. 952–61
30. Luo L, Yang Z, Yang P, Zhang Y, Wang L, Lin H, Wang J. An attention-based bilstm-crf approach to document-level chemical named entity recognition. Bioinformatics. 2018;34(8):1381–8.
31. Nasar Z, Jaffry SW, Malik MK. Named entity recognition and relation extraction: State-of-the-art. ACM Comput Surveys (CSUR). 2021;54(1):1–39.
32. Eisenstein J. Natural language processing; 2018.
33. Firth JR. A synopsis of linguistic theory, 1930–1955. Studies in Linguistic Analysis 1957.
34. Mikolov T, Sutskever I, Chen K, Corrado G, Dean J, Distributed representations of words and phrases and their compositionality. In Advances in neural information processing systems; 2013. , p. 3111–9.
35. Mikolov T, Chen K, Corrado G, Dean J. Efficient estimation of word representations in vector space; 2013. ArXiv preprint arXiv:1301.3781.
36. Le Q, Mikolov T. Distributed representations of sentences and documents. In: International conference on machine learning. PMLR; 2014, p. 1188–96
37. Ruder S. Neural transfer learning for natural language processing. PhD Thesis, NUI Galway; 2019.
38. Huh M, Agrawal P, Efros AA. What makes imagenet good for transfer learning? 2016. ArXiv preprint arXiv:1608.08614.
39. Vaswani A, Shazeer N, Parmar N, Uszkoreit J, Jones L, Gomez AN, Kaiser Ł, Polosukhin I. Attention is all you need. Adv Neural Inform Proc Syst. 2017;30.
40. Jurafsky D, Martin J. Speech and language processing: an introduction to speech recognition, computational linguistics and natural language processing, 3rd edn. Prentice Hall; 2021.
41. Devlin J, Chang M-W, Lee K, Toutanova K. Bert: pre-training of deep bidirectional transformers for language understanding. In: Proceedings of the 2019 conference of the North American chapter of the association for computational linguistics: human language technologies, Volume 1 (Long and Short Papers); 2019. p. 4171–86.
42. Wu Y, Schuster M, Chen Z, Le QV, Norouzi M, Macherey W, Krikun M, Cao Y, Gao Q, Macherey K. et al. Google's neural machine translation system: Bridging the gap between human and machine translation; 2016. ArXiv preprint arXiv:1609.08144.
43. Lee J, Yoon W, Kim S, Kim D, Kim S, So CH, Kang J. Biobert: a pre-trained biomedical language representation model for biomedical text mining. Bioinformatics. 2020;36(4):1234–40.
44. Alsentzer E, Murphy JR, Boag W, Weng W-H, Jin D, Naumann T, McDermott M. Publicly available clinical bert embeddings, 2019. ArXiv preprint arXiv:1904.03323
45. Barbieri F, Camacho-Collados J, Anke LE, Neves L. Tweeteval: Unified benchmark and comparative evaluation for tweet classification. Find Assoc Comput Linguist: EMNLP. 2020;2020:1644–50.
46. Liu F, hareghi E, Meng Z, Basaldella M, Collier N. Self-alignment pretraining for biomedical entity representations. In: Proceedings of the 2021 conference of the North American chapter of the association for computational linguistics: human language technologies, (Online), Association for Computational Linguistics; 2021. p. 4228–38

47. Dwork C, Roth A, et al. The algorithmic foundations of differential privacy. Found Trends® Theor Comput Sci. 2014;9(3–4):211–407.
48. Price WN, Cohen IG. Privacy in the age of medical big data. Nat Med. 2019;25(1):37–43.
49. Konečný J, McMahan HB, Yu FX, Richtárik P, Suresh AT, Bacon D. Federated learning: strategies for improving communication efficiency. In: NIPS Workshop; 2016.
50. Eigenschink P, Vamosi S, Vamosi R, Sun C, Reutterer T, Kalcher K. Deep generative models for synthetic data. ACM Comput Surv. 2021.
51. Obeid JS, Heider PM, Weeda ER, Matuskowitz AJ, Carr CM, Gagnon K, Crawford T, Meystre SM. Impact of de-identification on clinical text classification using traditional and deep learning classifiers. Stud Health Tech Inf. 2019;264:283.
52. Verberne S, D'hondt E, Oostdijk N, Koster C, Quantifying the challenges in parsing patent claims. In: Proceedings of the 1st international workshop on advances in patent information retrieval at ECIR 2010; 2010. p. 14–21
53. Johnson AE, Pollard TJ, Shen L, Lehman L-WH, Feng M, Ghassemi M, Moody B, Szolovits P, Anthony Celi L, Mark RG. Mimic-iii, a freely accessible critical care database. Sci. Data 2016;3(1):1–9.
54. Libbi CA, Trienes J, Trieschnigg D, Seifert C. Generating synthetic training data for supervised de-identification of electronic health records. Fut Internet. 2021;13(5):136.
55. Brown T, Mann B, Ryder N, Subbiah M, Kaplan JD, Dhariwal P, Neelakantan A, Shyam P, Sastry G, Askell A, et al. Language models are few-shot learners. Adv Neural Inform Proc Syst. 2020;33:1877–901.
56. Weissenbacher D, Banda J, Davydova V, Zavala DE, Sánchez LG, Ge Y, Guo Y, Klein A, Krallinger M, Leddin M, et al. Overview of the seventh social media mining for health applications (# smm4h) shared tasks at coling 2022. In: Proceedings of the seventh workshop on social media mining for health applications, workshop and shared task; 2022. p. 221–41.
57. Dirkson A, Verberne S, Sarker A, Kraaij W. Data-driven lexical normalization for medical social media. Multimodal Technol Inter. 2019;3(3):60.
58. van Buchem MM, Neve OM, Kant IM, Steyerberg EW, Boosman H, Hensen EF. Analyzing patient experiences using natural language processing: development and validation of the artificial intelligence patient reported experience measure (ai-prem). BMC Med Inf Dec Mak. 2022;22(1):1–11.
59. Bozik M. Aspect-based sentiment analysis on dutch patient experience survey data. Master's thesis, Master Computer Science, LIACS, Leiden University; 2022.
60. Hu Y, Verberne S. Named entity recognition for chinese biomedical patents. In: Proceedings of the 28th international conference on computational linguistics; 2020. p. 627–37.
61. Scells H, Zuccon G, Koopman B, Deacon A, Azzopardi L, Geva S. A test collection for evaluating retrieval of studies for inclusion in systematic reviews. In: Proceedings of the 40th international ACM SIGIR conference on research and development in information retrieval; 2017. p. 1237–40.
62. Scells H, Zuccon G, Koopman B. A comparison of automatic Boolean query formulation for systematic reviews. Inf Retrieval J. 2021;24(1):3–28.
63. Cormack GV, Grossman MR. Scalability of continuous active learning for reliable high-recall text classification. In: Proceedings of the 25th ACM international on conference on information and knowledge management; 2016. , p. 1039–48.
64. Paxton C, Niculescu-Mizil A, Saria S. Developing predictive models using electronic medical records: challenges and pitfalls. In: AMIA annual symposium proceedings, American medical informatics association, vol 2013. 2013, p. 1109.
65. Goldstein BA, Navar AM, Pencina MJ, Ioannidis J. Opportunities and challenges in developing risk prediction models with electronic health records data: a systematic review. J Am Med Inf Assoc. 2017;24(1):198–208.
66. Mullenbach J, Wiegreffe S, Duke J, Sun J, Eisenstein J. Explainable prediction of medical codes from clinical text. In: Proceedings of the 2018 conference of the North American chapter of the association for computational linguistics: human language technologies, Volume 1 (Long Papers), pp. 1101–1111, Association for Computational Linguistics, June 2018.
67. Beeksma M, Verberne S, van den Bosch A, Das E, Hendrickx I, Groenewoud S. Predicting life expectancy with a long short-term memory recurrent neural network using electronic medical records. BMC Med Inf Decision Mak. 2019;19(1):1–15.
68. Lucini FR, Fogliatto FS, da Silveira GJ, Neyeloff JL, Anzanello MJ, Kuchenbecker RS, Schaan BD. Text mining approach to predict hospital admissions using early medical records from the emergency department. Int J Med Inf. 2017;100:1–8.
69. Huang Y, Talwar A, Chatterjee S, Aparasu RR. Application of machine learning in predicting hospital readmissions: a scoping review of the literature. BMC Med Res Methodol. 2021;21(1):1–14.
70. De Lusignan S, Khunti K, Belsey J, Hattersley A, Van Vlymen J, Gallagher H, Millett C, Hague N, Tomson C, Harris K, et al. A method of identifying and correcting miscoding, misclassification and misdiagnosis in diabetes: a pilot and validation study of routinely collected data. Diabetic Med. 2010;27(2):203–9.
71. Tate AR, Martin AG, Ali A, Cassell JA. Using free text information to explore how and when gps code a diagnosis of ovarian cancer: an observational study using primary care records of patients with ovarian cancer. BMJ Open. 2011;1(1): e000025.

72. Zhou L, Cheng C, Ou D, Huang H. Construction of a semi-automatic icd-10 coding system. BMC Med Inf Decision Mak. 2020;20(1):1–12.
73. Magge A, Tutubalina E, Miftahutdinov Z, Alimova I, Dirkson A, Verberne S, Weissenbacher D, Gonzalez-Hernandez G. Deepademiner: a deep learning pharmacovigilance pipeline for extraction and normalization of adverse drug event mentions on twitter. J Am Med Inf Assoc. 2021;28(10):2184–92.
74. Dirkson A, Verberne S, Kraaij W, van Oortmerssen G, Gelderblom H. Automated gathering of real-world data from online patient forums can complement pharmacovigilance for rare cancers. Sci Rep. 2022;12(1):1–9.
75. Verberne S, Batenburg A, Sanders R, van Eenbergen M, Das E, Lambooij MS. Analyzing empowerment processes among cancer patients in an online community: a text mining approach. JMIR Cancer. 2019;5(1): e9887.
76. Gurulingappa H, Rajput AM, Roberts A, Fluck J, Hofmann-Apitius M, Toldo L. Development of a benchmark corpus to support the automatic extraction of drug-related adverse effects from medical case reports. J Biomed Inf. 2012;45(5):885–92.
77. Delgado-Rodríguez M, Llorca J. Bias J Epidemiol Commun Health. 2004;58:635–41.
78. Ribeiro MT, Singh S, Guestrin C. Why should i trust you? explaining the predictions of any classifier. In: Proceedings of the 22nd ACM SIGKDD international conference on knowledge discovery and data mining; 2016. p. 1135–44.
79. d'Alessandro B, O'Neil C, LaGatta T. Conscientious classification: A data scientist's guide to discrimination-aware classification. Big Data. 2017;5(2):120–34.
80. Mosteiro P, Kuiper J, Masthoff J, Scheepers F, Spruit M. Bias discovery in machine learning models for mental health. Information 2022;13(5).
81. Olfson M, King M, Schoenbaum M. Benzodiazepine Use in the United States. JAMA Psychiatry. 2015;72(2):136–42.
82. Federatie Medisch Specialisten. Angststoornissen. 2010. https://richtlijnendatabase.nl/richtlijn/angststoornissen/gegeneraliseerde_angststoornis_gas/farmacotherapie_bij_gas/enzodiazepine_gegeneraliseerde_angststoornis.html. (Accessed 18 Nov 2021)
83. Vinkers CH, Tijdink JK, Luykx JJ, Vis R. Kiezen voor de juiste benzodiazepine. Ned Tijdschr Geneeskd. 2012;156:A4900.
84. Singh H, Mhasawade V, Chunara R. Generalizability challenges of mortality risk prediction models: a retrospective analysis on a multi-center database. medRxiv (2021).
85. Baer T. Understand, manage, and prevent algorithmic bias. Berkeley, CA, USA: Apress; 2019.
86. Barocas S, Selbst AD. Big data's disparate impact. California Law Rev. 2016;104(3):671–732.
87. Bellamy RK, Dey K, Hind M, Hoffman SC, Houde S, Kannan K, Lohia P, Martino J, Mehta S, Mojsilović A, et al. Ai fairness 360: an extensible toolkit for detecting and mitigating algorithmic bias. IBM J Res Dev. 2019;63(4/5):4–1.
88. Lang WW, Nakamura LI. A model of redlining. J Urban Econ. 1993;33(2):223–34.
89. Ellenberg JH. Selection bias in observational and experimental studies. Statistics in Med. 1994;13:557–567. Place: England.
90. Geneviève LD, Martani A, Shaw D, Elger BS, Wangmo T. Structural racism in precision medicine: Leaving no one behind. Bmc Med Ethics. 2020;21(1):17.
91. Blodgett SL, Barocas S, Daumé III H, Wallach H. Language (Technology) is power: a critical survey of "Bias" in NLP. In: Proceedings of the 58th annual meeting of the association for computational linguistics, (Online) Association for Computational Linguistics, 2020, p. 5454–76.
92. Spruit M, Verkleij S, de Schepper K, Scheepers F. Exploring language markers of mental health in psychiatric stories. Appl Sci. 2022;12(4).
93. Mehrabi N, Morstatter F, Saxena N, Lerman K, Galstyan A. A survey on bias and fairness in machine learning. ACM Comput Surv. 2021;54.
94. Hardt M, Price E, Price E, Srebro N. Equality of opportunity in supervised learning. In: Lee D, Sugiyama M, Luxburg U, Guyon I, Garnett R. editors. Advances in neural information processing systems vol. 29, Curran Associates, Inc., 2016.
95. Saleiro P, Kuester B, Hinkson L, London J, Stevens A, Anisfeld A, Rodolfa KT, Ghani R. Aequitas: a bias and fairness audit toolkit, 2018.
96. Sogancioglu G, Kaya H. The effects of gender bias in word embeddings on depression prediction. In: Empowering communities: a participatory approach to AI for mental health, NeurIPS'22 Workshops, 2022.
97. Kamishima T, Akaho S, Asoh H, Sakuma J. Fairness-aware classifier with prejudice remover regularizer. In: Flach PA, De Bie T, Cristianini N, editors. Machine learning and knowledge discovery in databases. Springer, Berlin Heidelberg: Berlin, Heidelberg; 2012. p. 35–50.
98. Meng C, Trinh L, Xu N, Enouen J, Liu Y. Interpretability and fairness evaluation of deep learning models on mimic-iv dataset. Sci Rep. 2022;12(1):1–28.
99. Bender EM, Friedman B. Data statements for natural language processing: toward mitigating system bias and enabling better science. In: Transactions of the association for computational linguistics, vol. 6; 2018. p. 587–604.
100. van Lent M, Fisher W, Mancuso M. An explainable artificial intelligence system for small-unit tactical behavior. In: Proceedings of the 16th conference on innovative applications of artifical intelligence, IAAI'04. AAAI Press; 2004. p. 900–7.
101. Miller T. Explanation in artificial intelligence: insights from the social sciences. Artif Intell. 2019;267:1–38.

102. Gilpin LH, Bau D, Yuan BZ, Bajwa A, Specter M, Kagal L. Explaining explanations: an overview of interpretability of machine learning. In,. IEEE 5th international conference on data science and advanced analytics (DSAA). IEEE. 2018;2018:80–9.
103. Markus AF, Kors JA, Rijnbeek PR. The role of explainability in creating trustworthy artificial intelligence for health care: a comprehensive survey of the terminology, design choices, and evaluation strategies. J Biomed Informat. 2021;113: 103655.
104. Bhatt U, Xiang A, Sharma S, Weller A, Taly A, Jia Y, Ghosh J, Puri R, Moura JM, Eckersley P. Explainable machine learning in deployment. In: Proceedings of the 2020 conference on fairness, accountability, and transparency; 2020. p. 648–57.
105. Ahmad MA, Teredesai A, Eckert C. Interpretable machine learning in healthcare. In: 2018 IEEE international conference on healthcare informatics (ICHI); 2018. p. 447–7.
106. Adadi A, Berrada M. Peeking inside the black-box: a survey on explainable artificial intelligence (xai). IEEE Access. 2018;6:52138–60.
107. Liu N, Huang X, Li J, Hu X. On interpretation of network embedding via taxonomy induction. In: Proceedings of the 24th ACM SIGKDD international conference on knowledge discovery and data mining, KDD '18. Association for Computing Machinery; 2018. p. 1812–20
108. Lundberg SM, Lee S-I. A unified approach to interpreting model predictions. Adv Neural Inf Proc Syst. 2017;30
109. Rojas JC, Carey KA, Edelson DP, Venable LR, Howell MD, Churpek MM. Predicting intensive care unit readmission with machine learning using electronic health record data. Ann Am Thoracic Soc. 2018;15(7):846–53.
110. Shrikumar A, Greenside P, Kundaje A. Learning important features through propagating activation differences. In: Proceedings of the 34th international conference on machine learning, vol. 70, ICML'17, JMLR.org; 2017, p. 3145–53.
111. Selvaraju RR, Cogswell M, Das A, Vedantam R, Parikh D, Batra D. Grad-cam: visual explanations from deep networks via gradient-based localization. In: Proceedings of the IEEE international conference on computer vision; 2017, p. 618–26.
112. Jain S, Wallace BC. Attention is not explanation. In: Proceedings of NAACL-HLT; 2019, pp. 3543–56.
113. Wiegreffe S, Pinter Y. Attention is not not explanation. In: Proceedings of the 2019 conference on empirical methods in natural language processing and the 9th international joint conference on natural language processing (EMNLP-IJCNLP); 2019. p. 11–20.
114. Ross AS, Hughes MC, Doshi-Velez F. Right for the right reasons: training differentiable models by constraining their explanations. In: Proceedings of the 26th international joint conference on artificial intelligence, IJCAI'17, AAAI Press; 2017, p. 2662–70.
115. Rajani NF, McCann B, Xiong C, Socher R. Explain yourself! leveraging language models for commonsense reasoning. In: Proceedings of the 57th annual meeting of the association for computational linguistics; 2019, p. 4932–42.
116. Serrano S, Smith NA. Is attention interpretable? In: Proceedings of the 57th annual meeting of the association for computational linguistics; 2019, p. 2931–51.
117. Carvalho DV, Pereira EM, Cardoso JS. Machine learning interpretability: A survey on methods and metrics. Electronics. 2019;8(8):832.
118. Lertvittayakumjorn P, Toni F. Human-grounded evaluations of explanation methods for text classification. In: Proceedings of the 2019 conference on empirical methods in natural language processing and the 9th international joint conference on natural language processing (EMNLP-IJCNLP); 2019, p. 5195–205.
119. Holzinger A, Biemann C, Pattichis CS, Kell DB. What do we need to build explainable ai systems for the medical domain? 2017. ArXiv preprint arXiv:1712.09923.
120. Cabitza F, Rasoini R, Gensini GF. Unintended consequences of machine learning in medicine. Jama. 2017;318(6):517–8.
121. Payrovnaziri SN, Chen Z, Rengifo-Moreno P, Miller T, Bian J, Chen JH, Liu X, He Z. Explainable artificial intelligence models using real-world electronic health record data: a systematic scoping review. J Am Med Inf Assoc. 2020;27(7):1173–85.
122. Uddin MZ, Dysthe KK, Følstad A, Brandtzaeg PB. Deep learning for prediction of depressive symptoms in a large textual dataset. Neural Comput Appl. 2022;34(1):721–44.
123. Caicedo-Torres W, Gutierrez J. Iseeu2: Visually interpretable mortality prediction inside the icu using deep learning and free-text medical notes. Expert Syst Appl. 2022;202: 117190.
124. Hu S, Teng F, Huang L, Yan J, Zhang H. An explainable cnn approach for medical codes prediction from clinical text. BMC Med Inf Decis Mak. 2021;21(9):1–12.
125. Blanco A, Pérez A, Casillas A, Cobos D. Extracting cause of death from verbal autopsy with deep learning interpretable methods. IEEE J Biomed Health Inf. 2020;25(4):1315–25.
126. Arrieta AB, Díaz-Rodríguez N, Del Ser J, Bennetot A, Tabik S, Barbado A, García S, Gil-López S, Molina D, Benjamins R, et al. Explainable artificial intelligence (xai): Concepts, taxonomies, opportunities and challenges toward responsible ai. Inf Fusion. 2020;58:82–115.
127. Zhou J, Gandomi AH, Chen F, Holzinger A. Evaluating the quality of machine learning explanations: a survey on methods and metrics. Electronics. 2021;10(5):593.

Analytics

Statistical Analysis—Measurement Error

Timo B. Brakenhoff, Maarten van Smeden and Daniel L. Oberski

Abstract

An important aspect of data quality when conducting clinical analyses using real-world data is how variables in the data have been recorded or measured. The discrepancy between an observed value and the *true* value is called measurement error (also known as *noise* in the artificial intelligence and machine learning literature) and can have consequences for your analyses in all kinds of contexts. To properly assess the potential impact of measurement error it is essential to understand the relationship between the true and observed variables as well as the goal of the analysis and how it will be implemented in practice. Commonly, measurement error is distinguished as being classical, Berkson, systematic and/or differential. While it is clear that measurement error can have far-reaching consequences on analyses, the effect can differ depending on whether analyses are descriptive, explanatory or predictive. Validation studies can inform the estimation and characterization of measurement error as well as provide crucial information for correction methods that are available in several statistical programming languages such as SAS, R and Python.

Keywords

Measurement error · Misclassification · Noise · Correction · Bias · Modelling · Estimation

1 Introduction

Before applying an analytical method on data it is important to consider the quality of the data and how that quality might impact the results of the analysis. One important aspect of data quality is how variables in the data have been recorded or measured. There are many different situations in which the variable(s) that are measured or observed are different from what was intended to be measured. This discrepancy between an observed value and the *true* value is called **measurement error** and can have consequences for your analyses in all kinds of contexts (see Box 1 for two examples of the effect of measurement error in practice).

T. B. Brakenhoff (✉)
Julius Clinical, Zeist, The Netherlands
e-mail: timo.brakenhoff@juliusclinical.com

M. van Smeden · D. L. Oberski
Julius Center for Health Sciences and Primary Care, UMC Utrecht, Utrecht University, Utrecht, The Netherlands

D. L. Oberski
Dept. Methodology & Statistics, Utrecht University, Utrecht, The Netherlands

F. W. Asselbergs et al. (eds.), *Clinical Applications of Artificial Intelligence in Real-World Data*,
https://doi.org/10.1007/978-3-031-36678-9_6

Box 1: Examples of Measurement Error in Practice

- Measuring prevalence using different diagnostic tests
  - In Montreal, Canada a screening and treatment program for intestinal parasite infections was offered to newly arrived Southeast Asian refugees in Canada between July 1982 and February 1983. The 162 Cambodian refugees included in the sample were tested using two different diagnostic tests for the presence of Strongyloides Infection: enzyme-linked immunosorbent assay (immunoglobulin G) *serology* and *stool* examination (see table below for the amount of refugees that tested positive using each diagnostic test) [27, 28]. The observed sample prevalence based solely on serology was 77.2 percent, while it was 24.7 percent using information from stool examinations alone! This absolute difference of over 50 percentage points in prevalence demonstrates how crucial it is to consider the instrument that is being used to measure a quantity of interest, such as the prevalence. Note that these estimates also don't take into account other sources of uncertainty such as sampling variability (only 162 individuals of the whole population of Cambodian refugees were included in this sample) or the performance of the tests themselves (it is likely that several individuals may be false positives or false negatives as neither test has perfect sensitivity or specificity) [34].

	Stool +	Stool −	
Serology +	**38**	**87**	125
Serology −	**2**	**35**	37
	40	122	162

- Computer aided diagnosis of prostate cancer without gold standard outcome labels
  - Nir et al. [51] describe the automatic grading of prostate cancer in digitized histopathology images. They did this using various supervised machine and deep learning methods based on images labeled by pathologists. Just as in many medical image settings, this labeling is not perfect and specialists will not always agree when evaluating the same images. When these images act as important input for machine and deep learning algorithms meant for diagnostic or prognostic settings, this, often unavoidable, measurement error, or noise in the outcome labels can have significant consequences for the performance of the algorithms [35]. In the case of [51] multiple pathologists were asked to rate the same images and different methods were used to best account for the inter-observer variability in prostate cancer grading. While this may not always be possible to apply in practice, there are several other techniques that can help correct for measurement error in the outcome [35].

Where the term "measurement error" is frequently used with regards to errors in the measurement of continuous variables (such as an individual's age or height), the term "misclassification" is often used for discrete variables (such as an individual's preferences of received treatment). In Artificial intelligence and machine learning literature, errors in discrete or non-discrete variables are often called *noise* with noise existing either in the covariates (also known as predictors, features or attributes) or in the outcome(s) (also known as target variables, labels or classes). In this chapter, the term measurement error will be used to describe all these phenomena unless otherwise specified.

Errors in measurement can be caused through various mechanisms including, but not limited to, inaccuracy and imprecision of measurement instruments, errors due to self-reporting, errors in data coding or labeling, lack of data granularity, or when single measurements are taken of naturally fluctuating biological processes such as biomarkers. Common settings where such errors can occur include when measuring smoking [45], blood pressure [2, 53, 75], dietary intake [17, 18, 73], physical activity [16, 41], exposure to air pollutants [22, 69, 78], medical treatments received [5, 65, 71], diagnostic coding [15, 52, 77] and labels for medical images [12, 35, 55, 57].

All of the above mentioned measurement error mechanisms can lead to discrepancies between the sought after, perfectly measured and thus error-free *true* value of a variable and an imperfectly measured *observed* value of that same variable. In most cases we have not observed the former and we are in possession of the latter. This can have severe implications for the results of an analysis. Examples include the following:

- Brakenhoff et al. [7] demonstrate that even when the simplest form of measurement error, random error, is assumed when measuring blood pressure in routine care, this can have very divergent and unexpected consequences on the estimation of the effect of blood pressure on the possible risk of developing cardiovascular disease. The estimated relations can be severely biased positively or negatively depending on the amount of measurement error present in confounders and the relationship of those confounders with the observed blood pressure variable.
- When aiming for the best possible prediction performance using advanced artificial intelligence techniques such as deep learning for medical imaging, multiple authors [12, 35, 57] identify the need for large datasets of trustworthy labelled medical images (which are used as the outcome to be predicted) to train the desired model. The expertise required for this as well as regulations in the medical sector make this a challenging ask which can severely impact the performance of prediction models.

To properly assess the potential impact of measurement error it is essential to understand the relationship between the true and observed variables as well as the goal of the analysis (i.e. is the purpose to *describe*, *explain* or *predict?*) (See Box 3) and how it will be implemented in practice. However, the fact that measurement error may have far-reaching consequences on analyses in the field of statistics, epidemiology or artificial intelligence is nothing new [9, 26, 79]. Yet, despite this understanding and a plethora of recent literature on the subject [8, 36] there is still little attention paid to measurement error consequences and potential solutions in the medical literature [6, 67] and common myths [7, 74] are perpetuated. With the increasing availability of (big) data not collected for research purposes such as medical health records for explanation as well as the application of machine learning and deep learning algorithms for prediction, careful investigation of potential bias due to issues like measurement error is arguably more important than ever [21].

This chapter will provide an overview of the types of measurement error and why it is essential to keep this in consideration when conducting clinical data analysis. Subsequently the consequences of measurement error will be discussed and how this will differ depending on the goal of the analysis and the desired implementation. Lastly, an overview will be given of various tools for the estimation and correction of measurement error.

2 Types of Measurement Error

A common taxonomy to distinguish between types of measurement error differentiates between 4 types: classical, Berkson, systematic and differential. Each of these types can manifest differently in continuous or discrete data. They represent different ways in which true values and the observed variables relate to each other, which can have different consequences on the analysis being performed.

When considering ***continuous variables***, we can differentiate between multiple *measurement error models*. The simplest of these is called the *classical or random measurement error model* where the observed variable is equal to the true variable plus error, in this case a random variable with mean 0 which is independent of the true variable. This error model can be extended to accommodate *systematic error* or dependencies between the error and the observed variable, the true variable or other auxiliary variables. When the relations between the observed and true variable are non-linear, transformations can be used to make it linear. In specific circumstances it is more appropriate to model the true variable as equal to the observed variable plus a random variable with mean 0 which is independent of the observed variable. This is called *Berkson error*. Lastly, depending on if the error contains information on the outcome variable which you may be interested in or not, the error is referred to as *differential* or *nondifferential* respectively. Box 2 provides technical definitions of these measurement error models.

For ***categorical variables***, discrepancies between the true value of a variable and the observed value is often referred to as misclassification. While misclassification is closely related to measurement error in continuous variables, the categorical nature of the variables means that misclassification is often expressed in terms of mis*classification probabilities*. For example, in the case of a binary observed and true variable, regardless of the type of measurement error assumed, misclassification can best be described in terms of sensitivity, specificity and predictive values (namely positive predictive value and negative predictive value). Note that similar to measurement error models, misclassification can also be (non)differential and have a structure similar to Berkson error (while the latter is not often observed) [36].

Box 2: Technical Definitions of Types of Measurement Error in Continuous Variables

Suppose we are interested in the relationship between an outcome variable ***Y*** and a covariate of interest **X** given covariates **Z**. If a variable **X** is measured with error, the observed variable is denoted by **X***, with the true value of this variable (**X**) being unobserved. Note that notation differs across the literature and the notation chosen here is consistent with that of [36 and 68]. The following types of error are most commonly distinguished:

- **Classical measurement error:**
  $X^* = X + U$, where U is a random variable with mean 0 that is independent of X.
- **Linear measurement error**
  $X^* = \alpha_0 + \alpha_X X + U$, where U is a random variable with mean 0 that is independent of X, α_0 is an intercept term and α_X is the coefficient of X. Note that classical measurement error is a special case of linear measurement error where $\alpha_0 = 0$ and $\alpha_X = 1$.
- **Systematic error**
  $X^* = \alpha_0 + \alpha_X X$, where α_0 is an intercept term and α_X is the coefficient of X which each represent systematic error that may be dependent on X.
- **Nondifferential error**
  The distribution of Y given (X, Z, X*) depends only on (X, Z)
- **Berkson measurement error**
  $X = X^* + U$, where U is a random variable with mean 0 that is independent of X*.

3 Consequences of Measurement Error

3.1 Goal of the Analysis

Before discussing the consequences of measurement error it is important to clearly identify the goal of the analysis. A common framework used to distinguish between the goal of statistical modeling is whether it is used for **description**, **explanation** or **prediction** [70] (See Box 3). Shmueli [70] mostly disregards descriptive modelling as it is frequently used for characterization of the observed data structure and is not often used for theory building. In public health and healthcare research, however, descriptive modelling plays a crucial role, e.g. when estimating incidence rates or prevalences of disease. In the context of measurement error and its impact, this section will mostly focus on the distinction between explanatory and predictive modelling.

Box 3: Definitions of Types of Statistical Modelling

- **Descriptive modelling** is aimed at summarizing or representing the data. E.g. calculating an incidence rate for a disease over a particular time period, or by fitting a regression model to quantify the association between a covariate and an outcome, without causal inference or prediction intentions.
- **Explanatory modelling** is the application of models to data for the purpose of testing and quantifying causal relations. E.g. fitting a regression model to estimate the causal effect of a certain factor (e..g. a medical treatment, registered as a dispensed drug) on the occurrence of a certain outcome (e.g. a health outcome such as (cause-specific) mortality or hospital admission).
- **Predictive modelling** the application of models to data for the main purpose of predicting new or future observations. E.g. fitting a regression model to predict the probability of the occurrence of a certain health outcome (e.g. 5-year mortality) for future individuals taking into account various relevant covariates (e.g. medical history, demographics, laboratory tests, etcetera).

While often not clearly separated in literature, studies with explanation and prediction goals fundamentally differ due to the differences in aims and subsequent diverging choices at every step of the modelling process (designing the study, collecting data, preparing data, exploring data, selecting variables, selecting statistical models, evaluating models and using models in practice). Note that both types of modelling can be used in combination, each achieving a separate specific goal within an overarching analysis that may be of an explanatory or predictive nature. An example of this is the application of prediction models (including machine learning models [44]) to estimate propensity scores [58] that are used to adjust for confounding when estimating causal effects.

The measurement of variables for explanatory modelling generally focuses on obtaining measurements that are as reliable and accurate as possible to appropriately represent the underlying constructs. Conversely, for many predictive modelling studies priority goes towards reliably estimating the outcome/target variable (often called *labeling* [1, 19, 49, 50]), while the measurement quality of the covariates necessary for making predictions should ideally be of a similar quality when the model is constructed as when the model is applied to new patients. So far, however, much of the attention in the measurement error literature [9, 37] has been specifically devoted to explanatory modelling. More recently, attention is being given to the prediction setting, showing the impact of *heterogeneity* in how variables are measured in the training and implementation settings, also referred to as *transportability* [9], and how this impacts the performance of prediction models [42, 43, 54].

The above broad differentiation in modeling goals and the different role of errors in measurement exemplifies the importance of keeping in mind the goal of the analysis, how the results of the analysis will be generalized and in which settings the results will be applied.

3.2 The Impact of Measurement Error in Explanatory Modelling

Much of the health science measurement error literature has been focussed on the consequences of different types of measurement error when engaging in explanatory modelling. Carroll et al. [9], describe how the consequences of measurement error is a "triple whammy": covariate-outcome relationships can be biased, power to detect clinically meaningful relationships is diminished and important features of the data can be masked.

When assuming classical measurement error or misclassification in a single continuous or binary categorical covariate of interest, the estimated univariable covariate-outcome relation will be biased towards the null (also known as *attenuation*). However, when the covariate has more than two categories or when considering a multivariable model (models with more than one covariate) where at least 1 confounder measured with classical error, the estimated covariate-outcome relation can be biased in either direction, even if the covariate of interest is not measured with error [7]. This unpredictability of the magnitude and direction of bias and precision on the estimated effect is compounded if error is systematic or differential. Berkson error on the other hand often does not lead to bias in the estimated covariate-outcome relation, but can diminish precision. Regarding measurement error in the outcome of an explanatory model, classical error will generally not lead to bias in a covariate-outcome relation while other types of error like systematic or differential error can substantially bias estimators [46]. Table 1 of [37] provides a useful overview of the effects of measurement error according to the type of error and target of the analysis for explanatory modelling.

3.3 The Impact of Measurement Error in Predictive Modelling

Attention for the role of measurement error in predictive modelling is relatively recent. In particular, the concept of *measurement heterogeneity,* which means the covariates (predictors) are measured differently (i.e. have different measurement error) between training and external validation settings for prediction models, has been shown to have an important impact on the performance of prediction models. Measurement heterogeneity can, for instance, occur when different measurement protocols or different types of tests are used when developing a clinical prediction model as compared to the setting in which they are externally validated or applied. Various studies [42, 43, 54] have shown how in different measurement scenarios often leads to deteriorated performance of the calibration and discrimination of prediction models.

Regarding the impact of measurement error or noise in the development of machine learning or deep learning models, attribute (i.e. covariate) noise is often considered to have a less severe impact on predictive performance than label (i.e. outcome) noise [25, 66]. Label noise can diminish accuracy of predictions and classification performance as well as increase the amount of training samples required for model development [19, 50]. In addition, error prone outcomes can lead to prediction unfairness if the error differs over subgroups of interest [4]. For an overview of the impact of class and attribute noise, see [79].

Box 4: Five Myths About Measurement Error

van Smeden et al. [74] identifies and debunks 5 common myths about measurement error:

1. Measurement error can be compensated for by large numbers of observations
   a. No, a large number of observations does not resolve the most serious consequences of measurement error in epidemiological data analyses. These remain regardless of the sample size.
2. The effect of a covariate of interest on the outcome is underestimated when variables are measured with error

   a. No, the effect of a covariate of interest can be over- or underestimated in the presence of measurement error depending on which variables are affected, how measurement error is structured and the expression of other biasing and data sampling factors.
3. Covariate measurement error is non-differential if measurements are taken without knowledge of the outcome
   a. No, covariate measurement error can be differential even if the measurement is taken without knowledge of the outcome.
4. Measurement error can be prevented but not mitigated in data analyses
   a. No, statistical methods for measurement error bias corrections can be used in the presence of measurement error provided that data are available on the structure and magnitude of measurement error from an internal or external source. This often requires planning of a measurement error correction approach or quantitative bias analysis, which may require additional data to be collected.
5. Certain types of research are unaffected by measurement error
   a. No, measurement error can affect all types of research.

4 Correction of Measurement Error

Several approaches have been suggested to circumvent (or at least lower) the detrimental consequences of measurement error, in particular to reduce bias (one of the 3 whammies of measurement error). To understand the possible value of correction, the natural first step is in identifying potential error-prone variables. To quantify and correct for measurement error, additional information is required which can often be collected through validation studies.

4.1 Validation Studies

Validation studies (also referred to as ancillary studies) on the error-prone variables can aid the investigation into the structure, type and amount of measurement error present [37]. These studies can also be essential for the application of several correction methods discussed later in this section. Generally speaking, there are four types of validation studies: internal validation studies, calibration studies, replicates studies and external validation studies.

In an **internal validation study**, both the error-prone observed variable as well as (a reliable representation of) the true variable (i.e. gold standard measurement) are observed in a subset of the data. Measurement of a gold standard only in a subset can be motivated by a measurement procedure that is time-consuming, expensive, invasive or even impossible to obtain for the whole study sample. Usually an internal validation study is assumed to contain data from a *random* subset of the study sample, but alternative sampling strategies are available depending on the type of measurement error and the measurement error correction method that can be used [47]. With a suitable internal validation study, the relations between the error-prone observed variable and the true variable can directly be estimated, which can be used for measurement error correction. If the true variable or gold standard measurement is not available, but another variable (reference measurement) unbiased at the individual level is, it is sometimes called a **calibration study**. This type of study can be used as input for the measurement error correction method called regression calibration, if certain assumptions are met.

In a **replicates study,** multiple replicate measurements from the same instrument (e.g. multiple measurements of blood pressure during the same hospital visit) or different instruments that measure the same underlying construct (e.g. multiple diagnostic tests for the same disease) are collected. When the variable of interest contains random measurement error, having multiple measurements available can provide essential information on the amount and type of measurement error present.

Validation studies can also use data available from external sources such as similar cohorts from another country. For example, for separate individuals not included in the main study, both the error-prone variable as well as the true variable (or gold standard measurement) and necessary covariates might be available. This can then be used to inform measurement error correction methods. Note that for such **external validation studies** it is very important to assess the heterogeneity between the external and internal setting and how transportable the information is. More information on the design and desirable size of validation studies can be found in [37].

4.2 Correction Methods

Characterizing the amount and type of error is an important first step when applying strategies to correct for the measurement error. At the most basic level, common metrics such as the bias and variance or classification probabilities like sensitivity and specificity can be used to characterize how accurate and precise observed variables are compared to the true variables. The next step is to identify the type of measurement error observed (see Sect. 2) and use those models to further quantify various aspects of the error. In general, measurement error correction methods use information obtained through validation studies to take into account measurement error in the analyses by estimating the research results in the counterfactual situation where there was no measurement error.

Many different approaches have been proposed in the literature which characterize the error present as well as correct for the bias that may arise due to this error in the final analyses. Approaches include: regression calibration [11], simulation extrapolation [14, 37], likelihood methods [10], score function methods [3, 72], methods-of-moment correction [20], latent variable analysis [32], structural equation modelling [4, 63], multiple imputation for measurement error correction [13], inverse probability weighting [23], bayesian analyses [26], cluster-based correction [49].

More detailed information on the various types of error and how to correct for them can be found in extensive literature on the topic. Various measurement error text books exist, with [9] focussing on nonlinear models, [26] on Bayesian methods of adjustment and [8]) providing a more broad overview. Similarly, reviews such as the one by Guolo [24] give an overview of robust techniques to correct for measurement error in covariates. More recently, the STRATOS initiative wrote a two-part tutorial on the basic theory of measurement error and simple methods of adjustment [36] as well as on more complex methods of adjustment and advanced topics [68]. Literature focused on the impact of measurement error (referred to as noise) in both covariates and outcomes in the field of machine learning and how to deal with it includes [19, 50, 64, 79].

While several methods can be easily programmed using standard functionality of different software tools, specific packages, macros or procedures are available for more complex measurement error correction in different programming languages. In SAS, for example, macros include *%blinplus* [59], *%relibpls8* [60] and *%rrc* [40] which have been developed for various implementations of regression calibration. Similarly in STATA, procedures include *rcal* and *eivreg* for regression calibration [29], and *simex* and *simexplot* for simulation extrapolation [30]. For the R language, packages include *simex* [39] and *simexaft* [31] for simulation extrapolation approaches, *lavaan* [61] for latent variable analysis and structural equation modelling, as well as *mecor* [48] for measurement error correction in linear regression models. Also in Python, an increasing amount of relevant packages are being developed, such as *pyEMU* [76] for environmental model uncertainty analysis and *snorkel* [56] for rapid training data creation in the face of potential label noise.

An important alternative method to investigate the impact of measurement error on your study results if no suitable additional information is available, is to perform sensitivity analyses. Various amounts of measurement error can be assumed in hypothetical scenarios where the analysis is rerun and the results are compared against the original results. To assess multiple hypothetical scenarios with various amounts of measurement error simultaneously, probabilistic sensitivity analyses can be performed (see Chapter 19 of [62]). A similar technique applied to examine the impact of measurement error (and correct for it) when additional information is lacking in both explanatory and prediction modelling is quantitative bias analysis [33, 38].

References

1. Algan G, Ulusoy I. Label noise types and their effects on deep learning. 2020. ArXiv: https://arxiv.org/abs/2003.10471
2. Bauldry S, Bollen KA, Adair LS. Evaluating measurement error in readings of blood pressure for adolescents and young adults. Blood Press. 2015;24:96–102. https://doi.org/10.3109/08037051.2014.986952.
3. Boeschoten L, Oberski D, De Waal T. Estimating classification errors under edit restrictions in composite survey-register data using multiple imputation latent class modelling (MILC). J Off Stat. 2017;33:921–62. https://doi.org/10.1515/jos-2017-0044.
4. Boeschoten L, van Kesteren E-J, Bagheri A, Oberski DL. Achieving fair inference using error-prone outcomes. Int J Interact Multimed Artif Intell. 2021;6:9. https://doi.org/10.9781/ijimai.2021.02.007.
5. Boudreau DM, Daling JR, Malone KE, et al. A validation study of patient interview data and pharmacy records for antihypertensive, statin, and antidepressant medication use among older women. Am J Epidemiol. 2004;159:308–17. https://doi.org/10.1093/aje/kwh038.
6. Brakenhoff TB, Mitroiu M, Keogh RH, et al. Measurement error is often neglected in medical literature: a systematic review. J Clin Epidemiol. 2018;98:89–97. https://doi.org/10.1016/j.jclinepi.2018.02.023.
7. Brakenhoff TB, van Smeden M, Visseren FLJ, Groenwold RHH. Random measurement error: why worry? An example of cardiovascular risk factors. PLoS ONE. 2018;13: e0192298. https://doi.org/10.1371/journal.pone.0192298.
8. Buonaccorsi JP. Measurement error: models, methods, and applications. New York: Chapman and Hall/CRC; 2010.
9. Carroll RJ, Ruppert D, Stefanski LA, Crainiceanu CM. Measurement error in nonlinear models: a modern perspective. 2nd ed. New York: Chapman and Hall/CRC; 2006.
10. Carroll RJ, Spiegelman CH, Lan KKG, et al. On errors-in-variables for binary regression models. Biometrika. 1984;71:19–25. https://doi.org/10.1093/biomet/71.1.19.
11. Carroll RJ, Stefanski LA. Approximate quasi-likelihood estimation in models with surrogate predictors. J Am Stat Assoc. 1990;85:652–63. https://doi.org/10.1080/01621459.1990.10474925.
12. Ching T, Himmelstein DS, Beaulieu-Jones BK, et al. Opportunities and obstacles for deep learning in biology and medicine. J R Soc Interface. 2018;15:20170387. https://doi.org/10.1098/rsif.2017.0387.
13. Cole SR, Chu H, Greenland S. Multiple-imputation for measurement-error correction. Int J Epidemiol. 2006;35:1074–81. https://doi.org/10.1093/ije/dyl097.
14. Cook JR, Stefanski LA. Simulation-extrapolation estimation in parametric measurement error models. J Am Stat Assoc. 1994;89:1314–28. https://doi.org/10.1080/01621459.1994.10476871.
15. Delate T, Jones AE, Clark NP, Witt DM. Assessment of the coding accuracy of warfarin-related bleeding events. Thromb Res. 2017;159:86–90. https://doi.org/10.1016/j.thromres.2017.10.004.
16. Ferrari P, Friedenreich C, Matthews CE. The role of measurement error in estimating levels of physical activity. Am J Epidemiol. 2007;166:832–40. https://doi.org/10.1093/aje/kwm148.
17. Freedman LS, Commins JM, Willett W, et al. Evaluation of the 24-hour recall as a reference instrument for calibrating other self-report instruments in nutritional cohort studies: evidence from the validation studies pooling project. Am J Epidemiol. 2017;186:73–82. https://doi.org/10.1093/aje/kwx039.
18. Freedman LS, Schatzkin A, Midthune D, Kipnis V. Dealing with dietary measurement error in nutritional cohort studies. JNCI J Natl Cancer Inst. 2011;103:1086–92. https://doi.org/10.1093/jnci/djr189.
19. Frenay B, Verleysen M. Classification in the presence of label noise: a survey. IEEE Trans Neural Netw Learn Syst. 2014;25:845–69. https://doi.org/10.1109/TNNLS.2013.2292894.
20. Fuller WA. Measurement error models. New York: John Wiley & Sons; 1987.
21. Gianfrancesco MA, Tamang S, Yazdany J, Schmajuk G. Potential biases in machine learning algorithms using electronic health record data. JAMA Intern Med. 2018;178:1544. https://doi.org/10.1001/jamainternmed.2018.3763.
22. Goldman GT, Mulholland JA, Russell AG, et al. Impact of exposure measurement error in air

pollution epidemiology: effect of error type in time-series studies. Environ Health. 2011;10:61. https://doi.org/10.1186/1476-069X-10-61.
23. Gravel CA, Platt RW. Weighted estimation for confounded binary outcomes subject to misclassification. Stat Med. 2018;37:425–36. https://doi.org/10.1002/sim.7522.
24. Guolo A. Robust techniques for measurement error correction: a review. Stat Methods Med Res. 2008;17:555–80. https://doi.org/10.1177/0962280207081318.
25. Gupta S, Gupta A. Dealing with noise problem in machine learning data-sets: a systematic review. Procedia Comput Sci. 2019;161:466–74. https://doi.org/10.1016/j.procs.2019.11.146.
26. Gustafson P. Measurement error and misclassification in statistics and epidemiology: impacts and bayesian adjustments. CRC Press (2003)
27. Gyorkos TW, Frappier-Davignon L, Dick Maclean J, Viens P. Effect of screening and treatment on imported intestinal parasite infections: results from a randomized, Controlled Trial. Am J Epidemiol. 1989;129:753–61. https://doi.org/10.1093/oxfordjournals.aje.a115190
28. Gyorkos TW, Genta RM, Viens P, Maclean JD. Seroepidemiology of Strongyloides infection in the Southeast Asian refugee population in. Canada. Am. J. Epidemiol. 1990;257–64
29. Hardin JW, Schmiediche H, Carroll RJ. The regression-calibration method for fitting generalized linear models with additive measurement error. Stata J Promot Commun Stat Stata. 2003;3:361–72. https://doi.org/10.1177/1536867X0400300406.
30. Hardin JW, Schmiediche H, Carroll RJ. The simulation extrapolation method for fitting generalized linear models with additive measurement error. Stata J Promot Commun Stat Stata. 2003;3:373–85. https://doi.org/10.1177/1536867X0400300407.
31. He W, Xiong J, Yi GY, SIMEX R package for accelerated failure time models with covariate measurement error. J Stat Softw. 2012;46:1–14. https://doi.org/10.18637/jss.v046.c01
32. Hui SL, Walter SD. Estimating the error rates of diagnostic tests. Biometrics. 1980;36:167–71. https://doi.org/10.2307/2530508.
33. Jiang T, Gradus JL, Lash TL, Fox MP. Addressing measurement error in random forests using quantitative bias analysis. Am J Epidemiol. 2021. https://doi.org/10.1093/aje/kwab010.
34. Joseph L, Gyorkos TW, Coupal L. Bayesian estimation of disease prevalence and the parameters of diagnostic tests in the absence of a gold standard. Am J Epidemiol. 1995;141:263–72. https://doi.org/10.1093/oxfordjournals.aje.a117428.
35. Karimi D, Dou H, Warfield SK, Gholipour A. Deep learning with noisy labels: exploring techniques and remedies in medical image analysis. Med Image Anal. 2020;65: 101759. https://doi.org/10.1016/j.media.2020.101759.
36. Keogh RH, Shaw PA, Gustafson P, et al. STRATOS guidance document on measurement error and misclassification of variables in observational epidemiology: Part 1—Basic theory and simple methods of adjustment. Stat Med. 2020;39:2197–231. https://doi.org/10.1002/sim.8532.
37. https://onlinelibrary.wiley.com/doi/abs/10.1002/sim.8531
38. Lash TL, Fox MP, MacLehose RF, et al. Good practices for quantitative bias analysis. Int J Epidemiol. 2014;43:1969–85. https://doi.org/10.1093/ije/dyu149.
39. Lederer W, Küchenhoff H. A short introduction to the SIMEX and MCSIMEX. Newsl R Proj. 2006;6(4):26–31.
40. Liao X, Zucker DM, Li Y, Spiegelman D. Survival analysis with error-prone time-varying covariates: a risk set calibration approach. Biometrics. 2011;67:50–8. https://doi.org/10.1111/j.1541-0420.2010.01423.x.
41. Lim S, Wyker B, Bartley K, Eisenhower D. Measurement error of self-reported physical activity levels in New York City: assessment and correction. Am J Epidemiol. 2015;181:648–55. https://doi.org/10.1093/aje/kwu470.
42. Luijken K, Groenwold RHH, Calster BV, et al. Impact of predictor measurement heterogeneity across settings on the performance of prediction models: a measurement error perspective. Stat Med. 2019;38:3444–59. https://doi.org/10.1002/sim.8183.
43. Luijken K, Wynants L, van Smeden M, et al. Changing predictor measurement procedures affected the performance of prediction models in clinical examples. J Clin Epidemiol. 2020;119:7–18. https://doi.org/10.1016/j.jclinepi.2019.11.001.
44. McCaffrey DF, Griffin BA, Almirall D, et al. A tutorial on propensity score estimation for multiple treatments using generalized boosted models. Stat Med. 2013;32:3388–414. https://doi.org/10.1002/sim.5753.
45. Murray RP, Connett JE, Lauger GG, Voelker HT. Error in smoking measures: effects of intervention on relations of cotinine and carbon monoxide to self-reported smoking. The Lung Health Study Research Group. Am J Public Health. 1993;83:1251–7. https://doi.org/10.2105/AJPH.83.9.1251.
46. Nab L, Groenwold RHH., Welsing PMJ, van Smeden M. Measurement error in continuous endpoints in randomised trials: problems and solutions. Stat Med. 2019;38:5182–96. https://doi.org/10.1002/sim.8359.
47. Nab L, van Smeden M, de Mutsert R, et al. Sampling strategies for internal validation samples for exposure measurement error correction: a study of visceral adipose tissue measures replaced by waist circumference measures. Am J Epidemiol Kwab. 2021a;114. https://doi.org/10.1093/aje/kwab114
48. Nab L, van Smeden M, Keogh RH, Groenwold RHH. mecor: An R package for measurement error correction in linear regression models with a continuous outcome. Comput Methods Programs Biomed. 2021b;208:

49. Nicholson B, Sheng VS, Zhang J. Label noise correction and application in crowdsourcing. Expert Syst Appl. 2016;66:149–62. https://doi.org/10.1016/j.eswa.2016.09.003.
50. Nigam N, Dutta T, Gupta HP. Impact of noisy labels in learning techniques: a survey. In: Kolhe ML, Tiwari S, Trivedi MC, Mishra KK, editors. Advances in Data and Information Sciences. Singapore: Springer; 2020. p. 403–11.
51. Nir G, Hor S, Karimi D, et al. Automatic grading of prostate cancer in digitized histopathology images: learning from multiple experts. Med Image Anal. 2018;50:167–80. https://doi.org/10.1016/j.media.2018.09.005.
52. Nissen F, Morales DR, Mullerova H, et al. Validation of asthma recording in the clinical practice research datalink (CPRD). BMJ Open. 2017;7: e017474. https://doi.org/10.1136/bmjopen-2017-017474.
53. Nitzan M, Slotki I, Shavit L. More accurate systolic blood pressure measurement is required for improved hypertension management: a perspective. Med Devices Auckl NZ. 2017;10:157–63. https://doi.org/10.2147/MDER.S141599.
54. Pajouheshnia R, van Smeden M, Peelen LM, Groenwold RHH. How variation in predictor measurement affects the discriminative ability and transportability of a prediction model. J Clin Epidemiol. 2019;105:136–41. https://doi.org/10.1016/j.jclinepi.2018.09.001.
55. Pot M, Kieusseyan N, Prainsack B. Not all biases are bad: equitable and inequitable biases in machine learning and radiology. Insights Imag. 2021;12:13. https://doi.org/10.1186/s13244-020-00955-7.
56. Ratner A, Bach SH, Ehrenberg H, et al. Snorkel: rapid training data creation with weak supervision. Proc VLDB Endow Int Conf Very Large Data Bases 2017;11:269–282. https://doi.org/10.14778/3157794.3157797
57. Ravì D, Wong C, Deligianni F, et al. Deep learning for health informatics. IEEE J Biomed Health Inform. 2017;21:4–21. https://doi.org/10.1109/JBHI.2016.2636665.
58. Rosenbaum PR, Rubin DB. The central role of the propensity score in observational studies for causal effects. Biometrika. 1983;70:41–55.
59. Rosner B, Spiegelman D, Willett WC. Correction of logistic regression relative risk estimates and confidence intervals for measurement error: the case of multiple covariates measured with error. Am J Epidemiol. 1990;132:734–45. https://doi.org/10.1093/oxfordjournals.aje.a115715.
60. Rosner B, Spiegelman D, Willett WC. Correction of logistic regression relative risk estimates and confidence intervals for random within-person measurement error. Am J Epidemiol. 1992;136:1400–13. https://doi.org/10.1093/oxfordjournals.aje.a116453.
61. Rosseel, Y. lavaan: an R package for structural equation modeling. J Stat Softw. 2012;48:1–36. https://doi.org/10.18637/jss.v048.i02.
62. Rothman KJ, Greenland S, Lash TL. Modern epidemiology. Wolters Kluwer Health/Lippincott Williams & Wilkins Philadelphia; 2008.
63. Sánchez BN, Budtz-Jørgensen E, Ryan LM, Hu H. Structural equation models. J Am Stat Assoc. 2005;100:1443–55. https://doi.org/10.1198/016214505000001005.
64. Schnack, H. Bias, noise, and interpretability in machine learning. In: Machine Learning. Elsevier; 2020. p. 307–28
65. Schneeweiss S, Avorn J. A review of uses of health care utilization databases for epidemiologic research on therapeutics. J Clin Epidemiol. 2005;58:323–37. https://doi.org/10.1016/j.jclinepi.2004.10.012.
66. Shanthini A, Vinodhini G, Chandrasekaran RM, Supraja P. A taxonomy on impact of label noise and feature noise using machine learning techniques. Soft Comput. 2019;23:8597–607. https://doi.org/10.1007/s00500-019-03968-7.
67. Shaw PA, Deffner V, Keogh RH, et al. Epidemiologic analyses with error-prone exposures: review of current practice and recommendations. Ann Epidemiol. 2018;28:821–8. https://doi.org/10.1016/j.annepidem.2018.09.001.
68. Shaw PA, Gustafson P, Carroll RJ, et al. STRATOS guidance document on measurement error and misclassification of variables in observational epidemiology: Part 2—More complex methods of adjustment and advanced topics. Stat Med. 2020;39:2232–63. https://doi.org/10.1002/sim.8531.
69. Sheppard L, Burnett RT, Szpiro AA, et al. Confounding and exposure measurement error in air pollution epidemiology. Air Qual Atmosphere Health. 2012;5:203–16. https://doi.org/10.1007/s11869-011-0140-9.
70. Shmueli G. To Explain or to Predict? Stat Sci. 2010;25.https://doi.org/10.1214/10-STS330.
71. Smedt TD, Merrall E, Macina D, et al. Bias due to differential and non-differential disease- and exposure misclassification in studies of vaccine effectiveness. PLoS ONE. 2018;13: e0199180. https://doi.org/10.1371/journal.pone.0199180.
72. Stefanski LA. Unbiased estimation of a nonlinear function a normal mean with application to measurement err oorf models. Commun Stat - Theory Methods. 1989;18:4335–58. https://doi.org/10.1080/03610928908830159.
73. Thiébaut ACM, Freedman LS, Carroll RJ, Kipnis V. Is It necessary to correct for measurement error in nutritional epidemiology? Ann Intern Med. 2007;146:65. https://doi.org/10.7326/0003-4819-146-1-200701020-00012.
74. van Smeden M, Lash TL, Groenwold RHH. Reflection on modern methods: five myths about measurement error in epidemiological research. Int J Epidemiol. 2020;49:338–47. https://doi.org/10.1093/ije/dyz251.
75. van der Wel MC, Buunk IE, van Weel C, et al. A novel approach to office blood pressure measurement: 30-minute office blood pressure vs

daytime ambulatory blood pressure. Ann Fam Med. 2011;9:128–35. https://doi.org/10.1370/afm.1211.
76. White JT, Fienen MN, Doherty JE. A python framework for environmental model uncertainty analysis. Environ Model Softw. 2016;85:217–28. https://doi.org/10.1016/j.envsoft.2016.08.017.
77. Yu AYX, Quan H, McRae AD, et al. A cohort study on physician documentation and the accuracy of administrative data coding to improve passive surveillance of transient ischaemic attacks. BMJ Open. 2017;7: e015234. https://doi.org/10.1136/bmjopen-2016-015234.
78. Zeger SL, Thomas D, Dominici F, et al. Exposure measurement error in time-series studies of air pollution: concepts and consequences. Environ Health Perspect. 2000;108:419–26. https://doi.org/10.1289/ehp.00108419.
79. Zhu X, Wu X. Class noise vs. attribute noise: a quantitative study. Artif Intell Rev. 2004;22:177–210. https://doi.org/10.1007/s10462-004-0751-8.

Causal Inference and Non-randomized Experiments

Michail Katsoulis, Nandita Mitra and A. Floriaan Schmidt

Abstract

Traditionally, machine learning and artificial intelligence focus on problems of diagnosis or prognosis. Answering questions on whether a patient might have a certain disease (diagnosis) or is at risk of future disease (prognosis). In addition to these problems, one might be interested in identifying causal factors which can provide information on how to *change* disease onset or disease progression. In this chapter we introduce the potential outcomes framework, which provides a structured way of conceptualizing questions on causality. Using this framework we discuss how randomized and non-randomized experiments can be conducted, and analyzed, to obtain estimates of the likely causal effect an exposure may have on an outcome.

Keywords

Potential outcomes framework · Non-randomized study · Randomized controlled trials · G-formula · Inverse probability weighting

1 Causal Effects and Potential Outcomes

Researchers often conclude that a factor X is *associated* (or *correlated*) with an outcome Y. However, it may be of interest to be able to conclude that factor X *causes* outcome Y. Causal inference methods aim to answer questions such as: Do Covid masking restrictions reduce coronavirus rates? Does chemotherapy plus radiotherapy increase survival in women with endometrial cancer? Does physical therapy prevent back pain after surgery? Commonly used analytic designs and approaches may only allow one to conclude that these interventions are merely associated with the outcomes. For example, say a study concludes that prostatectomy (surgery to remove the prostate) is *associated* with increased survival among men over the age of 65 with stage III prostate cancer. One interpretation would be that elderly men who received a prostatectomy tended

M. Katsoulis
MRC Unit for Lifelong Health and Ageing, University College London,London, UK

N. Mitra
Division of Biostatistics, University of Pennsylvania, Philadelphia, USA

A. F. Schmidt (✉)
Department of Cardiology; Amsterdam University Medical Centres, Amsterdam, The Netherlands
e-mail: a.f.schmidt@amsterdamumc.nl

Institute of Cardiovascular Science; University College London, London, UK

Division of Heart and Lungs, University Medical Center Utrecht, Utrecht, Netherlands

F. W. Asselbergs et al. (eds.), *Clinical Applications of Artificial Intelligence in Real-World Data*,
https://doi.org/10.1007/978-3-031-36678-9_7

to have longer survival compared to elderly men who did not receive a prostatectomy. On the other hand, say a study concludes that tacrolimus (a skin ointment) *causes* a reduction in skin inflammation in patients with atopic dermatitis. A possible interpretation here would be that tacrolimus, if hypothetically applied to the entire patient population, results in a lower overall skin inflammation rate in this patient population as compared to the hypothetical setting in which no tacrolimus was administered. In the former example, we are making a comparison of outcomes on the basis of treatment actually received. In the latter example, we are making a comparison of two hypothetical scenarios, i.e., the entire population either taking or not taking the treatment. The latter example is what is called a *causal effect* and is the focus of the field of causal inference [1, 2].

Of note, whether association or causation is of importance is fully dependent on the research question at hand. For instance, in cardiovascular research, there is an interest in investigating gender differences in the occurrence of cardiovascular disease. This may have a partial causal explanation or may reflect historical and societal disparities in cardiovascular care between genders. Regardless, having knowledge on the association of gender and disease outcomes can help with clinical aspects of preventive care, diagnosis, and prognosis irrespective of causality. Many researchers feel that causal claims can only be made when the exposure of interest can be *intervened* upon (e.g. dosage of a medication) rather than inherent characteristics such as race or gender. For example, there is an ongoing discussion on whether one can consider race to be a cause since it is not manipulable [3].

Formal causal theory and methods are needed in order to obtain a causal interpretation. Let's first consider a simple linear regression model:

$$Y = \beta_0 + \beta_1 X + \varepsilon;\ \varepsilon \overset{iid}{\sim} N(0, \sigma^2)$$

In this model, we often interpret β_1 by saying "a one unit increase in X is expected to lead to an increase in Y of β_1 units". In reality, we simply observe some people with $X = x$ and other people with $X = x'$. Often we do not observe a change from x to x' in any single person. This then leads to the problem of how to infer causality. In order to define causal effects of interest there are two important components we must specify: (1) a model for the observed data and (2) causal assumptions (which we define in the next section). Causal assumptions are the link between our observed data and causal effects of interest; however, they are often not verifiable.

Here, we introduce the potential outcomes (counterfactual) framework first described by Rubin [4, 5] in order to aid in defining causal effects. We start with common notation. First, let A denote intervention. This can be defined as anything from a medical treatment, policy intervention, or exposure. Note that capital A is a random variable and lowercase a refers to a particular realization of the random variable A. For example, we can say $A = 1$ if a flu vaccine is received and $A = 0$ otherwise. A_i refers to the treatment status of subject i. Next, we let Y denote an outcome of interest which could be continuous (e.g. cholesterol levels), discrete (e.g. cancer remission or not), time to event (e.g. survival), or multidimensional (e.g. longitudinal measures of a biomarker). For example, we can say $Y = 1$ if you experience a recurrence of breast cancer within 5 years and $Y = 0$ otherwise.

We can think of potential outcomes as the outcomes we *would* see under each possible treatment option. For now, we consider the simplest scenario where treatments take place at one point in time; later in the chapter we address treatments over time. Here, Y^a is the outcome that would be observed if treatment was set to $A = a$. Each person has potential outcomes $\{Y^a; a \in \mathcal{A}\}$. For instance when the treatment is binary, Y^0 is the outcome if treated and Y^1 is the outcome if not treated.

Let's look at an example where the outcome is time to event. If treatment is influenza vaccine and the outcome is the time until the individual gets the flu, we would use the following notation:

Y^1: time until the individual would get the flu if they received the flu vaccine,

Y^0: time until the individual would get the flu if they did not receive the flu vaccine.

A second example, where the outcome is binary, is as follows. If treatment is local (A = 1) versus general (A = 0) anesthesia for hip fracture surgery and the outcome (Y) is major pulmonary complications we would use the notation:

Y^1: equal to 1 if major pulmonary complications and equal to 0 otherwise, if given local anesthesia,
Y^0: equal to 1 if major pulmonary complications and equal to 0 otherwise, if given general anesthesia.

Now, the *observed* outcome Y is the outcome under the treatment that a subject actually receives; that is, $Y = Y^A$. In most studies, where participants receive either an intervention treatment or a comparator treatment, for a single subject one can only observe Y^1 or Y^0, and the outcome under the complimentary treatment can be thought of as missing. Counterfactual outcomes are ones that would have been observed had the treatment been different. If a person's treatment was $A = 1$, then their counterfactual outcome is Y^0. If that person's treatment was $A = 0$, then their counterfactual outcome is Y^1.

Let's look at the influenza example again to understand counterfactual outcomes. The causal question we ask is "Did influenza vaccine prevent me from getting the flu?". What actually happened:

1. I got the vaccine and did not get sick.
2. My actual exposure was $A = 1$.
3. My observed outcome was $Y = Y^1$.

What would have happened (contrary to fact) had I not gotten the vaccine? Would I have gotten sick?

1. My counterfactual exposure is $A = 0$.
2. My counterfactual outcome is Y^0.

Before the treatment decision is made, any outcome is a potential outcome: Y^0 and Y^1. After the study, there is an observed outcome, $Y = Y^A$, and counterfactual outcomes Y^{1-A}. Counterfactual outcomes Y^0, Y^1 are typically assumed to be the same as potential outcomes Y^0, Y^1. Thus, these terms are often used interchangeably.

Note that so far we have implicitly assumed that the treatment given to one subject does not affect the outcome for another subject, i.e., $Y_i^{a_i,a_j} = Y_i^{a_i,a_j'}$. In other words, they are independent. If this assumption holds, we can simply write the potential outcome for subject i as only dependent on a_i (one index). However, in many situations, this assumption could be violated such as in the setting of infectious disease. For instance, vaccinating one person in a household might reduce risk of disease among others in the household. This is known as interference.

Now that we have defined potential outcomes, we can formally define causal effects. In general, we say that A has a causal effect on Y if Y^1 differs from Y^0. For example, let's say A is whether or not you take a cold medication (A = 1 you take it, A = 0 you don't) and Y is that your sore throat goes away after an hour (Y = 1 it goes away, Y = 0 it doesn't). Clearly, the statement "I took the cold medicine and my sore throat is gone, therefore the medicine worked" is not proper causal reasoning. This claim is equivalent to $Y^1 = 1$. But what would have happened had you not taken the medicine ($Y^0 =$)? There is only a causal effect if $Y^1 \neq Y^0$. This bring us to the "fundamental problem of causal inference" which stems from the issue that we can only observe one potential outcome for each person. However, with certain assumptions, we can estimate population level (average) causal effect which we will focus on next. In other words, it is possible to answer: What would the rate of sore throat cure be if everyone took the cold medicine versus if no one did? However, without very strong assumptions, we cannot identify individual causal effects that would allow us to answer: What would have happened to me if I had not taken the cold medicine?

Let's first consider individual causal effects. Consider a simple case of binary treatment ($A = 1$ if treated) and a binary outcome ($Y = 1$ if died). There are four types of individual causal effects [6].

Causal type	Y^0	Y^1	$\delta = Y^1 - Y^0$
Treatment fatal	0	1	1
Always live	0	0	0
Always die	1	1	0
Treatment curative	1	0	−1

Now, let's suppose we have a randomized study (A is randomized) with n participants and there is perfect compliance (all of the study participants adhere to the treatment they are randomized to). In this study, we never observe Y^0 *and* Y^1 for any individual. Instead, we have a random sample of Y^1's and a random sample of Y^0's. We cannot identify δ for any individual. However, we can identify the marginal probabilities $\mathbb{P}(Y^1 = 1)$ and $\mathbb{P}(Y^0 = 1)$. Importantly, We can also identify $\mathbb{E}(\delta)$.

Consider an example where we know that $\mathbb{P}(Y^1 = 1) = 0.1$ and $\mathbb{P}(Y^0 = 1) = 0.2$. In this example, the treatment reduces risk on average by 0.1. We can first write out these marginal probabilities in terms of joint probabilities:

$$\mathbb{P}(Y^1 = 1) = \mathbb{P}(Y^1 = 1, Y^0 = 1) + \mathbb{P}(Y^1 = 1, Y^0 = 0),$$
$$\mathbb{P}(Y^0 = 1) = \mathbb{P}(Y^1 = 1, Y^0 = 1) + \mathbb{P}(Y^1 = 0, Y^0 = 1).$$

We can then write out three examples of the potential outcomes distributions that are consistent with the observed data as follows:

Causal type	Ex1	Ex2	Ex3
Treatment fatal	0	0.05	0.1
Always live	0.8	0.75	0.7
Always die	0.1	0.05	0
Treatment curative	0.1	0.15	0.2

So, for instance, in Ex 1:

$$\begin{aligned}\mathbb{P}(Y^1 = 1) &= \mathbb{P}(Y^1 = 1, Y^0 = 1)\\ &\quad + \mathbb{P}(Y^1 = 1, Y^0 = 0)\\ &= 0.1(\text{always die})\\ &\quad + 0(\text{treatment fatal}) = 0.1,\\ \mathbb{P}(Y^0 = 1) &= \mathbb{P}(Y^1 = 1, Y^0 = 1)\\ &\quad + \mathbb{P}(Y^1 = 0, Y^0 = 1)\\ &= 0.1(\text{always die})\\ &\quad + 0.10\,(\text{treatment is curative}) = 0.2.\end{aligned}$$

The average causal effect (ACE) is one of the most common causal targets of inference used to compare treatments/exposures. The ACE is given by $\mathbb{E}(Y^1 - Y^0)$. This is the average outcome if everyone had been treated versus if no one had been treated; Fig. 1. Importantly, this is typically not equal to $\mathbb{E}(Y|A = 1) - \mathbb{E}(Y|A = 0)$ which is the average outcome in those who were treated versus the average outcome in those who were not treated; Fig. 2. Specifically, in non-randomized studies, patients who receive a treatment (say surgery) may be very different than those who do not. For instance, those who are deemed fit to withstand surgery may be younger, more healthy, and are less likely to smoke than those who are chosen not to receive surgery.

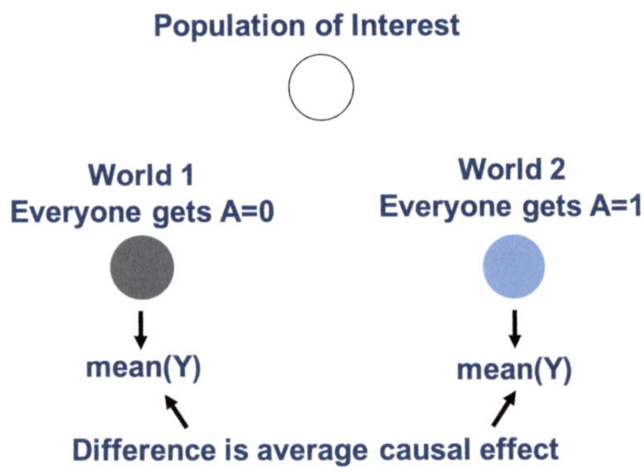

Fig. 1 The average causal effect

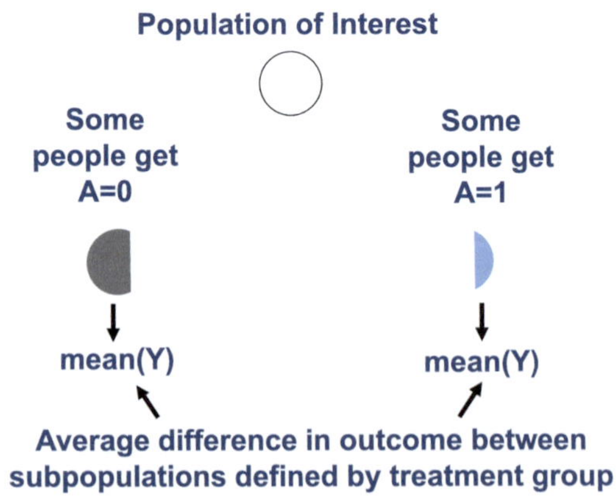

Fig. 2 Effect of a treatment in the real world

In addition to the ACE, $\mathbb{E}(Y^1 - Y^0)$, other causal estimands of interest may include the causal risk ratio, $\mathbb{E}(Y^1)/\mathbb{E}(Y^0)$, the average causal effect among a subgroup defined by V, $\mathbb{E}(Y^1 - Y^0|V = v)$, and the average treatment effect among the treated (ATT) given by $\mathbb{E}(Y^1 - Y^0|A = 1)$ [2]. The ATT, for instance, is a useful estimand when there is interest in the effect of an intervention (say, a treatment of hypertension) on those who received the intervention.

2 Necessary Conditions for Causality

2.1 Randomized Studies with Perfect Compliance

In Sect. 1, we formulated causal effects in terms of potential outcomes. Since potential outcomes are not fully observed we need to make some assumptions in order to be able to estimate (or identify) causal estimands of interest from the observed data. These are called identifying assumptions. Let's first consider a randomized study where there is perfect compliance. In other words, if R is the randomization indicator and A is an indicator of the treatment that is actually taken, then if there is perfect compliance in the trial, $R = A$. We will again consider the potential outcomes Y^0 and Y^1. In randomized trial with full compliance, clearly R is independent of the potential outcomes Y^0 and Y^1. We can express this independence in two different ways using the concepts of *ignorability* and *exchangeability* [6].

Ignorability is stated as $\mathbb{P}(R = 1|Y^0, Y^1) = \mathbb{P}(R = 1)$. In other words, treatment assignment does not depend on the potential outcomes. Say treatment assignment depends on the flip of a coin. Clearly the flip of the coin does not depend on the potential outcomes. Now, if everyone has some non-zero chance of being randomized to the treatment arm, we achieve *strong ignorability*. This assumption that $0 < \mathbb{P}(R = 1) < 1$ is called *positivity* and in this case refers to the fact that we have experimental treatment assignment. Another way to express independence is the concept of *exchangeability*. We can state exchangeability as $f(Y^0, Y^1|R = 1) = f(Y^0, Y^1|R = 0) = f(Y^0, Y^1)$ (where f is the distribution of the potential outcomes). In other words, subjects randomized to $R = 1$ or $R = 0$ are representative of all subjects with respect to the potential outcomes. They are exchangeable.

Exchangeability implies that $f(Y^1) = f(Y^1|R = 1) = f(Y|R = 1)$ and $f(Y^0) = f(Y^0|R = 0) = f(Y|R = 0)$. What we mean by this is that in a randomized trial with perfect compliance, the observed data (the observed outcome Y and the randomization indicator R) are enough to identify the distributions of the potential outcomes, allowing us to estimate causal effects.

Often exchangeability is denoted simply as $Y^a \amalg A$, which can be generalized to include conditional exchangeability $Y^a \amalg A|L$, for covariate L.

2.2 Observational Studies

Randomization allows us to assume, on average, that subjects in different treatment arms are similar to each other on all important factors, whether those factors are measured or not; see Sect. 3. In observational studies, the treatment, intervention or exposure is not controlled by the investigator and by definition is not randomized; although quasi-experiments may naturally occur [7]. Hence, subjects in the treatment group may look very different from those in the comparison group. For instance, men receiving surgery for prostrate cancer may be younger, more likely to be a nonsmoker, and have fewer comorbidities than men who do not receive surgery. The decision, made between the patient and physician, may be based in part by how well the patient is expected to tolerate the surgery. Without accounting for these differences in patient characteristics, the surgery group's survival after surgery may look better than the control group's merely because they were healthier to begin with. As mentioned before, factors that affect both the treatment decision and the outcome are called *confounders*.

Confounding is an important issue that must be addressed in the causal analysis of observational studies. Note that there may also be confounding in randomized trials where there is noncompliance (i.e., $R \neq A$) due to the fact that patients who do not comply with their treatment assignment maybe be different than those who stay on their assigned treatment and those factors may be related to their outcome. This is why RCTs typically do not directly assess treatment effects, but instead estimate the "Intention to Treat" effect; see Sect. 3. If confounders are measured, without meaningful error, we can use standard adjustment methods to control for confounding such as stratification on the confounder, regression adjustment or propensity score methods. Let L be a set of baseline (pre-treatment) covariates. Ignorability in this context means that there is no unmeasured confounding. In other words, if we condition on L, we can control for confounding (there's no hidden bias). If there is no unmeasured confounding, then if we, say, stratify on these covariates, within those strata, we would essentially have a randomized trial. Hence, ignorability can be thought of as conditional randomization where A is independent of the potential outcomes (Y^0, Y^1) given L.

Let's consider an example where treatment assignment depends on the potential outcomes where sicker patients are more likely to be treated. Hence, treated patients have a higher risk of a bad outcome. We need to account for these pre-treatment differences in health. Suppose L are measures of health such as family history of disease, age, weight, smoking status, alcohol, comorbidities, etc. Then within levels of L (i.e., people of the same age, with same co-morbid conditions, of same weight, with same smoking status, etc.), we hope that less healthy patients are not more likely to get treatment. This is the ignorability assumption.

The ignorability setting is comprised of the following three causal assumptions:

- (Condtional) *exchangeability*: treatment is as if randomized conditional on covariates (e.g. within covariate strata).
- *Positivity*: treatment is not assigned in a deterministic fashion (all subjects have a non-zero probability of being assigned to treatment regardless of their covariates). This can be violated when certain treatments are simply unavailable. For example, depending on the urgency, general anesthesia may be the only option available for women undergoing Cesarean section.
- *Consistency*: the potential outcomes are uniquely defined by each subject's own treatment level. This can be violated in situations such as a vaccine trial where one subject's vaccination status can affect another subject's potential outcomes. Other examples include *poorly* defined exposures such changes in BMI which may be occur due to causes such as diet, physical activity or disease.

These identifying assumptions allow us to estimate causal effects directly from the observed data Y, A, L.

3 Randomized Controlled Trials and Estimands of Treatment Effect

In the preceding sections we established a formal definition of causality, and discussed the necessary conditions to interpret a measure of association as an *estimate* of a causal effect.

Historically, discussions on causality have focused on choices in study design, or experiments, where randomized controlled trials (RCTs) remain the unequivocal paradigm. The developed mathematical framework allows for a more detailed discussion of why RCTs provide such a robust design to assess causality. Developing the necessary algebra to describe trial inference is important because it allows us to consider what additional step (analytical or design wise) are required to explore causality in non-randomized (i.e., observational) study designs. Before discussing these analytical methods, we will therefore first further introduce RCTs and touch upon some of the different estimands used in practice (i.e., the type of effect one attempts to estimate).

3.1 Why Association Does Not Imply Causation

Some key features of RCTs include (1) the presence of contemporary intervention and control groups, (2) random allocation of subjects to these groups, and (3) blinding of participants (and often the treating medical professionals) to the group allocations.

If we strip away these three features we are left with a single arm study of subjects who received an intervention. For example the left-panel in Fig. 3 illustrates the results of a hypothetical study assessing the concentration of low-density lipoprotein cholsterol (LDL-C) before ($T = 1$) and after ($T = 1$) subjects were offered treatment with PCSK9 monoclonal antibodies (mAb, a lipid lowering drug [8]). A single arm study would exclusively consider the treated group ($A = 1$). In contrast a "parallel group" design would also consider measurements in participants who did not (decide to) receive treatment ($A = 0$).

An obvious aim would be to attempt to quantify by how much *taking* PCSK9 mAb decreases LDL-C concentrations compared to *not taking* PCSK9 mAb over the same period of time. A relevant estimand would be the *average causal effect*: $\mathbb{E}(Y^0 - Y^1) = \alpha$.

A naive estimate of the treatment lowering effect of PCSK9 mAb would be to use the single arm study and simply take the difference in post- and pre-treatment LDL-C concentrations: $\mathbb{E}(Y|A = 1, T = 1) - \mathbb{E}(Y|A = 1, T = 0)$. Given that this is a hypothetical example we can also look at the otherwise unknown counterfactual pre- and post-treatment LDL-C concentrations, to clearly see that $\mathbb{E}(Y|A = 1, T = 1) - \mathbb{E}(Y|A = 1, T = 0) \neq \mathbb{E}(Y^0 - Y^1)$. Here we reiterate that by the exchangability assumption $\mathbb{E}(Y^0 - Y^1) = \mathbb{E}(Y^{1,t=1} - Y^{1,t=0})$, meaning that under exchangbility T is ignorable.

As is clear from Fig. 3 the difference in pre- and post-treatment LDL-C concentrations (in treated subjects) does not match the counterfactual difference. In practice this can be caused by a myriad of reasons, often closely linked to the study design and participant sample. In general, one would expect post-treatment concentrations to decrease whenever treatment initiation is (partially) based on a biomarker measurement being elevated (e.g., hypercholesterolemia). Measurements are always subject to (small) random fluctuations, as such the high value necessary to initiate treatment most likely reflects a degree of random upwards variation, which is unlikely to be of the same magnitude in subsequent measurements, hence resulting in a decrease. This well known phenomenon is often referred to as "regression to the mean" [13]. Furthermore, depending on the diagnosis it is not uncommon for a clinician to initiate multiple interventions at the same time. In our example, typically a prescription of lipid lowering therapy would coincide with (referral for) life-style counseling. Similarly, the simple act of prescribing a drug, will incentivse some patients to self-initiate life-style changes (e.g., start exercising more) which will (on average) decrease LDL-C independent of any effect of PCSK9 mAb.

Clearly a single arm study, comparing pre- and post-treatment LDL-C concentrations, will unlikely provide a good estimate of the causal effect of PCSK9 mAb lowering. Instead we could consider conducting a *cohort* study of contemporary participants initiating PCSK9 mAb (the treatment group), compared to a control group of participants who do not receive any treatment; Fig. 3. Assuming for the moment that the control group participants were "blinded" from the fact they did not receive any treatment, the difference in LDL-C concentration of the control group participants is identical to that of the counterfactual (i.e, comparing measurements at $T = 0$ to $T = 1$). However, because treatment was not initiated at random, we see that the control group measurements are substantially lower than that of the counterfactual; simply reflecting that medical professionals treat patients at risk. As such, despite having a control group, the difference between the treatment and control group will not equal our inferential target.

3.2 Treatment Estimands in Trials

While by itself inclusion of a control group does not typically result in a causal effect estimate of our inferential target $\mathbb{E}(Y^0 - Y^1) = \alpha$, it

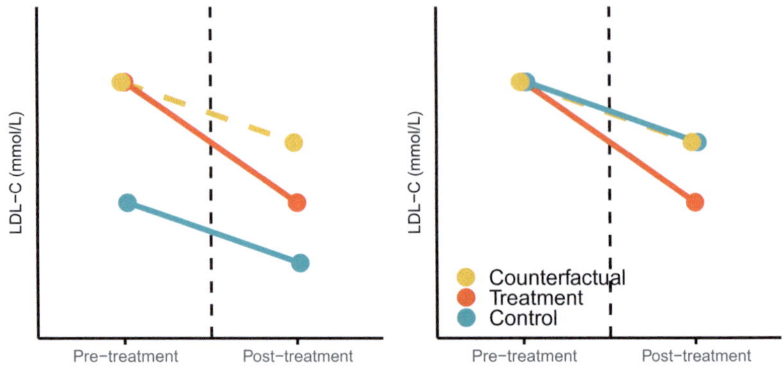

Fig. 3 Causal contrasts in a study evaluating changes in LDL-C concentration. The left-panel represents a possible *non-randomized* study, and the right-panel a possible scenario for a *randomized* study. Notice that the x-axis values are slightly dodged to help identify overlapping points and lines

does provide a suggestion how we could further improve our study – we could randomize treatment assignment! The right-panel of Fig. 3 illustrates this, showing agreement between the control group measurements and the counterfactual LDL-C measurements. In this setting we will have that $\mathbb{E}(Y|A=1, T=1) - \mathbb{E}(Y|A=0, T=1) = \mathbb{E}(Y^0 - Y^1)$, implying that stringently designed RCTs provide relevant causal estimates.

If we simply focus on time $T = 1$ the above estimator $\mathbb{E}(Y|A=1) - \mathbb{E}(Y|A=0)$ is often referred to as the "as-treated" (AT) estimator. Interestingly, and contrary to the above derivations, the AT estimator is considered to be a biased estimator. To see why, we will move a way from the hypothetical trial with perfect compliance (see Sect. 2.1), and expand our example to differentiate between treatment allocation Z, and the actual treatment taken A. To illustrate the difference, note that adherence is defined as

$$\mathbb{P}(A=1|Z=1) - \mathbb{P}(A=1|Z=0) = \phi$$

where values close to 1 indicate subjects generally took the allocated treatment, and smaller values indicate non-adherence to treatment allocation.

In the previous subsection we thus made the implicit and unrealistic, assumption of complete adherence. Worse, as shown in Fig. 4, in the presence of non-adherence the association between A and Y will be subject to confounding by common cause(s) L, violating the exchangeability assumption: $Y^a \not\perp\!\!\!\perp A$. Hence, in the presence of non-adherence, the AT-estimator will never equal the true causal treatment effect unless we are willing to assume there are no L at all. We could of course decide to condition on L and create a conditional AT-estimator, however knowledge of L is typically incomplete and above all it would be difficult to determine when such conditioning sufficiently addressed confounding - defeating the purpose of a trial: balancing on known *as well as* unknown confounders.

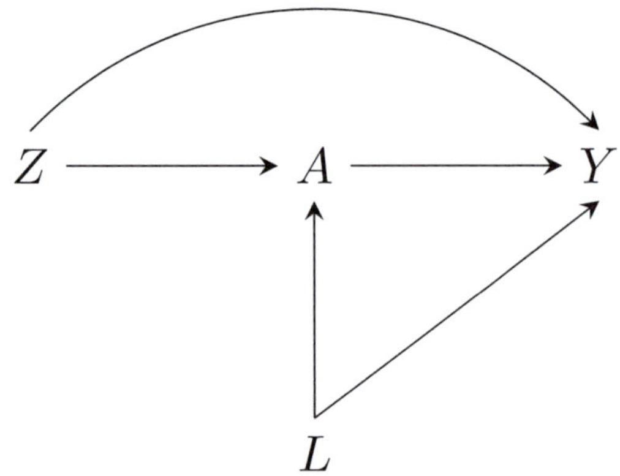

Fig. 4 A directed acyclic graph representation of a randomized control trial. Here Z represent treatment allocation, X treatment itself, Y the primary outcome, L measured and unmeasured common causes of X and Y. The directed paths (i.e., arrows) represents a cause and effect relation of unspecified magnitude which may also include zero (i.e., when there is no path)

Due to the frailty of associating A with Y, trials commonly forgo this estimand entirely and perform an "intention to treat" (ITT) analysis, with estimator

$$\mathbb{E}(Y|Z=1) - \mathbb{E}(Y|Z=0) = \alpha\phi + \tau.$$

Here α is the effect treatment allocation has on the outcome mediated through A. Additionally τ represents the possibility that treatment allocation may affect the outcome indirectly, sidestepping A. For example, subjects allocated to the untreated group may decide to exercise more. Inclusion of $\tau \neq 0$ is of course problematic because the ITT estimator no longer solely evaluates effects mediated through A, and a trial may incorrectly suggest treatment is beneficial.

By defining the ITT estimator as the sum of the true causal treatment effect (α) multiplied by adherence (ϕ) and the direct effect (τ) of treatment allocation, we can finally comment on the relevance of blinding in trial design. Blinding trial participant and staff, to knowledge of the allocated treatment ensures that, on average, enrolled subjects behave the same-way irrespective of Z, and thus that we can assume $\tau = 0$. The results of this is that $\mathbb{E}(Y|Z=1) - \mathbb{E}(Y|Z=0) \neq 0$ implies that $\alpha \neq 0$, irrespective of treatment adherence. In many ways randomization and blinding are complementary strategies to ensure participant groups are (on average) similar at baseline (*randomization*) and behave similar during follow-up (*blinding*).

Assuming blinding and randomization were conducted adequately the ITT estimator thus equals α only if participants completely adhered to treatment allocations. In all other settings the ITT estimator is a biased estimator of the causal treatment effect and will not equal α. The ITT estimator is thus a flawed *estimator*. Nevertheless, it does have desirable properties, 1) when sufficiently blinded the ITT estimator will (on average) be zero whenever $\alpha = 0$, and therefore 2) it often provides a robust indicator of effect direction (i.e., whether treatment is beneficial or not).

While the ITT estimator does not in general provide an estimate of our inferential target α, we can however use it to perform an instrumental variable (IV) analysis, which assuming $\tau = 0$, will on average equal our inferential target:

$$\frac{\mathbb{E}(Y|Z=1) - \mathbb{E}(Y|Z=0)}{\mathbb{P}(X=1|Z=1) - \mathbb{P}(X=1|Z=0)} = \frac{\alpha\phi}{\phi}, \\ = \alpha.$$

This IV estimator essentially corrects the ITT estimate for the amount of non-adherence, and in doing so obtains an estimate of $\alpha = \mathbb{E}(Y^1 - Y^0)$. Of course all this is under the assumption the trial has been appropriately randomized and blinded, which we can elegantly frame as ignorabililty. It is important to reiterate that the ignorabililty assumption refers to the randomized groups and as such all the previously discussed estimands will not generally hold for individuals, and do not represent *individual* causal effects unless there are convincing reasons to expect an absence of between-patient treatment heterogeneity [9]. Note Schmidt et al. 2018 [10] discusses IV analysis in the a setting of a meta-analysis of potentially unblinded trials, where $\tau \neq 0$.

4 Non-randomized Experiments of Time-Fixed Exposure and Confounders

As discussed RCTs are the gold standard to explore causal were design steps such as randomization and blinding are essential to ensure the three critical assumptions (exchangeability, positivity and consistency) are likely true. In many cases one may not be able to perform a RCT, for example an RCT may be prohibitively costly, or patients may be difficult to recruit. Moreover, randomisation may not always be ethical, for example when the comparator intervention can cause harm (e.g., shame surgeries). Because of these reasons only a small proportion (15–20%) clinical practice guidelines are based on an 'A' level of evidence (based on multiple RCTs), and most rely on evidence from non-randomized (observational) studies [11, 12]. It is therefore essential to be able to identify, and conduct, high quality analyses using non-randomised study designs.

Non-randomised studies, in contrast to RCTs, may be much less convincing to assess causal inferences for treatments/interventions. As an example, take an observational study from electronic health records where a researchers is interested in evaluating the effect statin prescription may elicit on the incidence of cardiovascular disease. Those who initiated statins are more likely to be in a worse health state compared to those who did not initiate statins. In other words, it is very likely that we have problems due to confounding by indication. If we have sufficiently detailed information from for example EHR capturing all the confounding variables, then there are many options to account for such confounding bias; otherwise, our analysis will suffer from unmeasured confounding. In the next paragraphs, we will explain in detail how to deal with non-randomised experiments of time-invariant exposures.

Let's focus on the following example: in the Table below, we have 12 patients with measured data on statin initiation X (0 = untreated, 1 = treated) and whether they developed cancer after 10 years, i.e. cancer incidence Y (0 = no cancer, 1 = cancer). The question of interest is: What is the effect of statin initiation on cancer incidence?

Participant	Other comorbidities L	Statin X	Cancer Y
Isabella	0	0	0
Oliver	0	0	1
Rachel	0	0	0
George	0	0	1
Rebecca	0	1	0
Oscar	0	1	1
Natalie	1	0	1
Tom	1	0	0
Margaret	1	0	0
Charles	1	1	1
Olivia	1	1	0
Harry	1	1	0

From these data, we observe that statin initiation (X) is associated with cancer incidence (Y): the probability of developing cancer among those who initiated statin therapy is $\mathbb{P}(Y = 1|X = 1) = 2/5 = 0.40$, while the probability of developing cancer among those who did not initiated statin therapy is $\mathbb{P}(Y = 1|X = 0) = 3/7 = 0.43$. The observed risk difference, is $\mathbb{P}(Y = 1|X = 1) - \mathbb{P}(Y = 1|X = 0) = -1/35$. At face value the observed difference in cancer incidence between statin initiators might be taken to imply statin prescription is carcinogenic. Depending on the plausibility of the in sect. 2.2 assumptions, the observed difference may be distinct from our inferential target estimand $\mathbb{P}(Y^{X=1} = 1) - \mathbb{P}(Y^{X=0} = 1)$

Let's assume that, in an over-simplistic scenario, the two groups have the same characteristics (age, sex socioeconomic status, family history of cancer etc.), apart from other comorbidities L. In other words, if we account for other comorbidities appropriately in this sample, we will emulate randomisation successfully.

Under the consistency, (conditional) exchangeability, and positivity assumptions (see sect. 2.2), we can estimate $\mathbb{P}(Y^{X=1} = 1) - \mathbb{P}(Y^{X=0} = 1)$ accounting for L, using standard regression modelling, standardisation or inverse probability of weighting.

4.1 Analytical Methods to Estimate the Effect of Time-Fixed Exposures

4.1.1 Regression Modelling

Standard regression modelling, in which we include all the (*likely*) confounders as covariates is a popular way of dealing with time-fixed confounders. In the example presented above, we could choose to create a logistic regression model, given that the outcome is binary. In that case, the estimand of interest would be the causal odds ratio, i.e.

$$\text{causal odds ratio} = \frac{\dfrac{\mathbb{P}(Y^{X=1} = 1)}{\mathbb{P}(Y^{X=1} = 0)}}{\dfrac{\mathbb{P}(Y^{X=0} = 1)}{\mathbb{P}(Y^{X=0} = 0)}}$$

which will be equal to the observed (conditional) odds ratio

$$\text{observed odds ratio} = \frac{\frac{\mathbb{P}(Y=1|X=1,L=l)}{\mathbb{P}(Y=0|X=1,L=l)}}{\frac{\mathbb{P}(Y=1|X=0,L=l)}{\mathbb{P}(Y=0|X=0,L=l)}}$$

under the assumptions described in sect. 2.2. Moreover, the observed odds ratio for X can be easily calculated from a logistic regression where the outcome is Y and we adjust for L, i.e.

$$\text{logit}(\mathbb{P}(Y=1|X,L)) = a_0 + a_1 X + a_2 L$$

In the example of Fig. 5, the odds ratio OR=e^{a_1} is equal to 1, which means that

$$\mathbb{P}\left(Y^{X=1}=1\right) = \mathbb{P}\left(Y^{X=0}=1\right).$$

4.1.2 Standardisation—G-Formula

The G-formula provide an alternative approach to account for possible confounding. Here we wish to obtain an unbiased estimate of the outcome risk under different interventions X leveraging the fact that conditional on L, the counterfactial outcome is independent of X, e.g. the conditional exchangeability assumption holds: $Y^x \amalg X|L$. Specifically, the observed conditional risk under treatment is equal to the counterfactual risks:

$$\mathbb{P}(Y=1|X=x,L=l) = \mathbb{P}\left(Y^{X=x}=1|L=l\right)$$

To calculate the $\mathbb{P}\left(Y^{X=x}=1\right)$, we will use the formula

$$\mathbb{P}\left(Y^{X=x}=1\right) = \sum_l \mathbb{P}(Y=1|X=x,L=l) \times \mathbb{P}(L=l), l \in \{0,1\}$$

In other words,

$$\mathbb{P}\left(Y^{X=1}=1\right) = \mathbb{P}(Y=1|X=1,L=0) \times \mathbb{P}(L=0) + \mathbb{P}(Y=1|X=1,L=1) \times \mathbb{P}(L=1)$$

and

$$\mathbb{P}\left(Y^{X=0}=1\right) = \mathbb{P}(Y=1|X=0,L=0) \times \mathbb{P}(L=0) + \mathbb{P}(Y=1|X=0,L=1) \times \mathbb{P}(L=1)$$

Risk had all individuals received treatment: $\mathbb{P}\left(Y^{X=1}=1\right)$

We know that the risk if all individuals had been treated is 1/2 in the 6 individuals with $L=0$ and 1/3 in the 6 individuals with $L=1$. Therefore, the risk if all individuals in the population had been treated will be a weighted average of 1/2 and 1/3 in which each group receives a weight proportional to its size. Since 50% of the individuals are in group $L=0$ and 50% of the individuals in $L=1$ The weighted average will be (1/2 × 0.5) + (1/3 × 0.5) = 0.42.

Risk had no individuals received treatment: $\mathbb{P}\left(Y^{X=0}=1\right)$

We know that the risk if all individuals had not been treated is 2/4 in the 6 individuals with $L=0$ and 1/3 in the 6 individuals with $L=1$. Therefore, the risk if all individuals in the population had not been treated will be a weighted average of 1/2 and 1/3 in which each group receives a weight proportional to its size. Since 50% of the individuals are in group $L=0$ and 50% of the individuals in $L=1$. The weighted average will be (2/4 × 0.5) + (1/3 × 0.5) = 0.42.

4.1.3 Inverse Probability Weighting

Inverse probability weighting (IPW) is a further alternative method to account for confounding, here one creates a pseudo-population in which treatment is independent of the covariates L. Treated and the untreated are (unconditionally) exchangeable in the pseudo-population because the X is independent of L. In other words, the arrow from the covariates L to the treatment X is removed (see Fig. 5).

Using IPW, we weight each individual by the inverse of the probability of receiving the treatment (exposure), conditional on the confounders.

$$\text{IPW} = \frac{1}{\mathbb{P}(X|L)}$$

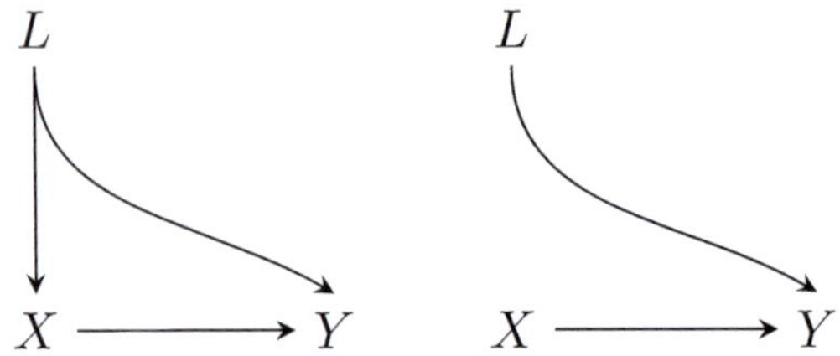

Fig. 5 Directed acyclic graphs in the population (right panel) and the pseudo-population (left panel) creates by inverse probability weights

In our example, the created pseudo-population will be twice as large as the original population (see Fig. 5 in the right). Under conditional exchangeability $Y^x \amalg X|L$ in the original population, treatment is randomized in the pseudo-population i.e. treated and the untreated are (unconditionally) exchangeable in the pseudo-population because the X is independent of L From the pseudo-population, we can calculate $\mathbb{P}(Y^{X=1} = 1)$ and $\mathbb{P}(Y^{X=0} = 1)$.

That is, the associational risk ratio in the pseudo-population is equal to the causal risk ratio in both the pseudo-population and the original population.

In the pseudo-population (see Fig. 6 we observe that a) among the untreated the expected number of cancer events are 5 in 12 individuals, i.e. $\mathbb{P}(Y^{X=0} = 1) = 5/12 = 0.42$, and b) among the treated the expected number of cancer events are 5 in 12 individuals, i.e. $\mathbb{P}(Y^{X=1} = 1) = 5/12 = 0.42$. We therefore find that there is no causal effect of treatment X on the outcome Y, i.e., $\mathbb{P}(Y^{X=0} = 1) = \mathbb{P}(Y^{X=0} = 1)$.

5 Non-randomized Experiments of Time-Dependent Exposure and Confounders

In this chapter, we will explain how to deal with non-randomised experiments of time-dependent exposures. We will first explain why standard methods (e.g., outcome regression models) fail to provide correct estimates of average causal exposure effect estimate correctly the causal effect when time-dependent confounders are affected by exposure (treatment) history.

5.1 Why Standard Methods May Fail

In Fig. 7 treatment A can change with time $t \in \{0, 1\}$, as do the confounders L. In this example, L_1 is both a confounder (between A_0 and Y) and a mediator (between A_1 and Y), in other words, we should both adjust for L_1 (because it is a confounder) and not adjust for L_1 (because it's a mediator). If we adjust for L_1, we induce bias because we block part of the effect of A_0 through L_1. However, if we do not adjust for L_1, the estimated effect will be biased through the back door pathway $A_1 \leftarrow L_1 \rightarrow Y$, which induces confounding bias.

5.2 Use of G-Methods to Overcome the Problem

Below, we will present an example we IPW is used account for time-varying confounding without removing exposure effects mediated by L_0 and L_1. IPW creates a pseudo-population in which the arrows headed to A_0 and A_1 do not exist and hence we do not need to adjust for L_0 and L_1 (Fig. 8).

For example, in the table below, if we want to estimate the causal contrast $\mathbb{E}(Y^{\bar{a}=(1,1)}) - \mathbb{E}(Y^{\bar{a}=(0,1)})$,when $\bar{a}$ is the treatment history, then we should estimate the associational risk difference in the pseudo-population $\mathbb{E}(Y|A_0 = 1, A_1 = 1) - \mathbb{E}(Y|A_0 = 0, A_1 = 1)$ created by the weights

$$\begin{aligned}\text{IPW} &= \frac{1}{\mathbb{P}(A_0|L_0) \times \mathbb{P}(A_1|L_0, A_0, L_1)} \\ &= 282.5 - 281.82 = 0.68.\end{aligned}$$

Please note, that we would not get the correct answer for the causal effect of A on Y if

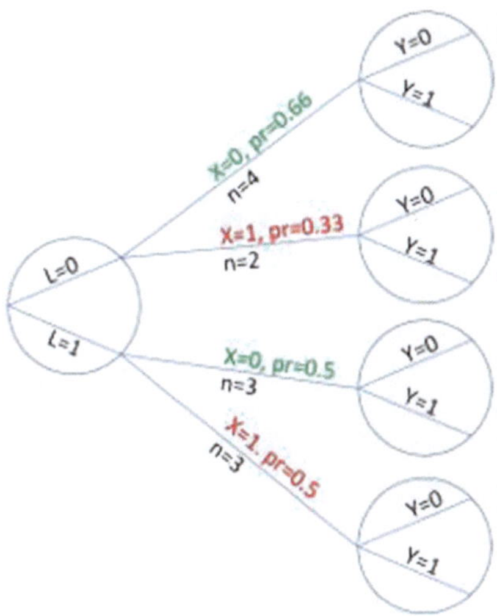

Observed people with Y=1	Pr(X/L)	$IPW = \frac{1}{pr(X/L)}$	Expected people with Y=1 in the pseudo-population
2	2/3=0.66	1/0.66=1.5	3
2	2/3=0.66	1/0.66=1.5	3
1	1/3=0.33	1/0.33=3	3
1	1/3=0.33	1/0.33=3	3
2	2/4=0.5	1/0.5=2	4
1	1/2=0.5	1/0.5=2	2
2	2/4=0.5	1/0.5=2	4
1	1/2=0.5	1/0.5=2	2

Fig. 6 Calculation of inverse probability weights (IPW)

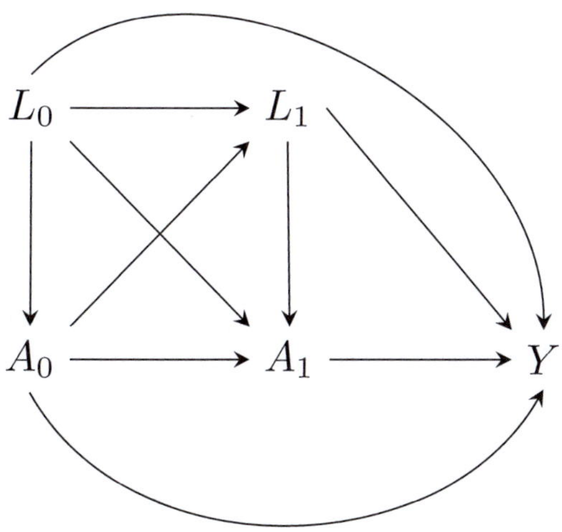

Fig. 7 A directed acyclic graph with time-dependent confounders L affected by treatment history

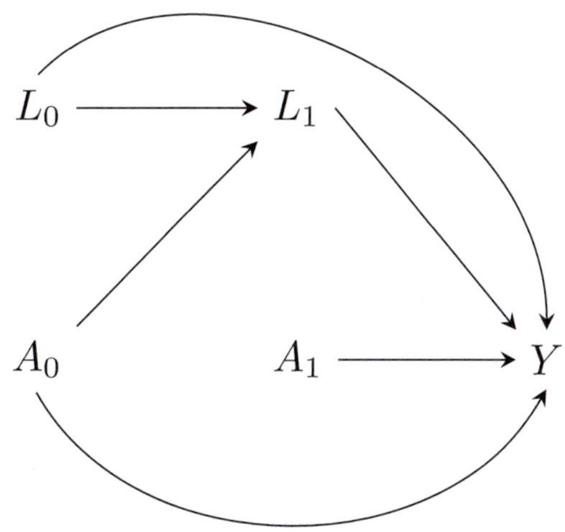

Fig. 8 A directed acyclic graph with time-dependent confounders L affected by treatment history in the pseudo-population, created by IPW

<table>
<tr><th>L_0</th><th>A_0</th><th>L_1</th><th>A_1</th><th>N</th><th>$E[Y \mid A_0, L_1, A_1]$</th><th>$P(A_0 \mid L_0)$</th><th>$P(A_1 \mid L_1, A_0, L_0)$</th><th>IPW*</th><th>$N_{ps}$</th><th>$E[Y \mid A_0, A_1]$</th><th>$E_{ps}[Y \mid A_0, A_1]$</th></tr>
<tr><td>0</td><td>0</td><td>0</td><td>0</td><td>3000</td><td>200</td><td>2/3</td><td>3/4</td><td>12/6=2</td><td>6000</td><td colspan="2">When A_0=0, A_1=0</td></tr>
<tr><td>0</td><td>0</td><td>0</td><td>1</td><td>1000</td><td>250</td><td>2/3</td><td>1/4</td><td>12/2=6</td><td>6000</td><td>221.67</td><td>227.27</td></tr>
<tr><td>0</td><td>0</td><td>1</td><td>0</td><td>1000</td><td>150</td><td>2/3</td><td>1/4</td><td>12/2=6</td><td>6000</td><td colspan="2">When A_0=1, A_1=0</td></tr>
<tr><td>0</td><td>0</td><td>1</td><td>1</td><td>3000</td><td>300</td><td>2/3</td><td>3/4</td><td>12/6=2</td><td>6000</td><td>243</td><td>247.5</td></tr>
<tr><td>0</td><td>1</td><td>0</td><td>0</td><td>1000</td><td>180</td><td>1/3</td><td>2/3</td><td>9/2</td><td>4500</td><td colspan="2">When A_0=0, A_1=1</td></tr>
<tr><td>0</td><td>1</td><td>0</td><td>1</td><td>500</td><td>280</td><td>1/3</td><td>1/3</td><td>9</td><td>4500</td><td>288.57</td><td>281.82</td></tr>
<tr><td>0</td><td>1</td><td>1</td><td>0</td><td>1250</td><td>220</td><td>1/3</td><td>1/2</td><td>6</td><td>7500</td><td colspan="2">When A_0=1, A_1=1</td></tr>
<tr><td>0</td><td>1</td><td>1</td><td>1</td><td>1250</td><td>240</td><td>1/3</td><td>1/2</td><td>6</td><td>7500</td><td>297</td><td>282.5</td></tr>
<tr><td>1</td><td>0</td><td>0</td><td>0</td><td>1000</td><td>260</td><td>1/2</td><td>2/5</td><td>5</td><td>5000</td><td colspan="2" rowspan="8">In general
$E[Y^{A_0=a_0,A_1=a_1}] = E_{ps}[Y \mid A_0, A_1]$

And

$E_{ps}[Y \mid A_0, A_1] \neq E[Y \mid A_0, A_1]$</td></tr>
<tr><td>1</td><td>0</td><td>0</td><td>1</td><td>1500</td><td>300</td><td>1/2</td><td>3/5</td><td>10/3</td><td>5000</td></tr>
<tr><td>1</td><td>0</td><td>1</td><td>0</td><td>1000</td><td>320</td><td>1/2</td><td>2/5</td><td>5</td><td>5000</td></tr>
<tr><td>1</td><td>0</td><td>1</td><td>1</td><td>1500</td><td>280</td><td>1/2</td><td>3/5</td><td>10/3</td><td>5000</td></tr>
<tr><td>1</td><td>1</td><td>0</td><td>0</td><td>2000</td><td>260</td><td>1/2</td><td>2/3</td><td>6/2=3</td><td>6000</td></tr>
<tr><td>1</td><td>1</td><td>0</td><td>1</td><td>1000</td><td>280</td><td>1/2</td><td>1/3</td><td>6</td><td>6000</td></tr>
<tr><td>1</td><td>1</td><td>1</td><td>0</td><td>750</td><td>320</td><td>1/2</td><td>1/4</td><td>8</td><td>6000</td></tr>
<tr><td>1</td><td>1</td><td>1</td><td>1</td><td>2250</td><td>340</td><td>1/2</td><td>3/4</td><td>8/3</td><td>6000</td></tr>
</table>

$$*\text{IPW} = \frac{1}{P(A_0 \mid L_0) * P(A_1 \mid L_1, A_0, L_0)}$$

1. we do not adjust for L_0 and L_1, because the associational risk difference in the actual population is not causal

$$\mathbb{E}(Y \mid A_0 = 1, A_1 = 1) - \mathbb{E}(Y \mid A_0 = 0, A_1 = 1) = 297 - 288.57 = 8.43$$

2. we adjust for L_0 and L_1 (e.g. through standardisation), because the standard methods fail in the context of time dependent confounding affected by prior treatment.

For example, within the strata defined by L_0 and L_1, we have that

$$L_0 = 0, L_1 = 0 : \mathbb{E}(Y \mid A_0 = 1, A_1 = 1) - \mathbb{E}(Y \mid A_0 = 0, A_1 = 1) = 280 - 250 = 30,$$
$$L_0 = 0, L_1 = 1 : \mathbb{E}(Y \mid A_0 = 1, A_1 = 1) - \mathbb{E}(Y \mid A_0 = 0.A_1 = 1) = 240 - 300 = -60,$$
$$L_0 = 1, L_1 = 0 : \mathbb{E}(Y \mid A_0 = 1, A_1 = 1) - \mathbb{E}(Y \mid A_0 = 0, A_1 = 1) = 280 - 300 = -20,$$
$$L_0 = 1, L_1 = 1 : \mathbb{E}(Y \mid A_0 = 1.A_1 = 1) - \mathbb{E}(Y \mid A_0 = 0.A_1 = 1) = 340 - 280 = 60.$$

Accounting for L_0 and L_1 (e.g., through regression adjustment) would give us an estimate of

$$\mathbb{E}(Y \mid A_0 = 1, A_1 = 1) - \mathbb{E}(Y \mid A_0 = 0, A_1 = 1)$$

which is equal to

$$30 \times \mathbb{P}(L_0 = 0, L_1 = 0) - 60 \times \mathbb{P}(L_0 = 0, L_1 = 1) - 20 \times \mathbb{P}(L_0 = 1, L_1 = 0) + 60 \times \mathbb{P}(L_0 = 1, L_1 = 1)$$
$$= \frac{30 \times 5500}{23000} - \frac{60 \times 5500}{23000} - \frac{20 \times 6500}{23000} + \frac{60 \times 5500}{23000} = -0.21,$$

which does not correspond to the causal risk difference.

We could also derive unbiased estimates when dealing with time-dependent confounders, affected by prior treatment (exposure) using the other g-methods (i.e. g-formula, g-estimation), however this is beyond the scope of this chapter.

References

1. Pearl J. Causality: models, reasoning, and inference. Cambridge University Press; 2009.
2. Hernan M, Robins J. Causal inference: what If. Chapman & Hall; 2020.
3. Kaufman J, Cooper R. Commentary: considerations for use of racial/ethnic classification in etiologic research. Am J Epidemiol. 2001;154(4):291–8.
4. Rubin DB. Estimating causal effects of treatments in randomized and nonrandomized studies. J Educ Psychol. 1974;66(5):688–701.
5. Rubin DB. Causal inference using potential outcomes. J Am Stat Assoc. 2005;100(469):322–31.

6. Greenland S, Robin J. Identifiability, exchangeability, and epidemiological confounding. Int J Epidemiol. 1986;15(3):413–9.
7. Meyer BD. Natural and quasi-experiments in economics. NBER Technical Working Papers 0170, National Bureau of Economic Research, Inc, Dec. 1994.
8. Schmidt AF, Carter JL, Pearce LS, Wilkins JT, Overington JP, Hingorani AD, Casas JP. Pcsk9 monoclonal antibodies for the primary and secondary prevention of cardiovascular disease. Cochrane Database of Syst Rev. 2020;10.
9. Schmidt A, Klungel O, Nielen M, De Boer A, Groenwold R, Hoes A. Tailoring treatments using treatment effect modification. Pharmacoepidemiology and drug safety. 2016;25(4):355–62.
10. Schmidt A, Groenwold R. Adjusting for bias in unblinded randomized controlled trials. Stat Methods Med Res. 2018;27(8):2413–27.
11. Lai AG, Chang WH, Parisinos CA, Katsoulis M, Blackburn RM, Shah AD, Nguyen V, Denaxas S, Davey Smith G, Gaunt TR, et al. An informatics consult approach for generating clinical evidence for treatment decisions. BMC Medical Inf Dec Making. 2021;21(1):1–14.
12. Fanaroff AC, Califf RM, Windecker S, Smith J, Sidney C, Lopes RD. Levels of evidence supporting American college of Cardiology/American Heart Association and European Society of Cardiology Guidelines, 2008–2018. JAMA. 2019;321:1069–80.
13. Bland JM, Altman DG. Statistic notes: regression towards the mean BMJ 1994; 308(6942):1499 https://pubmed.ncbi.nlm.nih.gov/8019287/

Statistical Analysis—Meta-Analysis/Reproducibility

Mackenzie J. Edmondson, Chongliang Luo and Yong Chen

Abstract

Federated learning has gained great popularities in the last decade for its capability of collaboratively building models on data from multiple datasets. However, in real-world biomedical settings, practical challenges remain, including the needs to protect privacy of the patients, the capability of accounting for between-site heterogeneity in patient characteristics, and, from operational point of view, the number of needed communications across data partners. In this chapter, we describe and provide examples of multi-database data-sharing mechanisms in the healthcare data context and highlight the primary methods available for performing statistical regression analysis in each setting. For each method, we discuss the advantages and disadvantages in terms of data privacy, data communication efficiency, heterogeneity awareness, and statistical accuracy. Our goal is to provide researchers with the insight necessary to choose among the available algorithms for a given setting of conducting regression analysis using multi-site data.

1 Introduction

Following passage of the 21st Century Cures Act in 2015, the Food and Drug Administration (FDA) has placed additional focus on using real-world data (RWD) to support regulatory decision-making. This has resulted in an increase in the number of observational studies using RWD conducted by researchers in the United States to generate real-world evidence [1, 2].Kindly note, in order to maintain consistency with other chapters in this book, Keywords are required for this chapter. Please provide if possible. A study using RWD may seek to examine the benefits or risks of a particular medical product or intervention, such as whether patients taking a particular drug are more susceptible to serious adverse events than those who are not. Alternatively, many studies featuring RWD are epidemiological, focused on identifying risk factors most strongly associated with an adverse outcome of particular interest. In many of these studies, regression analyses are often conducted to

M. J. Edmondson
Biostatistics at Merck, 707 S Smedley St., Philadelphia, PA 19146, USA

C. Luo
Division of Public Health Sciences, Washington University School of Medicine in St Louis, 600 S Taylor Ave, St Louis, MO 63110, USA
e-mail: chongliang@wustl.edu

Y. Chen (✉)
Division of Biostatistics, The University of Pennsylvania, 423 Guardian Dr, Blockley Hall 602, Philadelphia, USA
e-mail: ychen123@upenn.edu

F. W. Asselbergs et al. (eds.), *Clinical Applications of Artificial Intelligence in Real-World Data*,
https://doi.org/10.1007/978-3-031-36678-9_8

investigate the question of interest. Regression allows for modeling an outcome as a function of a collection of treatments, exposures, or covariates and enables quantification of associations between covariates and the outcome through estimated regression coefficients. Several types of regression models can be used for modeling a variety of health outcomes. For example, continuous outcomes such as blood pressure can be analyzed by linear regression, binary outcomes such as mortality status can be analyzed by logistic regression, count outcomes such as number of hospital visits can be analyzed by Poisson regression, and time-to-event outcomes such as cancer survival time can be analyzed by Cox regression.

Real-world observational studies often benefit from their ability to include large amounts of patient data from a variety of sources. Observational RWD, compared to patient data collected in clinical trials or other types of interventional studies, are relatively inexpensive to obtain. RWD are frequently extracted from patients' electronic health records, insurance claims, or other written records of patient data. Recent improvements in techniques for data standardization, phenotype definition, and large-scale data analysis have made multi-institution collaborations for observational studies easier than ever, allowing for large sample sizes from a variety of heterogeneous sources to generate robust real-world evidence and increase generalizability of results. Studies of rare outcomes or exposures can also benefit from multi-institution collaboration, with larger collections of patient data resulting in increased power to detect significant associations.

Large-scale RWD observational studies often require multiple institutions to contribute data to achieve more generalizable results. The two main mechanisms for 'sharing' data include centralized data repositories and distributed data-sharing. The granularity of data shared depends on the data use agreements (DUA) among participating institutions. Some DUAs allow for all individual patient data (IPD) to be centralized, resulting in a pooling of all patient data within a cloud or at the coordinating center for the study. Other agreements prohibit sharing of IPD, instead only allow summary-level aggregate data (AD) to be shared by each institution. With this distributed or federated data sharing mechanism, individual databases maintain control over their own data and conduct analyses locally before sharing results with collaborating institutions. Each of these data-sharing arrangements permits a distinct set of methods to be used to conduct multi-database regression. A popular nationwide example of a centralized data repository is the Nationwide Inpatient Sample (NIS) from the Healthcare Cost and Utilization Project (HCUP) and a popular example of international, distributed or federated data network is the Observational Health Data Sciences and Informatics (OHDSI) network (ohdsi.org). In the context of COVID-19, a popular centralized data repository is the National COVID Cohort Collaborative or N3C (https://ncats.nih.gov/n3c) and a popular distributed or federated data network method is the Consortium for Clinical Characterization of COVID-19 by EHR or 4CE (https://covidclinical.net/). Both networks have large nationwide and international collaborators. N3C has 73 sites within the USA approved to share data centrally as of May 2021 [3] and 4CE has 20 sites within the USA approved to collaborate and run similar models locally while pooling results for meta-analysis purposes [4]. The choice of data sharing mechanism, i.e. centrally or distributively, is often made at the institutional level, with some institutions being risk averse and preferring to run models only locally. The potential risk of privacy leakage could hinder some institutions from sharing essential IPD data and thus limit the study to cover a broader population.

The purpose of this review is to describe and provide examples of multi-database data-sharing mechanisms in the healthcare data context and highlight the primary methods available for performing statistical regression analysis in each setting. For each regression method, we discuss the advantages and disadvantages in terms of data privacy, data communication efficiency, heterogeneity awareness, and statistical accuracy. Our goal is to provide researchers with the insight necessary to choose the data-sharing arrangement and corresponding regression method most appropriate for any particular real-world multi-database study.

2 Data Sharing Arrangements in Multi-database Studies

Before data from different databases can be shared either with a centralized or distributed mechanism, they need to be standardized to ensure that naming conventions and coding systems are common across institutions. This data standardization or harmonization usually requires data to be transformed into a common data model (CDM) and a common representation. Examples of CDMs include the Informatics for Integrating Biology and the Bedside (i2b2, https://www.i2b2.org/) developed by Harvard Medical School and funded by the National Institute of Health (NIH) in 2004, the Observational Medical Outcomes Partnership (OMOP, https://www.ohdsi.org/data-standardization/the-common-data-model/) by OHDSI in 2007, the Sentinel CDM (https://www.sentinelinitiative.org/methods-data-tools/sentinel-common-data-model) launched by FDA in 2008, and the PCORnet CDM (https://pcornet.org/data/) started by the patient Centered Outcomes Research Institute (PCORI) in 2014 [5]. The data standardization can either be done within each participating institution or at the coordinating center, depending on the data-sharing mechanism.

2.1 Centralized Data

When data within multi-database studies are centralized, IPD are pooled together from all participating institutions within some central entity and managed by a coordinating center. This type of data sharing arrangement offers the largest analytic flexibility, allowing for modeling using data at any level of granularity (individual- or summary-level). Due to this very advantage, centralized data sharing is usually preferred by researchers.

Several multi-database collaborations using centralized data currently exist. A recent example is the N3C, a centralized enclave of IPD derived from the EHRs of people who tested positive for COVID-19 or who had related symptoms [6]. Currently, N3C has patient-level information for nearly 5 million patients contributed by several participating institutions. The data are centralized in a cloud-based analytics platform, accessible for analysis within the cloud in the form of limited or de-identified datasets. Another example is the rise of all-payer claims databases (APCDs), which are large databases in many states including medical, pharmacy, and dental claims collected from both public and private payers [7]. APCDs are designed to make de-identified patient claims data available for analyzing healthcare outcomes and costs at a large scale.

While appealing to many researchers, the flexibility of centralized patient data comes at a cost in terms of security and data privacy. Information shared across institutions under a centralized data sharing mechanism often consists of large amounts of potentially identifiable health information, such as records indicating patients' medication and diagnosis history. In an effort to protect sensitive patient information, privacy regulations such as those stipulated in the Health Insurance Portability and Accountability Act (HIPAA) or the General Data Protection Regulation (GDPR) prohibit sharing of raw patient-level data across institutions [8, 9]. For example, in the USA, HIPAA sets 18 identifiers such as name, date of birth, and home address, etc. that can be used to identify a single individual. If collaborating institutions agree to centralize data, these data must be transformed into HIPPA-approved "limited datasets," which are "de-identified" by stripping off any of these identifiers. In de-identified datasets, longitudinal data are often date-shifted to further protect patient privacy. While less sensitive than raw data, limited datasets have been shown to be susceptible to patient reidentification, so there is some degree of patient-level privacy risk associated with multi-database studies using centralized data [10, 11]. In addition to patient privacy, there are also concerns about privacy at the institution level, with some institutions concerned about being identified and deemed lower quality than their peer institutions as a consequence of sharing patient-level data [12]. Sharing of patient-level data also often requires contractual agreements among collaborating institutions and approval from institutional review boards, both of which can be time-consuming.

2.2 Distributed Data

With a distributed data sharing mechanism, collaborating institutions maintain control over their own IPD and only share summary-level AD with other institutions. No central data repository is required; instead, IPD analysis is performed locally at each institution to calculate summary measures, which are then aggregated and further analyzed at a coordinating center. This allows for data quality checks and analysis via statistical programs that can be shared across institutions, resulting in greater protection of sensitive patient data relative to the centralized data setting.

The additional security offered by using a distributed data network is considered valuable by many stakeholders in multi-database studies, including patients, researchers, and health care system leaders. However, there are questions from these same stakeholders regarding whether the additional privacy protection is worth the costs of data standardization and any potential analysis limitations due to reducing the granularity of data that can be shared across institutions [6]. While standardizing data at each institution can initially be time-consuming, data can be updated in accordance with the latest uniform specifications relatively quickly. This also avoids having to transfer and standardize data repeatedly at a central data repository in a centralized data setting. Additionally, many of the distributed regression methods detailed later in this review have been shown to produce results either closely approximating or identical to those obtained when one analyzes pooled patient-level data, suggesting a need for improved education for stakeholders regarding the utility of distributed regression methods.

There are several examples of distributed data networks being used to conduct multi-database studies. One example is the OHDSI program, an international network of researchers and observational health databases which standardize their data in accordance with the OMOP CDM [13]. The OHDSI network makes use of 600 million unique patient records without sharing any patient-level data, allowing for large-scale collaborative analyses to generate quality real-world evidence without risking patient privacy [14]. Another example is the Sentinel System, a distributed data network led by the FDA for post-market surveillance of approved drugs, vaccines, and medical devices [15]. The Sentinel System is made up of a collection of health care organizations which analyze their own medical billing and electronic health records data using a common statistical program, sending summary-level information to a coordinating center for further analysis. Many other distributed data networks currently exist, including the 4CE, the PCORnet [16], the Vaccine Safety Datalink run by Centers for Disease Control and Prevention [17], and the Health Care Systems Research Network [18]. With the increasing prominence of distributed data networks comes the desire for more advanced distributed regression methods to better analyze data in these distributed data networks.

3 Regression Methods for Multi-database Studies

We next review a variety of regression methods that have been used in multi-database studies. We first describe a set of conventional methods which have been used frequently in practice to analyze data in either centralized or distributed data settings. We then highlight a collection of contemporary methods primarily designed for multi-database studies with a distributed data sharing mechanism. The reviewed methods are evaluated regarding preservation of patient privacy, communication efficiency of summary-level AD, and statistical estimation accuracy. We also review distributed regression methods that take account of heterogeneity across databases.

3.1 Pooled Regression

When data from multiple databases are centralized, this allows for pooled regression to be performed. We consider the outcome that is from the generalized linear model (GLM) family (e.g. continuous, binary and count) or the survival analysis (i.e. time-to-event), which are commonly seen in healthcare studies. Assume we have pooled IPD for N patients and denote the p -dimensional covariate vector as $\boldsymbol{x}_i$ and the outcome as y_i for the i-th patient, $i = 1, \ldots, N$. The regression coefficients (e.g. association effect sizes) β are estimated by minimizing the negative log-likelihood function (or loss function),

$$\hat{\beta} = \arg\min_{\beta} L(\beta).$$

For example, if the outcome is from GLM family, then $L(\beta)$ is the negative log-likelihood function of GLM [19], and if the outcome is time-to-event, then $L(\beta)$ is the negative log partial likelihood of the Cox proportional hazard model [20].

The pooled analysis provides the most analytical flexibility and allows for finer statistical modeling that accounts for rare features (e.g. covariates or outcome), missing data, interaction effects estimation, and heterogeneity, etc. Pooled regression is frequently viewed as the gold standard when evaluating distributed regression methods in multi-database studies [21]. Estimated regression coefficients produced by other methods are often compared to those from pooled regression. We refer to the discrepancy as estimation bias. The best distributed methods are expected to produce accurate estimates with small bias, and a "lossless" estimate is one with zero bias. Treating pooled regression as the gold standard without treating the data source as a fixed or random effect implicitly assumes that there is not substantial heterogeneity by database. This assumption can be met in practice if a multi-database study is designed in such a way that minimizes any potential sources of heterogeneity. If treatment-effect heterogeneity by institution is apparent and cannot be properly accounted for, the validity of results produced by pooled analysis is more questionable.

3.2 Meta-Analysis of Database-Specific Regression Coefficients

If only summary-level data can be shared among collaborating institutions under a distributed data sharing agreement, a distributed regression method often used is the meta-analysis approach. We assume each of K databases holds IPD for n_j patients, $j = 1, \ldots, K$, and $N = \sum_{j=1}^{K} n_j$. We denote the covariate vector as $\boldsymbol{x}_{ij}$ and the outcome as y_{ij} for the i-th patient in the j-th database, $i = 1, \ldots, n_j, j = 1, \ldots, K$. Using the data from each individual database, i.e. $\boldsymbol{X}_j = \left(\boldsymbol{x}_{1j}, \ldots, \boldsymbol{x}_{n_j j}\right)^T$, and $\boldsymbol{Y}_j = \left(y_{1j}, \ldots, y_{n_j j}\right)^T$, we obtain individual estimates from each database as

$$\hat{\beta}_j = argmin_{\beta} L_j(\beta), j = 1, \ldots, K,$$

where $L_j(\beta)$ is the negative log likelihood of the regression model using the j-th database data only. The variance of $\widehat{\beta}_j$ is also estimated as $\widehat{V}_j$.

To conduct a meta-analysis and obtain a common estimate of the regression coefficient, each institution shares the coefficient estimate and its variance estimate with the coordinating center. These individual estimates, i.e. $\widehat{\beta}_j$ and $\widehat{V}_j$ are p -dimensional vectors and are considered privacy-preserving summary-level AD. The coordinating center can then perform meta-analysis using each institution's estimates, e.g. inverse variance weighted average to produce a common estimate and variance for the regression coefficient,

$$\hat{\beta}_M = \left\{\sum_{j=1}^{K} \hat{V}_j^{-1}\right\}^{-1} \left\{\sum_{j=1}^{K} \hat{V}_j^{-1} \hat{\beta}_j\right\}, \hat{V}_M = \left\{\sum_{j=1}^{K} \hat{V}_j^{-1}\right\}^{-1},$$

where $\widehat{\beta}_M$ is the "meta-estimator" and $\widehat{V}_M$ is its variance estimate.

The above averaging approach assumes fixed effects, that is, for each coefficient estimated by a regression model, there is one true effect shared by all databases included in the analysis. If this assumption cannot be met due to apparent heterogeneity in effects by database, random-effects meta-analysis can instead be used [22]. Random-effects meta-analysis allows coefficients to vary by database, with each database's respective coefficient assumed to be a random sample of some distribution of effects. Rather than estimating assumed underlying true effects, random-effects meta-analysis estimates the mean of each effect's assumed distribution. Whether fixed- or random-effects meta-analysis is more appropriate in a given multi-database study depends on the setting. A study where substantial efforts are made to limit any database-driven heterogeneity can likely provide a strong case for using fixed-effects meta-analysis. Random-effects meta-analysis is a more conservative option, producing overall coefficient estimates with greater uncertainty. In the presence of database-level covariates, meta-regression can be used to better explain the between-database heterogeneity.

Several published multi-database studies have used meta-analysis to estimate overall regression coefficients. You et al. compared platelet inhibitors ticagrelor and clopidogrel in terms of their association with ischemic and hemorrhagic events in acute coronary syndrome patients undergoing percutaneous coronary intervention [23]. Suchard et al. conducted a large-scale comparative effectiveness and safety evaluation in an effort to determine the optimal monotherapy for hypertension among a collection of first-line drug classes [14]. Vashisht et al. compared a number of second-line treatment options for type 2 diabetes in terms of their associations with a collection of adverse events [24]. All three studies calculated database-specific hazard ratios (HRs), aggregating them via random-effects meta-analysis to produce an overall HR estimate.

Meta-analysis of database-specific regression coefficients is a commonly used method for multi-database studies due to its convenience of data communication (i.e. minimum requirement of AD by $\widehat{\beta}_j$ and $\widehat{V}_j$) and good accuracy (i.e. asymptotically unbiased, [25]) [26, 27]. However, meta-analysis has also been shown to result in biased estimation relative to pooled estimates, especially in settings with small sample sizes or rare outcomes [28, 29]. The detrimental bias induced by small samples may not be diluted by averaging in meta-analysis when most collaborative databases have limited size. In the case that the outcome or some covariates lack variation in certain databases, some individual estimates may be unavailable. Consequently, these databases must be excluded from the collaborative study, resulting in potential loss of valuable samples. Moreover, meta-analytical approaches, e.g. meta-regression is known to suffer from aggregation bias (or ecological bias) and hence problematic when used for studying treatment-covariate interaction [30–32].

3.3 Contemporary Distributed Regression Methods: Homogeneous Data

Recent years have seen development of various distributed regression methods for multi-database studies without sharing IPD across institutions. These methods achieve a balance between IPD data privacy and estimation accuracy by requiring more AD (or a combination of IPD and AD) than meta-analysis (but still privacy-preserving) to obtain estimates closer to those from pooled analysis compared to those from meta-analysis. We now review these methods and evaluate their data communication efficiency (e.g. iterative or non-iterative) and estimation accuracy (i.e. bias to the pooled analysis as compared to the meta-analysis). We consider homogeneous databases in this section.

We start with linear regression which is used for continuous outcomes. The availability of the closed form solution (i.e. ordinary least-square estimation) makes divide-and-conquer a simple yet insightful idea for distributed regression [33]. The least square solution can be written as

$$\hat{\beta} = \left(\sum_{j=1}^{K} X_j^T X_j\right)^{-1} \left(\sum_{j=1}^{K} X_j^T Y_j\right), \hat{V} = \left(\sum_{j=1}^{K} X_j^T X_j\right)^{-1} \hat{\sigma}^2,$$

where $\hat{\sigma}^2 = \left(\sum_{j=1}^{K} n_j\right)^{-1} \sum_j^K \{Y_j^T Y_j - 2Y_j^T X_j \hat{\beta} + \hat{\beta}^T X_j^T X_j \hat{\beta}\}$ is the estimate of the random error variance.

It is easy to see that the required AD from the j-th database are the $p \times p$ matrix $X_j^T X_j$, the $p \times p$ matrix $X_j^T X_j$, p-dimensional vector $X_j^T Y_j$, and scalars $Y_j^T Y_j$ and n_j. This divide-and-conquer approach reconstructs pooled regression estimates using summary-level AD supplied by each participating database and obtains lossless (i.e. identical) estimates relative to pooled regression.

Linear regression is unique among other types of regression in that the estimated coefficients have closed-form solutions. For other types of regression, such as logistic regression for binary outcomes or Poisson regression for count outcomes, there are no closed-form solutions for estimating coefficients. Rather, coefficients are estimated using iteratively reweighted least squares, an algorithm also known as the Newton–Raphson algorithm which requires repeated evaluations of derivatives at potential solutions until convergence is reached [34]. In a centralized data setting, this procedure can be completed relatively simply with access to all patient data. In a distributed data setting, this is no longer trivial, as derivatives need to be evaluated by each participating institution using their respective patient-level data. Wu et al. extended the divide-and-conquer idea in distributed linear regression for performing distributed logistic regression, by aggregating derivative evaluations from each participating database at a coordinating center within each of the algorithm iterations [35]. Specifically, at the s-th iteration

$$\hat{\beta}^{(s+1)} = \hat{\beta}^{(s)} + \left(\sum_{j=1}^{K} X_j^T diag\left\{\pi_j^{(s)}\left(1 - \pi_j^{(s)}\right)\right\} X_j\right)^{-1} \left(\sum_{j=1}^{K} X_j^T (Y_j - \pi_j^{(s)})\right),$$

$$\hat{V} = \left(\sum_{j=1}^{K} X_j^T diag\{\pi_j(1 - \pi_j)\} X_j\right)^{-1},$$

where $\pi_j^{(s)} = e^{X_j \hat{\beta}^{(s)}} / (1 + e^{X_j \hat{\beta}^{(s)}})$. The AD required from the j-th institute at the s-th iteration is the $p \times p$ matrix $X_j^T diag\left\{\pi_j^{(s)}\left(1 - \pi_j^{(s)}\right)\right\} X_j$ and the p-dim vector $X_j^T (Y_j - \pi_j^{(s)})$. Lu et al. proposed a similar iterative algorithm for fitting Cox model for time-to-event outcomes [36]. Each of these iterative methods for distributed regression is also lossless, producing estimates that have been shown to be identical to those produced by pooled analysis if all data were centralized.

While lossless, the above iterative distributed regression procedures can incur significant communication costs. Depending on the particular study, reaching convergence can require a large number of iterations. In the context of a multi-database study, each iteration requires a round of communication between the coordinating center and each collaborating institution. Sharing AD between institutions is most often not automatic and can delay completion of multi-database studies. In recent years, communication-efficient alternatives to iterative algorithms have been proposed to address this issue. Huang and Huo [37] proposed a Distributed One-Step Estimator (denoted as DOSE in this review) to improve upon the basis of the meta-estimator,

$$\hat{\beta}_{DOSE} = \hat{\beta}_M - \left\{\sum_{j=1}^{K} \nabla^2 L_j\left(\hat{\beta}_M\right)\right\}^{-1} \left\{\sum_{j=1}^{K} \nabla L_j\left(\hat{\beta}_M\right)\right\}.$$

Here $\nabla L_j\left(\hat{\beta}_M\right)$ and $\nabla^2 L_j\left(\hat{\beta}_M\right)$ are the first and second derivatives (i.e. gradient and hessian) of the likelihood function at the j-th database, evaluated at the meta-estimator $\hat{\beta}_M$. This method is thus a non-iterative distributed regression method. It requires the above derivatives (p-dim vector and $p \times p$ matrix) from the j-th database as AD, and improves the meta-estimator towards pooled regression. The DOSE applies to any regression models in the GLM family. Shu et al. proposed a distributed method for inverse probability weighted Cox regression model [38]. The method provides lossless estimation of the marginal hazard ratio, given the risk set tables from all databases as the summary-level AD.

In some situations, we may have IPD available from some databases and AD from others. Multilevel regression methods that combine

IPD and AD are potentially advantageous over two-stage methods [39]. This line of multilevel meta-analysis models has been discussed by several researchers but deserves more exploration. Duan et al. proposed a one-shot distributed algorithm for performing logistic regression (ODAL) requiring only one round of communication among participating institutions [40]. The ODAL method assumes a lead institution and constructs a surrogate likelihood [41] that combines IPD from the lead institution and AD from other collaborative institutions. The surrogate likelihood serves as a good approximation of the pooled likelihood and thus improves the meta-estimator towards the pooled estimation. The surrogate likelihood assuming the first institute as the lead institute is constructed as

$$\tilde{L}(\beta) = L_1(\beta) + \left\{\nabla L\left(\hat{\beta}_M\right) - \nabla L\left(\hat{\beta}_M\right)\right\}^T \beta,$$

and the ODAL surrogate estimator is

$$\tilde{\beta} = \arg\min_{\beta}\tilde{L}(\beta).$$

Here $\nabla L\left(\widehat{\beta}_M\right) = N^{-1}\sum_{j=1}^{K} n_j \nabla L_j\left(\widehat{\beta}_M\right)$ is the gradient of the pooled likelihood evaluated at the meta-estimator $\widehat{\beta}_M$. Similar surrogate likelihood ideas have been applied to Cox regression (ODAC, [28]), Poisson regression (ODAP, [42]), and hurdle regression (ODAH, [43]). These "ODAX" algorithms, while not lossless, have been shown to produce estimates nearly matching those produced by pooled regression, sacrificing an often-negligible amount of accuracy for a reduction in required communication among collaborating institutions. These methods are considered "one-shot" approaches for distributed regression since they only require sharing of AD from each site once.

The above reviewed distributed regression methods are summarized in Table 1. We also illustrate the data communication for multi-database logistic regression using a simulated data example in Fig. 1. In this example, both the GLORE and ODAL methods use the meta-estimator as initial value and obtains estimates towards the pooled analysis. The GLORE method is lossless but requires communicating AD from all databases in multiple iterations, while in ODAL method the lead database requires AD from other databases only once but obtains estimates very close to the pooled analysis. In general, all distributed methods are subject to the trade-off between performance (accuracy) and operational convenience (communication-efficiency). This is displayed in Fig. 2, which also includes the distributed regression methods that are robust to heterogeneity, reviewed in the next section.

3.4 Contemporary Distributed Regression Methods: Heterogeneous Data

A major challenge in multi-database studies is modeling heterogeneity, which is especially difficult in distributed regression due to the restriction to the accessibility of IPD. We review some recently developed distributed regression methods that are heterogeneity-aware. Many of them have connection with the homogeneous methods reviewed in last section. See Table 2 for a summary of these methods and refer to the original papers for technical details.

For linear regression, each database may have its own specific effects (associations between covariates and outcome). The linear mixed-effects model (LMM) is used to model continuous outcomes with heterogeneous, database-specific regression coefficients (including intercepts). LMM also does not have a closed form solution; however, the pooled likelihood can be reconstructed using the same required AD as in DLM, and hence a lossless one-shot distributed linear mixed-effects model (DLMM) is available [45].

For other types of outcomes in the GLM family, heterogeneous database-specific regression coefficients can be modeled by a generalized linear mixed-effects model (GLMM). Due to the computational complexity, few distributed methods exist for fitting GLMM, including the collaborative GLMM (cGLMM) proposed by

Table 1 Comparison of available distributed regression methods for homogeneous multi-database studies

Outcome type	Distributed method	Literature	Data Sharing	AD required	Communication efficiency	Accuracy
Continuous	DLM	Chen et al. [33]	All AD	$p \times p$ matrix, p -dim vector, scalars	Non-iterative	Lossless
Binary	GLORE	Wu et al. [35]	All AD	$p \times p$ matrix, p-dim vector	Iterative	Lossless
Time-to-event	WebDISCO	Lu et al. [36]	All AD	$p \times p$ matrix, p-dim vector	Iterative	Lossless
[a]GLM family	DOSE	Huang et al. [37]	All AD	$p \times p$ matrix, p-dim vector	Non-iterative	[b]> meta
Time-to-event	D-IPW Cox	Shu et al. [38]	All AD	Risk set tables	Non-iterative	Lossless (marginal HR)
GLM family	Multilevel modeling	Riley et al. [39], Sutton et al. [44],	IPD+AD	p-dim vectors	Non-iterative	>meta
Binary	ODAL	Duan et al. [28]	IPD+AD	$p \times p$ matrix, p-dim vector	Non-iterative	>meta
Time-to-event	ODAC	Duan et al. [40]	IPD+AD	Risk set tables, $p \times p$ matrix, p-dim vector	Non-iterative	>meta
Count	ODAP, ODAH	Edmondson et al. [42], Edmondson et al. [43]	IPD+AD	$p \times p$ matrix, p-dim vector	Non-iterative	>meta

[a]GLM family contains continuous, binary, count and other types of outcomes. [b]>meta: more accurate than meta-estimator (smaller bias relative to pooled regression)

Zhu et al. [46]. The cGLMM decomposes the Expectation–Maximization (EM) algorithm and is privacy-preserving. However, it is communication-extensive due to the slow convergence nature of the EM algorithm. Recently, inspired by the DLMM, Luo et al. proposed an alternative distributed method for fitting GLMM [47]. It adopts the DLMM method to decompose each iteration of the penalized quasi-likelihood (PQL) estimation algorithm, and thus is called the distributed PQL (dPQL) algorithm. The PQL is a common and fast-converging algorithm for fitting GLMM, and hence the dPQL algorithm is considered communication-efficient as only a few rounds of AD communication are required. For example, the dPQL algorithm achieves convergence within 5 iterations in a study profiling 929 hospitals regarding rates of COVID-19 mortality or referral to hospice. Both cGLMM and dPQL are lossless and iterative.

There are also several heterogeneity-aware distributed methods using the surrogate likelihood approach. Recently, Tong et al. proposed robust-ODAL for performing distributed logistic regression which accounts for potential heterogeneity by database, designed to be more robust in the event of any outlying collaborating institutions [48]. Luo et al. proposed ODACH for fitting stratified Cox regression where the nuisance baseline hazard functions at institutions are assumed heterogeneous [49]. Nuisance parameter heterogeneity may also exist in the GLM family and can be modeled by the proportional likelihood ratio (PLR) model [50]. Luo et al. adopted the surrogate likelihood

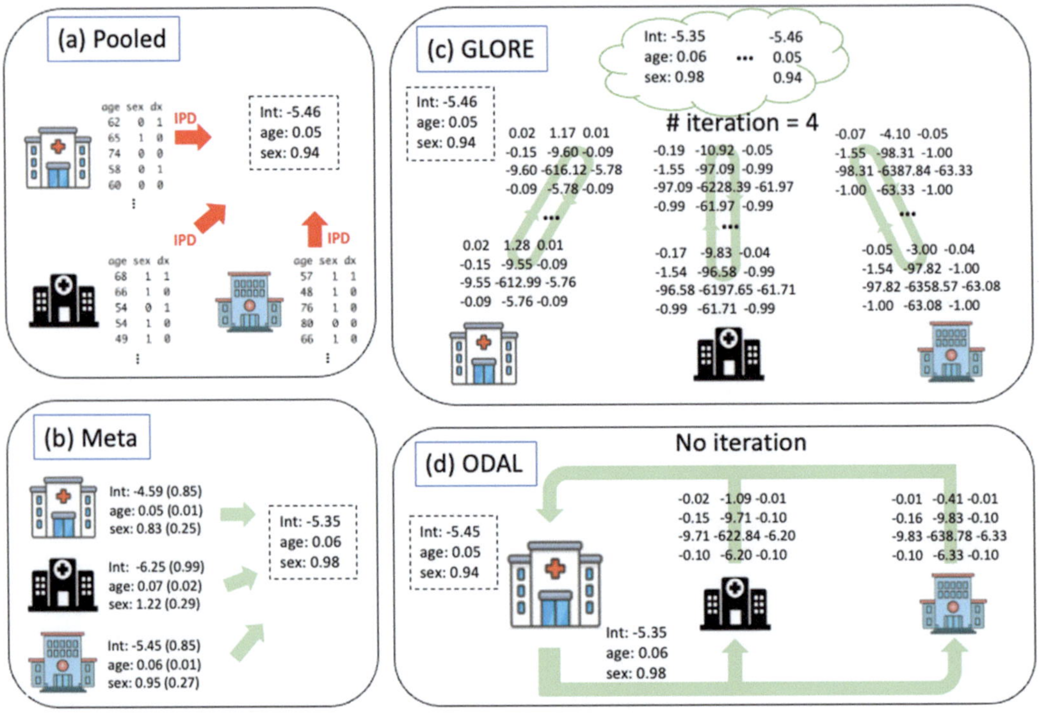

Fig. 1 An example for multi-database logistic regression with pooled or distributed methods. The purpose of the regression is to identify associations of patient age, sex with certain disease diagnosis. The IPD data from three databases (hospitals) were simulated. (a) Pooled regression is considered the "gold-standard" but requires communicating sensitive IPD from all databased. (b) Meta-analysis aggregate individual estimates from each database to obtain a meta-estimator. (c) Grid Binary LOgistic REgression (GLORE) is a lossless (i.e. obtains identical result as pooled analysis) but iterative distributed logistic regression method. The coordinate center sends out updated estimates and require each database to return corresponding aggregate data (i.e. gradients and hessian). The number of iterations is 4. (d) One-shot Distributed Algorithm for Logistic regression (ODAL) is a non-iterative distributed method. The lead database combines its own IPD with aggregate data (i.e. gradients and hessian) from other databases to obtain almost identical estimates as the pooled analysis

idea and proposed a distributed PLR (DPLR) method for heterogeneity of nuisance parameters in the GLM family [53]. Similarly, Tong et al. proposed a distributed conditional logistic regression (dCLR, [51]) algorithm accounting for baseline rate heterogeneity of binary outcomes across databases. Another approach to account for nuisance parameter heterogeneity is via density ratio tilting (DRT) model. Duan et al. proposed a distributed DRT (DDRT, [52]) method which relies on the surrogate efficient score function for estimation. The non-asymptotic error bound for the proposed distributed estimator was established as well as its limiting distribution when both sample size per institution and the number of institutions go to infinity.

4 Discussion

Real-world data analysis has gained more attention in recent years, for example, in the area of drug/vaccine safety surveillance, discovering risk factors for rare diseases, and aiding clinical trial design. Integrating data from multiple sources is essential for gaining statistical power and increasing the generalizability of the distilled real-world evidence. A larger and more diverse collection of data sources benefits common knowledge discovery as well as understanding the heterogeneity of populations. Large-scale observational studies are often conducted by researchers from clinical research networks that have the resources to bring all the

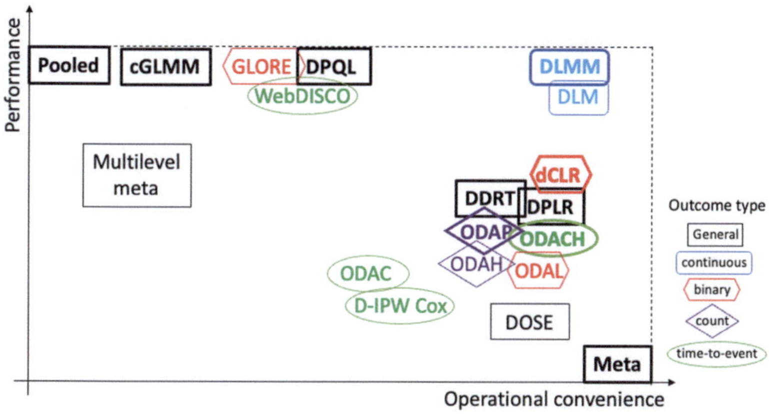

Fig. 2 Multi-database regression methods: trade-off between performance (accuracy) and operational convenience (communication-efficiency). A method is considered more accurate if it produces estimates closer to pooled regression, and more communication efficient if it requires less IPD or AD and is less iterative. Pooled regression is considered the "gold-standard" but requires communicating IPD. Meta-analysis is considered the most communication efficient but may not be accurate in the case of rare outcome or heterogeneity. The details of the reviewed methods are in Tables 1 and 2. Methods in bold boxes are more robust to database heterogeneity. Box shape and color indicate the outcome type for the method, while methods in black boxes are for general types of outcomes (e.g. GLM family)

Table 2 Comparison of available distributed regression methods for heterogeneous multi-database studies

Outcome Type	Distributed method	Literature	Data Sharing Arrangement	AD required	Communication efficiency	Accuracy
Continuous	DLMM	Luo et al. [45]	All AD	$p \times p$ matrix, p-dim vector, scalars	Non-iterative	Lossless
[a]GLM family	cGLMM	Zhu et al. [46]	All AD	$p \times p$ matrix, p-dim vector, scalars	Iterative (slow convergence; > 1000 iterations)	Approximately lossless
GLM family	dPQL	Luo et al. [47]	All AD	$p \times p$ matrix	Iterative (5–10 iterations)	Lossless
Binary	Robust-ODAL	Tong et al. [48]	IPD+AD	$p \times p$ matrix, p -dim vector	Non-iterative	[b]>meta
Time-to-event	ODACH	Luo et al. [49]	IPD+AD	$p \times p$ matrix, p -dim vector	Non-iterative	>meta
GLM family	dPLR	Luo et al. [50]	IPD+AD	$p \times p$ matrix, p -dim vector	Non-iterative	>meta
Binary	dCLR	Tong et al. [51]	IPD+AD	$p \times p$ matrix, p -dim vector	Non-iterative	>meta
GLM family	DDRT	Duan et al. [52]	IPD+AD	$p \times p$ matrix, p -dim vector	Non-iterative	>meta

[a]GLM family contains continuous, binary, count and other types of outcomes. [b]>meta: more accurate than meta-estimator (smaller bias relative to pooled regression)

subject-level data together. Though the collaboration within clinical research networks makes centralized data possible, the communicational and infrastructural burdens are often excessive. The meta-analysis approach only requires small pieces of AD, and hence is a convenient evidence synthesis approach used in many multi-database studies. Despite its communication efficiency, meta-analysis has shown to be suboptimal when the outcome is rare.

The distributed regression methods that are reviewed in this chapter are mostly developed within the past decade. Most of them show the tradeoff between operational convenience and performance benefit (see Fig. 2 for an illustration). A distributed regression method usually requires more AD and more iterations of AD communication to obtain an estimate that is closer to that from pooled analysis. Some one-shot methods (e.g. ODAL, ODAC) could be further improved by running more iterations (e.g. use the ODAL estimator as the initial estimate and repeat ODAL). Moreover, when heterogeneity is considered, the design of distributed regression usually becomes more difficult, as the pooled model also becomes increasingly complicated. DLMM is perhaps an exception, which adds no extra operational burden (i.e. the same AD requirement as DLM) when heterogeneity (i.e. random effects) is considered.

All the reviewed distributed regression methods rely on AD for protecting data privacy. This is generally accepted in biomedical research; meta-analysis, for example, requires sharing AD and is commonly used in practice. One advantage of using AD for privacy-preserving is that the ADs are task-specific. For example, AD for conducting distributed logistic regression cannot be used for conducting distributed Poisson regression, and AD for studying acute myocardial infarction can't be used for studying stroke. This provides an extra layer of protection when sharing AD across databases. The non-iterative distributed regression methods (e.g. DOSE, ODAL, ODAC, DLMM) are appreciated as they minimize the communicational and infrastructural burden.

Privacy-preserving distributed algorithms have also been extensively studied in domains other than data integration in healthcare clinical research networks. The development of these algorithms is generally referred to as federated learning in machine learning research. Data privacy frameworks have been developed to rigorously quantify the risk of adversarial attacks. The attacks, such as the membership inference attack (MIA [54, 55]), may cause privacy leakage when the data are repeatedly queried. To this end, the AD release mechanism in the reviewed distributed regression methods has not been rigorously studied to meet privacy-preserving criteria such as k-anonymity or differential privacy (DP, [56, 57]). Specifically, the k-anonymity criterion prevents a distributed algorithm from the risk of re-identification, which arises from linking potential quasi-identifiers (e.g. combinations of patient characteristics) to external sources [58]. The reviewed distributed regression methods can potentially meet the k-anonymity requirement. Special care needs to be taken when communicating AD according to data privacy regulations and data characteristics (e.g. rare predictors) [59, 60].

Barriers also exist when using distributed regression methods for practical multi-database collaboration. Data standardization or harmonization is essential for a high-quality multi-database study. Open-source CDMs, such as the OHDSI OMOP, play an important role in harmonizing data from various nations, institutions and coding systems. Secure and convenient data communication software and platforms are also essential for encouraging collaboration across databases. Researchers have developed software and platforms to promote the usage of their specific or general distributed regression methods [61–63]. Large clinical research networks such as OHDSI are also devoted to developing the infrastructures for more collaborative and accessible distributed learning across databases.

Real-world data such as EHR and claims data are not collected for research purposes. The second use of these data for real-world evidence thus often faces data quality problems such as missingness or mismeasurement and population heterogeneity. Besides the classical regression methods reviewed in this chapter, novel statistical learning methods may be necessary for addressing these problems. Combining RWD with clinical trials is also a popular research area and requires novel method development. Finally, implementation of the distributed algorithms and embedding them with clinical research networks for translation to clinical practices also require future work.

References

1. Sherman RE, Anderson SA, Dal Pan GJ, Gray GW, Gross T, Hunter NL, LaVange L, Marinac-Dabic D, Marks PW, Robb MA, Shuren J. Real-world evidence—what is it and what can it tell us. N Engl J Med. 2016;375(23):2293–7.
2. Jarow JP, LaVange L, Woodcock J. Multidimensional evidence generation and FDA regulatory decision making: defining and using "real-world" data. JAMA. 2017;318(8):703–4.
3. NIH. *Announcement: Access to the COVID-19 Data Analytics Platform is Open.* 2021. https://ncats.nih.gov/news/releases/2020/access-to-N3C-COVID-19-data-analytics-platform-now-open (visited on 05/06/2021).
4. 4CE. *Consortium for Clinical Characterization of COVID-19 by EHR: Members.* 2021. https://covidclinical.net/members.index.html (visited on 05/06/2021).
5. Weeks J, Pardee R. Learning to share health care data: a brief timeline of influential common data models and distributed health data networks in U.S. health care research. *eGEMs (Generating Evidence & Methods to improve patient outcomes).* 2019;7(1): 4, p. 1–7. https://doi.org/10.5334/egems.279.
6. Haendel MA, Chute CG, Bennett TD, Eichmann DA, Guinney J, Kibbe WA, Payne PR, Pfaff ER, Robinson PN, Saltz JH, Spratt H. The National COVID Cohort Collaborative (N3C): rationale, design, infrastructure, and deployment. J Am Med Inform Assoc. 2021;28(3):427–43.
7. Love D, Custer W. Miller P, 2010. All-payer claims databases: state initiatives to improve health care transparency. New York (NY): Commonwealth Fund.
8. Centers for Disease Control and Prevention. HIPAA privacy rule and public health. Guidance from CDC and the US Department of Health and Human Services. *MMWR: Morbidity and Mortality Weekly Report*, 2003;52(Suppl 1):1–17.
9. Voigt P, Von dem Bussche A. The EU general data protection regulation (GDPR). A Practical Guide, vol. 10. no. 3152676, 1st ed. Cham: Springer International Publishing; 2017. p. 10–5555.
10. D. McGraw, Building public trust in uses of Health Insurance. Portability and Accountability Act de-identified data. J Am Med Inform Assoc. 2012; https://doi.org/10.1136/amiajnl-2012-000936
11. Benitez K, Malin B. Evaluating re-identification risks with respect to the HIPAA privacy rule. J Am Med Inform Assoc. 2010;17(2):169–77. https://doi.org/10.1136/jamia.2009.000026.
12. Mazor KM, Richards A, Gallagher M, Arterburn DE, Raebel MA, Nowell WB, Curtis JR, Paolino AR, Toh S. Stakeholders' views on data sharing in multicenter studies. J Comparat Effectiveness Res. 2017;6(6):537–47.
13. Hripcsak G, Duke JD, Shah NH, Reich CG, Huser V, Schuemie MJ, Suchard MA, Park RW, Wong ICK, Rijnbeek PR, Van Der Lei J. Observational health data sciences and informatics (OHDSI): opportunities for observational researchers. Stud Health Technol Inf. 2015;216:574.
14. Suchard MA, Schuemie MJ, Krumholz HM, You SC, Chen R, Pratt N, Reich CG, Duke J, Madigan D, Hripcsak G, Ryan PB. Comprehensive comparative effectiveness and safety of first-line antihypertensive drug classes: a systematic, multinational, large-scale analysis. The Lancet. 2019;394(10211):1816–26.
15. Ball R, Robb M, Anderson SA, Dal Pan G. The FDA's sentinel initiative—a comprehensive approach to medical product surveillance. Clin Pharmacol Ther. 2016;99(3):265–8.
16. Fleurence RL, Curtis LH, Califf RM, Platt R, Selby JV, Brown JS. Launching PCORnet, a national patient-centered clinical research network. J Am Med Inform Assoc. 2014;21(4):578–82.
17. Chen RT, Glasser JW, Rhodes PH, Davis RL, Barlow WE, Thompson RS, Mullooly JP, Black SB, Shinefield HR, Vadheim CM, Marcy SM. Vaccine safety datalink project: a new tool for improving vaccine safety monitoring in the United States. Pediatrics. 1997;99(6):765–73.
18. Vogt TM, Lafata JE, Tolsma DD, Greene SM. The role of research in integrated health care systems: the HMO Research Network. Permanente J. 2004;8(4):10.
19. Nelder JA, Wedderburn RW. Generalized linear models. J Royal Stat Soc: Series A (General). 1972;135(3):370–84.
20. Cox DR. Regression models and life-tables. J Roy Stat Soc: Ser B (Methodol). 1972;34(2):187–202.
21. Oxman AD, Clarke MJ, Stewart LA. From science to practice: meta-analyses using individual patient data are needed. JAMA. 1995;274(10):845–6. https://doi.org/10.1001/jama.1995.03530100085040.
22. Riley RD, Higgins JP. Deeks JJ. 2011. Interpretation of random effects meta-analyses. BMJ, 342.
23. You SC, Rho Y, Bikdeli B, Kim J, Siapos A, Weaver J, Londhe A, Cho J, Park J, Schuemie M, Suchard MA. Association of ticagrelor vs clopidogrel with net adverse clinical events in patients with acute coronary syndrome undergoing percutaneous coronary intervention. JAMA. 2020;324(16):1640–50.
24. Vashisht R, Jung K, Schuler A, Banda JM, Park RW, Jin S, Li L, Dudley JT, Johnson KW, Shervey MM, Xu H. Association of hemoglobin A1c levels with use of sulfonylureas, dipeptidyl peptidase 4 inhibitors, and thiazolidinediones in patients with type 2 diabetes treated with metformin: analysis from the observational health data sciences and informatics initiative. JAMA Netw Open. 2018;1(4):e181755–e181755.
25. Zeng D, Lin DY. On random-effects meta-analysis. Biometrika. 2015;102(2):281–94.
26. Rassen JA, Avorn J, Schneeweiss S. Multivariate-adjusted pharmacoepidemiologic analyses of confidential information pooled from multiple health care

utilization databases. Pharmacoepidemiol Drug Saf. 2010;19(8):848–57.

27. Toh S, Reichman ME, Houstoun M, Ding X, Fireman BH, Gravel E, Levenson M, Li L, Moyneur E, Shoaibi A, Zornberg G, Hennessy S. Multivariable confounding adjustment in distributed data networks without sharing of patient-level data. Pharmacoepidemiol Drug Saf. 2013;22(11):1171–7. https://doi.org/10.1002/pds.3483. Epub 2013 Jul 23 PMID: 23878013.
28. Duan R, Luo C, Schuemie MJ, Tong J, Liang CJ, Chang HH, Boland MR, Bian J, Xu H, Holmes JH, Forrest CB. Learning from local to global: an efficient distributed algorithm for modeling time-to-event data. J Am Med Inform Assoc. 2020;27(7):1028–36.
29. Firth D. Bias reduction of maximum likelihood estimates. Biometrika. 1993;80(1):27–38.
30. Berlin JA, Santanna J, Schmid CH, Szczech LA, Feldman HI. Individual patient-versus group-level data meta-regressions for the investigation of treatment effect modifiers: ecological bias rears its ugly head. Stat Med. 2002;21(3):371–87.
31. Riley RD, Debray TP, Fisher D, Hattle M, Marlin N, Hoogland J, Gueyffier F, Staessen JA, Wang J, Moons KG, Reitsma JB. Individual participant data meta-analysis to examine interactions between treatment effect and participant-level covariates: statistical recommendations for conduct and planning. Stat Med. 2020;39(15):2115–37.
32. Fisher DJ, Carpenter JR, Morris TP, Freeman SC, Tierney JF. Meta-analytical methods to identify who benefits most from treatments: daft, deluded, or deft approach? BMJ. 2017;356: j573. https://doi.org/10.1136/bmj.j573.
33. Chen Y, Dong G, Han J, Pei J, Wah BW, Wang J. Regression cubes with lossless compression and aggregation. IEEE Trans Knowl Data Eng. 2006;18(12):1585–99.
34. Ben-Israel A. A Newton-Raphson method for the solution of systems of equations. J Math Anal Appl. 1966;15(2):243–52.
35. Wu Y, Jiang X, Kim J, Ohno-Machado L. G rid Binary LO gistic RE gression (GLORE): building shared models without sharing data. J Am Med Inform Assoc. 2012;19(5):758–64.
36. Lu CL, Wang S, Ji Z, Wu Y, Xiong L, Jiang X, Ohno-Machado L. WebDISCO: a web service for distributed cox model learning without patient-level data sharing. J Am Med Inform Assoc. 2015;22(6):1212–9.
37. Huang C, Huo X. A distributed one-step estimator. Math Program. 2019;174:41–76. https://doi.org/10.1007/s10107-019-01369-0.
38. Shu D, Yoshida K, Fireman BH, Toh S. Inverse probability weighted Cox model in multi-site studies without sharing individual-level data. Stat Methods Med Res. 2020;29(6):1668–81.
39. Riley RD, Simmonds MC, Look MP. Evidence synthesis combining individual patient data and aggregate data: a systematic review identified current practice and possible methods. J Clin Epidemiol. 2007;60(5):431–9. https://doi.org/10.1016/j.jclinepi.2006.09.009. Epub 2007 Feb 5 PMID: 17419953.
40. Duan R, Boland MR, Liu Z, Liu Y, Chang HH, Xu H, Chu H, Schmid CH, Forrest CB, Holmes JH, Schuemie MJ. Learning from electronic health records across multiple sites: a communication-efficient and privacy-preserving distributed algorithm. J Am Med Inform Assoc. 2020;27(3):376–85.
41. Jordan MI, Lee JD, Yang Y. Communication-efficient distributed statistical inference. J Am Stat Assoc. 2019;114(526):668–81. https://doi.org/10.1080/01621459.2018.1429274.
42. Edmondson MJ, Luo C, Islam MN, Sheils NE, Buresh J, Chen Z, Bian J, Chen Y. Distributed quasi-Poisson regression algorithm for modeling multi-site count outcomes in distributed data networks. J Biomed Inf. 2022;104097.
43. Edmondson MJ, Luo C, Duan R, Maltenfort M, Chen Z, Locke K, Shults J, Bian J, Ryan PB, Forrest CB, Chen Y. An efficient and accurate distributed learning algorithm for modeling multi-site zero-inflated count outcomes. Sci Rep. 2021;11(1):1–17.
44. Sutton AJ, Kendrick D, Coupland CA. Meta-analysis of individual-and aggregate-level data. Stat Med. 2008;27(5):651–69.
45. Luo C, Islam M, Sheils NE, Buresh J, Reps J, Schuemie MJ, Ryan PB, Edmondson M, Duan R, Tong J, Marks-Anglin A. DLMM as a lossless one-shot algorithm for collaborative multi-site distributed linear mixed models. Nat Commun. 2022;13(1):1–10.
46. Zhu R, Jiang C, Wang X, Wang S, Zheng H, Tang H. Privacy-preserving construction of generalized linear mixed model for biomedical computation. Bioinformatics, 2020:36(Supplement_1);i128–35.
47. Luo C, Islam MN, Sheils NE, Buresh J, Schuemie MJ, Doshi JA, Werner RM, Asch DA, Chen Y. dPQL: a lossless distributed algorithm for generalized linear mixed model with application to privacy-preserving hospital profiling. J Am Med Inf Assoc. 2022; ocac067. https://doi.org/10.1093/jamia/ocac067.
48. Tong J, Duan R, Li R, Scheuemie MJ, Moore JH, Chen Y. Robust-ODAL: learning from heterogeneous health systems without sharing patient-level data. In: Pacific symposium on biocomputing 2020, 2019; 695–706.
49. Luo C, Duan R, Naj AC, et al. ODACH: a one-shot distributed algorithm for Cox model with heterogeneous multi-center data. Sci Rep. 2022;12:6627. https://doi.org/10.1038/s41598-022-09069-0.
50. Luo X, Tsai WY. A proportional likelihood ratio model. Biometrika. 2012;99(1):211–22.
51. Tong J, Luo C, Islam MN, Sheils NE, Buresh J, Edmondson M, Merkel PA, Lautenbach E, Duan R,

Chen Y. Distributed learning for heterogeneous clinical data with application to integrating COVID-19 data across 230 sites. NPJ Dig Med. 2022;5(1):1–8.
52. Duan R, Ning Y, Chen Y. Heterogeneity-aware and communication-efficient distributed statistical inference. Biometrika. 2022;109(1):67–83.
53. Luo C, Duan R, Edmondson M, Shi J, Maltenfort M, Morris J, Forrest C, Hubbard R, Chen Y. Distributed proportional likelihood ratio model with application to data integration across clinical sites 2020.
54. Shokri R, Stronati M, Song C, Shmatikov V. Membership inference attacks against machine learning models. In 2017 IEEE symposium on security and privacy (SP). IEEE; 2017. p. 3–18.
55. Pyrgelis A, Troncoso C, De Cristofaro E. Knock knock, who's there? Membership inference on aggregate location data. 2017. ArXiv Prepr. https://arxiv.org/abs/1708.06145.
56. Dwork C, McSherry F, Nissim K, Smith A. Calibrating noise to sensitivity in private data analysis. J Priv Confidentiality. 2017;7:17–51.
57. Wasserman L, Zhou S. A statistical framework for differential privacy. J Am Stat Assoc. 2010;105:375–89.
58. Sweeney L. k-anonymity: a model for protecting privacy. Int J Uncertainty, Fuzziness Knowledge-Based Syst. 10, 557–570 (2002).
59. CMS Cell Suppression Policy, accessed April 15th, 2022. https://www.hhs.gov/guidance/document/cms-cell-suppression-policy.
60. Froelicher D, et al. Truly privacy-preserving federated analytics for precision medicine with multiparty homomorphic encryption. bioRxiv 2021.
61. Ohno-Machado L, et al. pSCANNER: patient-centered scalable national network for effectiveness research. J Am Med Inform Assoc. 2014;21:621–6.
62. Luo C, Duan R, Edmondson M, Tong J, Chen Y. pda: privacy-preserving distributed algorithms. R package version 1.0–2 2020. https://CRAN.R-project.org/package=pda.
63. Luo C, et al. pda: Privacy-Preserving Distributed Algorithms (v 1.2–4). Github. https://github.com/Penncil/pda. (Accessed on 20 Mar 2021).

Machine Learning—Basic Unsupervised Methods (Cluster Analysis Methods, t-SNE)

M. Espadoto, S. B. Martins, W. Branderhorst and A. Telea

Abstract

Understanding how trained deep neural networks achieve their inferred results is challenging but important for relating how patterns in the input data affect other patterns in the output results. We present a visual analytics approach to this problem that consists of two mappings. The so-called forward mapping shows the relative impact of user-selected input patterns to all elements of the output. The backward mapping shows the relative impact of all input elements to user-selected patterns in the output. Our approach is generically applicable to any regressor mapping between two multidimensional real-valued spaces (input to output), is simple to implement, and requires no specific knowledge of the regressor's internals. We demonstrate our method for two applications using image data—a MRI T1-to-T2 generator and a MRI-to-pseudo-CT generator.

M. Espadoto (✉)
Institute of Mathematics and Statistics, University of São Paulo, Sao Paulo, Brazil
e-mail: mespadot@ime.usp.br

S. B. Martins
Federal Institute of São Paulo, Sao Paulo, Brazil
e-mail: samuel.martins@ifsp.edu.br

W. Branderhorst
University Medical Center Utrecht, Utrecht, The Netherlands
e-mail: w.j.branderhorst@umcutrecht.nl

A. Telea
Department of Information and Computing Science, Utrecht University, Utrecht, The Netherlands
e-mail: a.c.telea@uu.nl

Keywords

Explainable AI · Sensitivity analysis · Medical image synthesis · Image-to-image transformation · Deep learning regression · Visual analytics

1 Introduction

In recent years, machine learning and in particular deep learning methods have been used in increasingly many applications. However, understanding how such trained models work is challenging, especially for the case of deep learning architectures [1, 2]. In certain domains, such as medical science, it is particularly important to gain such understanding, both for increasing the confidence and interpretability of the inferred results and also for increasing their acceptance by a wider public [3, 4].

Visual analytics (VA) tools and techniques have emerged as one of the approaches of choice in the field of Explainable Artificial Intelligence (XAI) [5–7]. However, while such methods have

F. W. Asselbergs et al. (eds.), *Clinical Applications of Artificial Intelligence in Real-World Data*,
https://doi.org/10.1007/978-3-031-36678-9_9

proven to be effective in improving training and explaining how deep learning architectures work, they have addressed comparatively far less the task of explaining how trained models achieve their inference. Moreover, such VA tools have mainly focused on explaining classifiers rather than the more general regressor models.

In this paper, we aim to fill the above gaps by proposing Instance-Based Inference Explainers (IBIX). In contrast to other VA techniques, which aim to explain how a trained model treats an entire dataset, our method focuses on explaining individual instances in such a dataset, and even user-selected parts of such instances, such as parts of images. To do this, IBIX offers two operation modes that explain (a) which parts of the inferred result (output) are most strongly affected by a user-specified part of the input; and (b) which parts of the input most strongly affect a user-selected part of the output. IBIX operates generically, requiring no knowledge of the architecture, hyperparameters, or training of a deep learned model, can be applied to any n-dimensional to m-dimensional data regressor, is simple to implement and use, and is computationally scalable. We demonstrate the use of IBIX for two deep learned regressors—a MR T1-to-T2 image synthesizer and an MRI-to-CT image synthesizer.

The structure of this paper is as follows. Section 2 discusses related work in VA techniques for deep learning engineering explanation and positions our contribution in this domain. Section 3 explains our method. Section 4 presents two applications of our method related to medical image synthesis. Section 5 discusses our contributions. Finally, Sect. 6 concludes the paper.

2 Related Work

Consider a dataset $\mathcal{D} = \{(\mathbf{x}_1, \mathbf{y}_1), \ldots, (\mathbf{x}_n, \mathbf{y}_n)\}$, where $\mathbf{x}_i \in \mathbb{R}^n$ is a sample of some high-dimensional data, e.g., an image, text document, or row in a data table; and $\mathbf{y}_i \in \mathbb{R}^m$ is a value associated with $\mathbf{x}_i$. In supervised machine learning, one typically wants to construct a function $f : \mathbb{R}^n \rightarrow \mathbb{R}^m$ so that, for a training or test set $\mathcal{D}$, $f(\mathbf{x}_i) \simeq \mathbf{y}_i, \forall (\mathbf{x}_i, \mathbf{y}_i) \in \mathcal{D}$. If we replace $\mathbb{R}^m$ by a set C of categorical labels, f becomes a *classifier*. In the general case, when the codomain f is a subset of $\mathbb{R}^m$, we speak of a *regressor*.

Deep learning (DL) is one of the (supervised) methods aiming to build models f following the above pattern. While deep neural networks (DNNs) has been advancing the state-of-the-art in a variety of domains [8–10], their nature of being *black-boxes* results in a lack of interpretability concerning their learned representations and predictions (outputs) [11]. While our methodology for explaining inference, next presented in Sect. 3, can be applied equally well to any regressor f, we limit its discussion in this paper—and thus the discussion of related work next—to DL applications.

Several visual analytics (VA) solutions have been proposed [11–15] to help practitioners understand, interpret, and improve, the working of such a model. Following a recent survey on VA methods for deep learning model engineering [6], visual explanations aim to explain one of the following parts of the common deep learning pipeline: *training*, *model*, or *inference*. We review methods in all these classes next, observing already that most such methods have been designed to help with classification models [12, 14]. Using VA tools to interpret deep generative models—the proposal of this paper—has attracted only limited attention.

2.1 Explaining Training

Using visualization during the *training process* aims to explore the training data and their learned representations, to answer questions such as which classes did train suboptimally, how are classes separable in the learned feature space, and which are hard-to-process observations. We also note that most VA work we are aware of for explaining training focuses on *classifier* models.

A common visual approach to investigate a dataset is to project its learned deep representations (feature vectors) onto two dimensions [12, 15] by a dimensionality reduction technique (e.g., t-SNE [16]). One can then plot all projected data instances as points in a scatter plot and assign a different color for each class [17–19]. This approach is also used to explain the trained model (Sect. 2.2).

Rauber et al. [17] show that the visual separability of classes in a t-SNE projection is highly correlated with the ability of a classifier to separate classes in the original feature space. Consequently, the visual inspection supports understanding poor predictions in two ways: (i) a pair of classes grouped in the 2D space can indicate class imbalance or the need for more data; and (ii) all classes mixed can indicate that the learned representations are not good enough for the addressed problem. In this sense, some methods also provide visual tools to assign labels to new data examples [19–21], especially in applications in which high-quality annotated data is absent, such as medical image analysis.

Some methods investigate the examples that the model is most uncertain or unsure about [20, 22, 23]. When analyzing these so-called *hard examples*, one can have insights on the model's inference (e.g., misprediction). For example, a hard example may have been incorrectly labeled, or it may have different patterns than others in its class, or it may be an outlier. To improve the model's accuracy, one can then retrain the model, for example, by assigning a different weight for each training example [24].

One common approach to visually investigate hard examples is to retrieve the original data (e.g., images) associated to specific projected data points in a 2D scatter plot [12, 15, 18, 25]. The user may then visually inspect the original data of points from different classes which are grouped in the projected space. On the other hand, *active learning* (AL) strategies automatically search for hard examples by selecting those near the model's decision boundaries and asking the user for feedback (e.g., labels) to improve the learning model [22, 23, 26]. Bernard et al. [20] proposes a visual-interactive labeling (VIAL) that unifies both approaches to make labeling more efficient. VIAL uses AL-based methods to leverage visual interactive interfaces for the analysis, for example, presenting hard examples to the user.

2.2 Explaining the Model

This class of visual methods enables users to explore intrinsic characteristics of the learned model such as its learned parameters [13, 27, 28] and architecture [29–31]. Visualizing such information helps model developers troubleshoot and further improve their models [11, 13, 29, 32]. Explaining the model consists of answering questions such as: How do the weight patterns correlate with specific architecture layers? How do activations (for each class) look? What types of latent features are learned by specific model layers?

VA solutions visualize model architectures commonly using a *computational graph* in which nodes represent neurons and weighted edges represent connections between a pair of neurons [29–31, 33]. One can also encode the weight magnitude using color or link thickness [12]. This design is taken by TensorBoard [31], a popular VA tool that visualizes learning curves during training and displays images generated by the trained model. Wongsuphasawat et al. [30] present a design study of the network architecture visualization from TensorBoard. Drawing computational graphs does not scale well for production-size architectures having millions of links. To address this, Liu et al. [29] use a bi-clustering-based edge bundling technique to reduce visual clutter caused by too many links.

Visualizing the learned filters (weights) allows investigating what a deep model has learned for a given problem—e.g., which filters are responsible for separating a class from others [27, 33]. SUMMIT [34] analyzes activation patterns by visualizing the interaction between the learned features and the model's predictions.

Other methods aim to investigate how *neuron activations* respond to particular classes throughout the network [13, 33, 35]. ActiVis [36] represents the model architecture as a graph (nodes are operations) from which users can visualize activation patterns at each layer and for each class by an interactive table view (columns are neurons and rows are activation instances). The tool displays also a 2D projection of instance activations colored according to their classes. Rauber et al. [13] also project activations to investigate the relationships between neurons. Other techniques map neuron activations to the input pixel space to display patterns recognized by the deep model [33, 35, 37].

Several techniques aim to explain what is the role of each network layer in the model inference [14]. Using such techniques, one could find that, in deep learning images, lower layers create representations of simple features (e.g., edges) while higher layers contain specific information about classes [38–40]. Other VA tools support finding stable layers—that learned a stable set of patterns—and layers that do not contribute to solving a given classification problem [28].

A few VA tools have aimed to explain generative adversarial networks (GANs) by exploring their internal structures. Gan Lab [41] is an interactive tool designed for non-experts to learn and experiment with GAN models. DGMTracker [42] and GANViz [43] aim to explain the training dynamics of GANs, e.g., by visualizing their neural activations, to help developers better train the models.

2.3 Explaining the Inference

The third and final class of VA methods, to which our proposal also belongs, aims to explain how outputs $f(\mathbf{x})$ of a trained model f depend on the input instances $\mathbf{x}$.

Saliency maps [27, 39, 44–47] are likely the most used and best known visual tool for inference explanation. For models whose inputs $\mathbf{x}$ are images, they mark each pixel $\mathbf{p} \in \mathbf{x}$ with a value indicating $\mathbf{p}$'s contribution, or influence, to the decision $f(\mathbf{x})$.

Also for image-processing networks, Zeiler and Fergus [27] used *deconvolutional networks*, as proposed in [35], to project learned feature activations to the input image space. This allows users to debug the deep model by visualizing the learned features from specific layers, with multiple variations of the technique being proposed afterwards [12]. Zhou et al. [44] propose Class Activation Mapping (CAM), a technique that shows the discriminative active region in an image for a given label. Selvaraju et al. [45] presented its relaxed generalization, Grad-CAM, which uses label-specific gradients to calculate the importance of spatial locations in convolutional layers.

All methods so far presented generate visual explanations based on components of the learned DNNs, such as their architectures and activations. Despite presenting impressive results for many problems [12], these visual methods are designed for a restricted class of DNNs. In contrast, a different approach, referred as *reverse engineering* [48], only uses the input $\mathbf{x}$ and inference $f(\mathbf{x})$ of the deep model without exploiting any model internals. For a learned deep model, this approach applies a *random perturbation* to the input and compares its inference with the unperturbed one [48]. One can then create visual explanations, e.g., a heatmap, from this comparison. Note that this approach is independent of the kind of DNN.

Bazzani et al. [49] use the reverse engineering approach for weakly supervised object detection. Given a pre-trained deep model designed for image classification, their method analyzes the degeneration in classification scores when artificially perturbing different regions of the image by masking them out. The masked regions that significantly drop the classification scores are considered as including the target objects. Other object detection methods use a similar strategy [50, 51].

Our proposed framework follows the reverse engineering approach when creating a heatmap from comparing the original inference and the perturbed one. This heatmap shows which parts of the inference—e.g., a reconstructed image by a generative neural network—have been influenced by input variables selected by the user and vice versa. This allows for a fine-grained study of how specific sets of output variables are affected by perturbations to input variables.

A distinctive attribute of our framework is that it enables the study of black-box models having continuous multivariate *inputs and outputs*, such as autoencoders and GANs. This is in stark contrast with most existing techniques described earlier, that either seek to explain single-output classification models, or require the use of internal structures of the network to derive an explanation of the model. This makes our framework particularly suitable for understanding models created for image transformation, for example, but not limited to those. Our framework can work with different types of models, regardless of their internal structure, as long as they have n inputs and m outputs, both real-valued, as detailed next.

3 IBIX Method

3.1 Definitions

Let $\mathbf{x} \in \mathbb{R}^n$ be an input sample, such as a n-dimensional feature vector or a grayscale image having n pixels. Let $f : \mathbb{R}^n \to \mathbb{R}^m$ be the learned model by a deep neural network. Note that the output space (and its dimensionality m) need not be identical to the input space (and its dimensionality n). We next denote $\mathbf{x} = (x_1, \ldots, x_n)$, i.e., $x_i \in \mathbb{R}$ is the ith component of the n-dimensional vector $\mathbf{x}$. Similarly, if $f(\mathbf{x}) = (y_1, \ldots, y_m)$, then let $f_i : \mathbb{R}^n \to \mathbb{R}$, $f_i(\mathbf{x}) = y_i$, be the ith component of the function f. Note that f_i is a real-valued function with n variables.

Let $M^{\mathbf{x}}$ be a region in $\mathbf{x}$, i.e., a subset of components of $\mathbf{x}$ that we are next interested to analyze. For example, if $\mathbf{x}$ is a 2D image, then $M^{\mathbf{x}}$ is a mask that we draw on the image to select some of its pixels. Formally, $M^{\mathbf{x}}$ can be modeled as an indicator with ones for the selected variables (pixels) x_i and zero elsewhere. That is, $M^{\mathbf{x}} \in \{0, 1\}^n$. Hence, $M = (M_1^{\mathbf{x}}, \ldots M_n^{\mathbf{x}})$ so that $M_i^{\mathbf{x}} = 1$ if variable x_i is selected and zero otherwise. Similarly, for the output, let M^f be a region in $f(I)$. Intuitively, M^f allows us to mark components of $f(\mathbf{x})$ that we want to 'trace back' to the input $\mathbf{x}$. Just as $M^{\mathbf{x}}, M^f \in \{0, 1\}^m$ can be modeled as an indicator. That is, $M^f = (M_1^f, \ldots M_m^f)$ so that M_i^f is one if output component $f_i(\mathbf{x})$ is selected for analysis and zero otherwise.

3.2 Forward Mapping

As outlined in Sect. 1, the first goal of out IBIX method is to visually explain how much specific parts of the input $\mathbf{x}$—more precisely, those marked by the user in a mask $M^{\mathbf{x}}$—affect the output $f(\mathbf{x})$. We call this a *forward mapping* and denote it as $F(M^{\mathbf{x}})$. Formally put, $F(M^{\mathbf{x}}) = (F_1, \ldots, F_m)$ with $F_j \in [0, 1]$, $1 \le j \le m$. That is, $F(M^{\mathbf{x}})$ is a weight vector, with one value F_j per output dimension.

We compute $F(M^{\mathbf{x}})$ by perturbing, or jittering, the marked part $M^{\mathbf{x}}$ of the input sample $\mathbf{x}$, passing the perturbed data through f, and seeing how much $f(\mathbf{x})$ has changed. The intuition behind this idea is simple: If changing the marked area of $\mathbf{x}$ does not affect the inferred value $f(\mathbf{x})$, then the respective input part can be seen as neglected by the regressor. Conversely, if a small change to the marked area strongly affects $f(\mathbf{x})$, then the regressor has somehow learned to be very sensitive to the respective input part. When the two above situations occur, it is the user who has to decide if neglect or high-sensitivity are desirable behavior or not for the regressor, depending on the actual location of $M^{\mathbf{x}}$ and variation of $F(M^{\mathbf{x}})$.

Computing $F(M^{\mathbf{x}})$ consists of two steps, as follows.

Single perturbation: Consider a (small) jitter value $h \in \mathbb{R}$. Let $\Delta\mathbf{x} = hM^{\mathbf{x}}$, that is, a vector which is zero outside the region $M^{\mathbf{x}}$ and equal to h inside $M^{\mathbf{x}}$, respectively. With it, we compute $f(\mathbf{x} + \Delta\mathbf{x})$, i.e., the model's response to the input $\mathbf{x}$ jittered by $\Delta\mathbf{x}$, normalized by the change size. We denote this normalized change by a vector $F^h(M^{\mathbf{x}}) = (F_1^h, \ldots, F_m^h)$, where

$$F_j^h = \frac{f_j(\mathbf{x} + \Delta\mathbf{x}) - f_j(\mathbf{x})}{h}, \quad 1 \le j \le m. \quad (1)$$

If h is small, F_j^h is the sum of the components of the forward finite-difference-approximated gradient of f_j that considers only the variables selected by $M^{\mathbf{x}}$. This is analogous to taking the derivative of f_j in the direction given by the n-dimensional unit vector corresponding to the ones in $M^{\mathbf{x}}$, i.e.

$$F_j^h \simeq \frac{\partial f_j}{\partial M^{\mathbf{x}}}. \quad (2)$$

As the directional derivative is linked to the gradient of a function by the dot product

$$\frac{\partial f_j}{\partial M^{\mathbf{x}}} = \nabla f_j \cdot M^{\mathbf{x}}, \quad (3)$$

it follows that

$$F_j^h \simeq \sum_{1 \le i \le n | M_i^{\mathbf{x}}=1} \frac{\partial f_j}{\partial x_i}. \quad (4)$$

where $\frac{\partial f_j}{\partial x_i}$ is the partial derivative of f_j with respect to the variable x_i.

Multiscale perturbation: To eliminate the effect of the choice of the jitter size h, we evaluate Eq. 1 for a N zero-centered, uniformly-spaced, jitters $h_k = kH/N$, with $-N \le k \le N$, where H is an application-dependent parameter specifying the maximum jitter, set typically to 10 to 20% of the norm of the input signal $\mathbf{x}$. The final forward mapping is then computed as

$$F(M^{\mathbf{x}}) = \frac{1}{2N} \sum_{-N \le k \le N} F^{h_k}(M^{\mathbf{x}}), \quad (5)$$

that is, the average of the responses for all perturbations h_k. Note that, conceptually, Eq. 5 is equivalent to computing a scale-space version of the directional derivative in Eq. 2. Intuitively, $F(M^{\mathbf{x}})$ will be large for output components of f which are strongly affected by changes in input variables selected in $M^{\mathbf{x}}$, and conversely.

3.3 Backward Mapping

The second goal of our IBIX method is to visually explain how much all variables in $\mathbf{x}$ affect a part of $f(\mathbf{x})$ that is selected by some mask M^f. By analogy to the forward mapping $F(M^{\mathbf{x}})$ in Sect. 3.2, we call this the *backward mapping* and denote it by $B(M^f)$. Formally put, $B(M^f) = (B_1, \ldots, B_n)$ with $B_j \in [0, 1]$, $1 \le j \le n$. That is, $B(M^f)$ is a weight vector, with one value B_j per input variable.

Unlike $F(M^{\mathbf{x}})$, we cannot compute $B(M^f)$ directly since we do not have the inverse function f^{-1} of our deep learned model. Hence, we proceed differently: We partition the input space of n variables into a set of K block regions D_k, $1 \le k \le K$. Intuitively, if $\mathbf{x}$ is an image, the blocks D_k can be seen as a tessellation of $\mathbf{x}$ into so-called superpixels. Each block D_k acts as a region mask $M^{\mathbf{x}}$ for the input $\mathbf{x}$. Next, we compute for each block D_k the forward mapping $F(D_k)$ using Eq. 5. Subsequently, we define the backward mapping from the mask M^f in the output space to block D_k in the input space, denoted as B_{D_k}, as the fraction of the integral of the forward mapping $F(B_k)$ that falls within M_f, i.e.,

$$B_{D_k} = \frac{\sum_{1 \le i \le m | M_i^f=1} F(D_k)_i}{\sum_{1 \le i \le m} F(D_k)_i}, \quad 1 \le k \le K. \quad (6)$$

Note that, if the blocks D_k are of unit size, i.e., the input space is partitioned into $K = n$ blocks, one per input variable x_k, and we consider a single scale h in Eq. 5, then $F(D_k)_i = \frac{\partial f_i}{\partial x_k}$. Then, for x_k, we get the backward mapping expression as

$$B_k = \sum_{1 \le i \le m | M_i^f=1} \frac{\partial f_i}{\partial x_k}. \quad (7)$$

That is, the value of the inverse mapping B at input variable k is the sum of all partial derivatives of f with respect to x_k for all components that are marked one in the mask M^f.

The forward mapping (Eq. 4) and the backward mapping (Eq. 7) have similar expressions—both are sums of partial derivatives, the difference being the indices that vary and the ones that are fixed. However, evaluating the backward mapping is more costly, since, in Eqs. 6 and 7, we sum over all dimensions i selected in the output-mask M^f. For each such dimension, we need to evaluate the full forward mapping F (Eq. 6) or, if we use the notation in Eq. 7, a partial derivative. The problem is that a typical DL model implementation does not let one 'selectively' evaluate a single output component f_i; we need to evaluate *all* the m output components even if some fall outside the mask M^f. In contrast, for the forward mapping (Eq. 4), we sum over all input variables marked as one in the input mask $M^{\mathbf{x}}$. This can be done very efficiently simply by changing the respective inputs of the neural network.

Following the above, computing the backward mapping is K times more expensive than computing the forward mapping, where K is the number of blocks used to represent the input space. Using fewer blocks (low K) accelerates computing this mapping but creates a low resolution understanding of how input variables affect the output region M^f—all variables in a block are seen as 'acting together' to influence the output. Conversely, using more blocks is slower, but gives a fine-grained understanding of how output dimensions in M^f depend on input variables—in the limit, for $K = n$, we see how how every single variable of $\mathbf{x}$ contributes to outputs in M^f. We discuss efficient ways to trade off computational speed *vs* insight resolution further in Sect. 4.1.2.

4 Explainer Applications

Our IBIX framework (Sect. 3) can be used to explain any $\mathbb{R}^n$ to $\mathbb{R}^m$ regressor, whether implemented by deep learning or not. The required adaptations for this are (1) defining ways to select the regions of interest $M^{\mathbf{x}}$ and M^f; (2) defining the jitter range H (Sect. 3.2); and (3) suitably visualizing the direct and inverse mappings F and B. We next illustrate IBIX on different deep learning applications: two image-to-image regressors for medical data (Sects. 4.1 and 4.2).

4.1 Explaining Autoencoders

We considered the generation of MR-T2 brain images (Fig. 1b) from MR-T1 brain images (Fig. 1a) using convolutional autoencoders (CAEs) [52]. This use-case is of interest when one wants to simulate the effect of a T2 scan but only avails of T1 scans as input data.

Figure 1a presents the CAE architecture we used, having three 2D convolutional layers with 16, 8, and 8 filters of 3×3 weights each, followed by ReLU activation [53] and 2D max-pooling in the encoder. The decoder contains the corresponding reconstruction operations. The model is trained to minimize mean squared error (MSE) between the generated and target T2 images using the *nadam* gradient optimizer [54].

We trained the CAE using the CamCan public dataset [55], which has 653 pairs of 3D MR-T1 brain images of 3 Tesla from healthy men and women between 18 and 88 years. For each 3D MR-T1 image, CamCan also has a corresponding 3D MR-T2 image. To our knowledge, CamCan is the largest public dataset with 3D images of healthy subjects acquired from different scanners.

We applied typical MRI noise reduction and bias field correction to all MR-T1 and MR-T2 images. Next, we registered the images to the same MNI template [56]. Since the considered CAE only supports 2D images, we extracted the central 2D axial slice from all 3D images to build our final training set (Fig. 1b, c). Each training instance is therefore an 8-bit grayscale 2D image: pixels' intensities within [0, 255]. Training the CAE reached mean squared errors around 0.0052 in the training set after 500 epochs with a batch size of 32. The trained model and preprocessed data are available online for replication purposes (https://github.com/hisamuka/IBIX-CAE).

4.1.1 Visual Explanation of CAE

We next used IBIX to explain the CAE MR-T1 to MR-T2 autoencoder. In this case, both inputs and outputs of the CAE function f are grayscale images, both of $m = n = 232 \times 200$ pixels. Hence, the masks $M^{\mathbf{x}}$ and M^f are binary images of the same size. To view and manipulate such images, we designed the user interface (Fig. 2) which is based on the *napari* image viewer [57]. The tool allows users to select an input MR-T1 image $\mathbf{x}$, run it through the trained CAE f, display the output MR-T2 $f(\mathbf{x})$, and, most importantly, paint regions $M^{\mathbf{x}}$ (in the input), respectively M^f (in the output), and next compute and visualize the forward and backward mappings F and B as heatmaps.

Figure 3 shows how IBIX works for the CAE problem. Images (a1) and (a2) show an MR-T1 input $\mathbf{x}$ and its CAE-synthesized MR-T2 output $f(\mathbf{x})$, respectively. In (b1), the user selected a single pixel region $M^{\mathbf{x}}$ in the input (marked red, see also inset). Image (b2) shows the *forward mapping F* of this single pixel using a heat colormap: Warm regions are output pixels which strongly change upon small changes of the (red) input pixel.

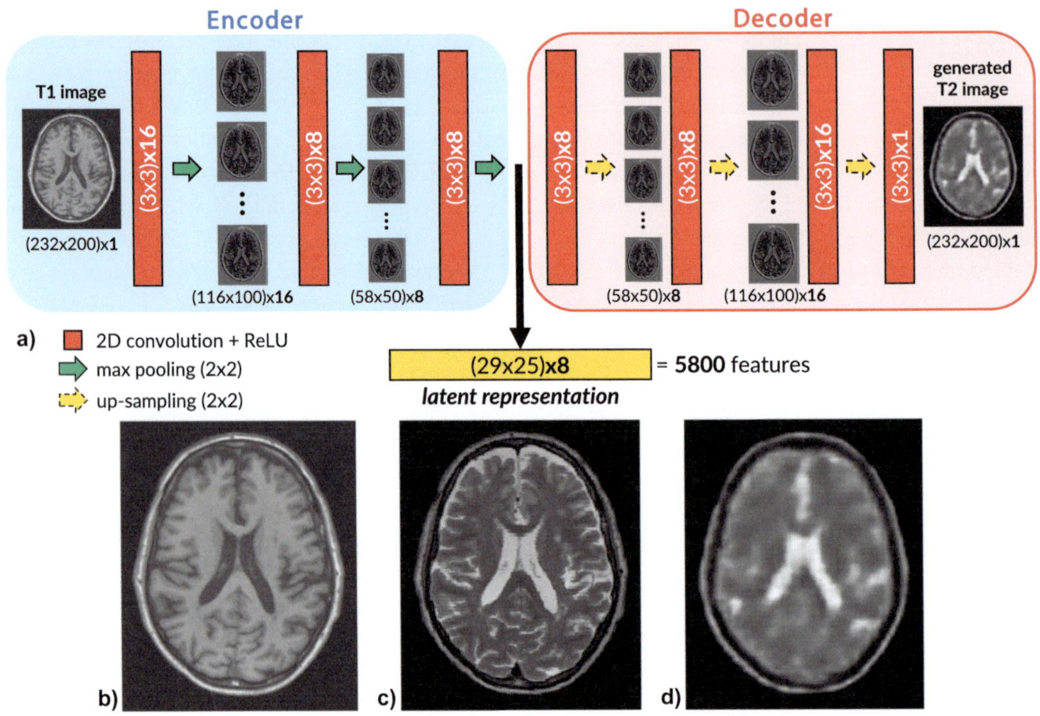

Fig. 1 **a** Architecture of the MR-T1 to MR-T2 convolutional autoencoder. The autoencoder is trained to generate the target MR-T2 brain image (**b**) from the input MR-T1 brain image (**a**). Output generated MR-T2 image shown in (**c**). See Sect. 4.1

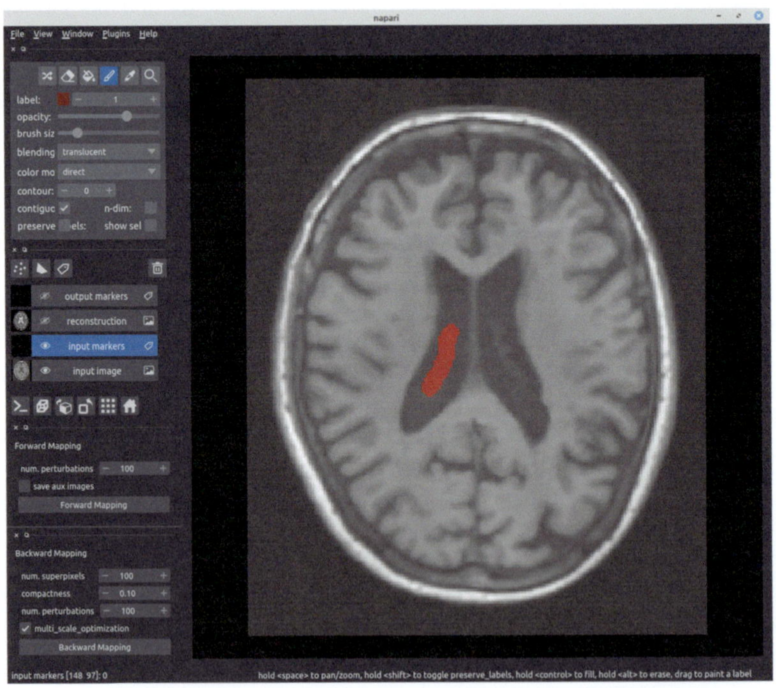

Fig. 2 User interface for the IBIX explainer with user-marked region in red

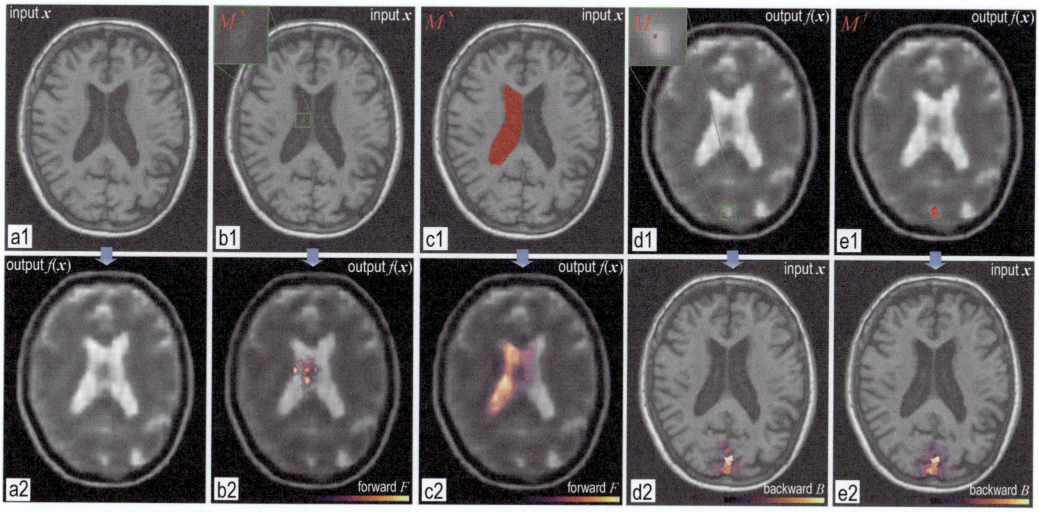

Fig. 3 Images (a1) and (a2) show an MR-T1 input and its CAE-synthesized MR-T2 output image, respectively. Images (b–c) and (d–e) show next the CAE forward, respectively backward, mappings (Sect. 4.1.1)

We see that these are close to the location of the red input—which is desired, since the MR-T1 to MR-T2 mapping should be *spatially coherent*. That is, a region **x** in the MR-T1 input is supposed to influence only *close* regions in the MR-T2 output. However, the forward mapping F (image b2) shows a non-linear 'response' shape to the single-selected input pixel in (b1) consisting of roughly six closely-packed peaks. This indicates some potential problems of the CAE training. Image (c1) shows a more complex input selection $M^{\mathbf{x}}$ consisting of the left ventricle. Image (c2) shows that this input region affects mostly left-ventricle pixels in the output, albeit with a limited 'leak' to the right ventricle. This is definitely desirable, since large-scale structures such as the ventricle are not supposed to appear fundamentally differently in MR-T1 and MR-T2 images. For both forward mapping examples, we considered 100 zero-centered, uniformly-spaced, jitters within $[-100, 100]$; that is, $N = H = 100$ for multiscale perturbation (Sect. 3.2).

Image (d1) shows the *backward mapping*: Here, we selected a single pixel (red, M^f) in the MR-T2 output. Image (d2) shows the regions in the corresponding MR-T1 input, as defined by *superpixels*, that strongly influenced the selected output region. As desired, these regions are located close to and around the selected pixel. Image (e1) extends this test by selecting a larger output region. In image (e2) we see that the backward mapping highlights input pixels close to and around the selected structure, which is desirable. In both examples, we used the popular SLIC algorithm [58] for superpixel segmentation due to its robustness and simplicity. We extracted $K = 500$ superpixels for evaluation with compactness value of 0.1. These numbers guarantee reasonable small-scale superpixels—which are desirable for a fine-grained understanding (Sect. 3.3)—but demands considerable processing times. We considered the same 100 jitters used for forwarding mapping.

Summarizing the use of IBIX for this example: Ideally, we want both the forward (F) and backward (B) mappings to be *localized*, i.e., when selecting a region in one of the (input or output) spaces, we see that a similar-location-and-shape region is responsible for that. If not, the CAE would have learned to 'couple' anatomically unrelated regions, which is clearly undesirable. Still, images (b1-b2) show that the CAE exhibits a certain amount of *diffusion*—small-scale structures can have a relatively strong effect at a certain distance from them in the output.

We tested the speed of IBIX on an AMD Ryzen 7 3700X 8-Core PC with 16 GB RAM with an NVIDIA Titan XP 12 GB GPU. Performing a for-

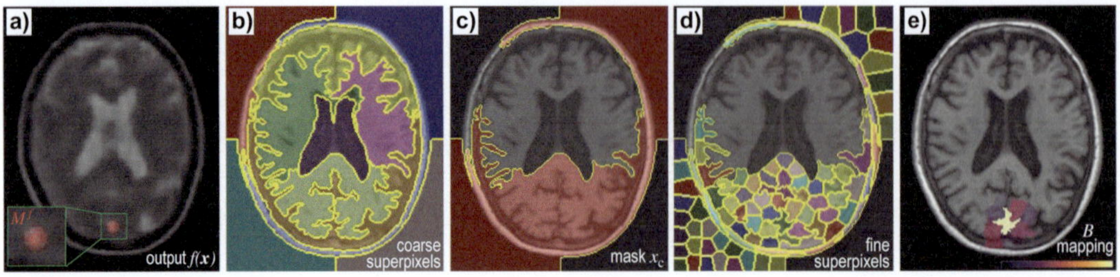

Fig. 4 Multiscale CAE optimization. From markers (M^f) drawn on the output (**a**), we first perform backward mapping on a coarse scale using just a few superpixels (**b**). We next locate superpixels having high B values (**c**) and refine the computation by segmenting only these on a finer-scale (**d**). Figure (**e**) shows the final backward mapping

ward mapping is *fast*, taking about 0.33 sec regardless the input selection size (i.e., the number of painted pixels in $M^{\mathbf{x}}$). Using $K = 500$ superpixels, performing a backward mapping takes about 174 seconds, roughly 500 times more than forward mapping (see also Sect. 3.3). This high processing time makes an interactive user experience unfeasible. When parallelizing the backward mapping—i.e., running its K forward mappings (500 in our case) in parallel (see Sect. 3.3)—computing is nearly halved: 97 s. Section 4.1.2 presents another optimization strategy to further speed up backward mapping.

4.1.2 Optimizing Backward Mapping

The standard superpixel segmentation method we use [58] allows one to control the size of superpixels but typically produces similar-size superpixels for an entire image. Hence, to get a high resolution of the backward mapping, we need to segment the input image $\mathbf{x}$ in a high number of superpixels, e.g., $K = 500$, each of which is next forward-mapped, yielding an overall slow method, as mentioned in Sect. 4.1.1. We observe that several of these superpixels are far from the markers M^f or even out of the brain. We also observe that, in general, the backward mapping is *localized*, i.e., B has high values over $\mathbf{x}$ only over *small* image extents, which are also typically close to M^f.

We use the above observations to accelerate the backward mapping B computation by a multiscale strategy, as follows. Consider Fig. 4, where image (a) shows the region M^f marked in the output. We first compute the backward mapping B using a coarse segmentation of the input $\mathbf{x}$ into a few superpixels $K_c \ll K$, where K is the number of fine-scale superpixels deemed small enough by the user for a good resolution. In our example, we use $K_c = 10$ coarse-scale superpixels, shown in Fig. 4b. We next compute B on these K_s superpixels as outlined in Sect. 3.3. Let $\mathbf{x}^c$ be the subset of the image $\mathbf{x}$ covered by coarse-scale superpixels having a B value over a user-specified threshold (Fig. 4c, red area). We next segment $\mathbf{x}_c$ into K_f fine-scale superpixels (Fig. 4d) and use these to compute the final backward mapping (Fig. 4e).

Several remarks are due, as follows. The total processing time of this multiscale strategy depends on the total superpixel count $K_c + K_f$ used for the coarse, respective fine, scales. Note that $K_f < K$ where K would be the number of superpixels used by the single-scale strategy (Sect. 3.3), since only a *subset* of the input $\mathbf{x}$ is segmented on the fine scale—red area in Fig. 4. In the example in Fig. 4, the fine-scale superpixels are roughly of the same size as the $K = 500$ superpixels needed to cover the entire image with the single-scale strategy. However, $K_f = 100$ and $K_c = 10$, so we have only 110 superpixels to treat instead of the 500 ones in the single-scale strategy. Using parallelization of the forward mapping (Sect. 3.3), the multiscale computation scheme needs only 24 seconds instead of 174 seconds (single-scale, sequential) or 94 seconds (single-scale, parallelized).

4.2 Explaining MRI-to-CT Generators

Besides MR-to-MR image generators (Sect. 4.1), medical imaging scientists have also been concerned with generating synthetic CT images from

MRI scans [59, 60]. This is useful e.g. in the context of MR-guided radiotherapy where one needs to examine the anatomy (typically best seen in a CT scan) for online position verification and dose planning of the radiotherapy [61]. Such applications are an important beneficiary of explainable AI (XAI) methods such as ours [7].

For MRI-to-CT generation for pelvis scans, Maspero et al. [62] have recently shown good results using Generative Adversarial Networks (GANs). GANs are a class of generative models that train by framing the problem as a supervised learning one with two sub-models: A *generator* model is trained to generate new examples; a *discriminator* model tries to classify examples as either real (from the domain) or fake (generated) ones. The two models are trained together in a zero-sum (adversarial) game until the discriminator model is fooled about half the time, meaning that the generator model can create plausible examples. For their task, Maspero et al. have used the Pix2Pix model [63], which is a GAN originally proposed for transferring image styles between two different domains, e.g., real picture to cartoons or satellite maps to blueprint maps.

In our work, we used a similar model to Maspero et al. to synthesize CT images from the head-and-neck and pelvis regions, as follows. The input image $\mathbf{x}$ is a set of 3 transaxial 2D image slices (480^2 pixels) obtained by taking the water, fat and in-phase images from a T2 TSE mDixon MRI sequence. Similar to [62], we did not use the fourth channel (out-phase) in this study. From each slice, a 256^2 pixel sub-image was extracted at a random location, clipped to the range between 0 and the 95% percentile, and then normalized to $[-1, 1]$. These images are further used for training our network. Figure 5a, c show two examples of such images. The scans are registered using Elastix [64, 65] to the ground-truth (GT), which are CT scans of the same patients. CT values are clipped to the $[-1024, 1250]$ HU range and then normalized to $[-1, 1]$. Figure 5b, d show two examples corresponding to the MRI scans in images (a,c). Two separate models are trained for the head-and-neck (60 scans) and pelvis (13 scans) regions, respectively. The *generator* model uses a U-NET architecture [66] using, for the encoder, 8 convolutional layers with 64, 128, 256, and 512 (last 5 layers) filters, each being a 4×4 filter applied with stride 2, and downsampling factor of 2; and for the decoder 8 convolutional layers with 512 (first 5 layers), 256, 128, and 64 filters and corresponding upsampling parameters to the encoder. The model is trained with L1 loss. The *discriminator* uses the Markov PatchGAN [63] that only penalizes structure at the scale of $N \times N$ pixel patches, with $N = 70$ pixels. As in Pix2Pix, the discriminator is run convolutionally across patches over the entire image, averaging all local responses to provide the final output, i.e., whether the generator creates real or fake images. Convolutions are 4×4 spatial filters applied with a stride of 2 and downsample factor of 2.

The above GAN achieves good results—a mean average error (MAE) between the predicted and ground-truth CT of 271.22 HU for air (< -200 HU), 56.67 HU for soft tissue ($-200 \ldots +200$ HU) and 311.74 HU for bone ($> +200$ HU) and a mean structural similarity index (SSIM [67]) between the two images of 0.89. However, subtle errors occur in the prediction. Figure 5e, h show two ground-truth CT scans of the head-and-neck region, with corresponding predicted images in (f, i) and ground-truth-*vs*-prediction errors color-coded in images (g, j)—white indicates no difference; blue indicates predicted value lower than GT value; and red indicates predicted value higher than GT value, respectively. Soft-tissue regions are, overall, predicted well. Yet, we see some 'bone loss' (blue arrows). We also see some 'fake bone' tissues being created by the prediction (red arrow A, image (i)) as well as small-scale cavities being filled up with tissue (other three red arrows, image (i)). Apart from that, we see a more general smoothing (or loss) of small-scale details.

Although we experimented with various ways of tuning of the GAN to decrease such artifacts, including hyperparameter grid search, we could not consistently eliminate them. As such, obtaining insights how the output (CT) structures depend on the input ones and, more importantly, on the

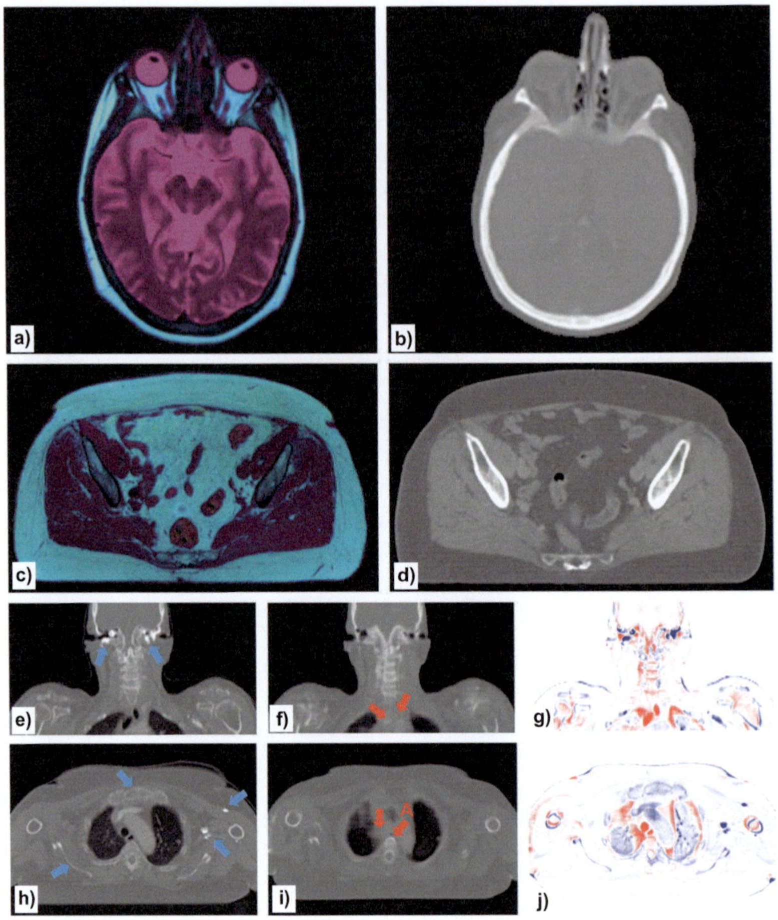

Fig. 5 Training data for the MRI to CT generation. **a**, **c** MRI 3-channel scans (water, fat, in phase) coded as RGB images; **b**, **d** CT scans of the same patients. **e**, **h** True CT scans with **f**, **i** synthetic CT reconstructions and **g**, **j** differences between the two (white = no difference; blue = pseudo-CT lower than true CT, see also blue arrows in (**e**, **h**); red = pseudo-CT higher than true CT, see also red arrows in (**f**, **i**). See Sect. 4.2

actual underlying anatomical details, is an important step to further tuning the prediction. For this, we use IBIX (see next Fig. 6).

We proceed as follows. Since the prediction errors are *small-scale* structures, we only select a few pixels in $M^{\mathbf{x}}$, respectively M^f. Also, we repeat the selection for close spatial locations in the input, respectively output, e.g., images (a–c) and (d–f). By comparing the obtained mappings F and B, we can better understand how the model learned the inference for such structures. For the forward mapping F, e.g., images (a–c), we show the region in the MRI input around the selection $M^{\mathbf{x}}$ as a small inset top-right in the respective images. The main image shows the output CT scan, overlaid by F, color-coded by a heatmap. For clarity, we also show F in the top-left inset. For the backward mapping, e.g., images (d–f), we use the same selection as in the corresponding forward mapping, i.e., $M^f = M^{\mathbf{x}}$, so we do not need to show this selection again. The main image shows the input MRI scan, overlaid by B, color-coded by a blue-to-yellow colormap. For clarity, we also show B in the top-left inset.

We next examine four different situations observed during the CT prediction, as follows.

Well-predicted bone: For this case, we want to understand how the model proceeded when achieving good prediction. Images (a-c) show three closely located selected pixel areas (yellow in the top-right insets) inside a vertebra structure, the latter seen as dark blue in the MR images in the insets. This structure is quite well predicted visible as the V-shaped light-gray area in the predicted images. The first (a) and last (c) selected areas are smaller than the middle one (b). We see that the forward mappings F match very well the expected shape of the bone—the hot-colored areas do not 'leak' out of the light-gray area, meaning that the selected bone pixels are used, indeed, only to predict bone in the same structure. Also, we see that the middle mapping F (image (b)) has a larger hot-spot than the other two. This is expected, since its selection—yellow in image (b)—is larger and more intense. If we look at the inverse mappings B for the same selections, we see a few bright-colored (yellow) superpixels in images (d–f). These are also quite closely located to the selected pixels. Hence, the predicted bone pixels are caused mainly by bone pixels in the same structure in the input MRI. In other words, the prediction is *localized* and follows the expected bone anatomy.

Poorly-predicted bone: As shown in Fig. 5e, h, some small-scale bone structures in the GT are missed by the model. To explain why this is the case, we select three pixel zones close to such a bone structure, visible as the dark ring in the MRI insets in Fig. 6g–i. Again, the middle selection (h) is larger than the other two. The forward mappings in images (g–i) show heatmaps that are located close to the ring structure, but do not closely follow its shape, being rather blurry. In all three maps, the region inside the ring is also marked by the heatmaps as being predicted by the small (yellow) selected areas which are on the bone proper. Hence, the model 'blurs out' the small-scale bone information. As a result, the bone itself is not visible in the output CTs. Again, the mapping for the larger selection (h) is stronger than the other two. This is an expected effect, since a larger selected input zone will affect a larger zone in the output. The backward mappings (images j–l) show a similar effect—the selected output pixels are affected by the entire area around the selected zone—that is, both by the elements marked dark in the MRI insets in (g–i) but also surrounding, brighter, pixels. Since the bone structure there is very thin, blurring occurs, i.e., the model 'averages' the bone with the surrounding softer tissues in its prediction. In other words, both the forward and backward mappings show that the trained model apparently understands that the pixels inside the ring pattern belong to the same structure, but it does not apply the same intensity value as in the well predicted bone. We conclude that the network looks at local structure, and could be improved if it would be trained to use information from other similar bones in a different and/or more distant location.

Well-predicted cavities: As shown in Fig. 5e–i, air-filled cavities inside the tissue—black in those images—are well predicted. It is interesting to examine this further. Images (m–o) show such a cavity in the MRI input (insets) in which we, again, selected three pixel areas with the middle one (n) larger than the other two. The forward mappings show heatmaps which are very high close to the selected pixels (central pink dot in the respective heatmaps) but also contain a 'ring' of high F values close to the air-tissue interface, i.e., where the black hole touches the surrounding gray pixels. This means that the model used the selected air pixels to predict both air pixels but also the *borders* of the entire air cavity. Interestingly, the heatmaps are black (zero) in the cavity outside the selected pixels themselves. By definition of F (Sect. 3.2), this means that small changes in the air values in the input MRI will not affect the prediction of air in the output CT. This is a desirable result as it shows that the model is resistant to noise present in the input in low-HU areas. In other words, if the network had been sensitive to small-scale variations of the acquired intensity in low-HU areas, it would have had a hard time predicting the air cavity as all being the same tissue type—air, that is. However, our forward mapping show that this was not the case since the perturbations IBIX applies only affect a subset of the local pixels *inside* the cavity and the homogeneous HU value of air was apparently not due to deviating noisy pixels being constrained by the prediction of other pixels in the cavity. The backward mappings (p,r) show a similar insight: In the insets, we see a value slightly higher than the surroundings in for the cavity, visible as the whitish-light-blue color surrounded by dark blue. This shows (1) that predicted CT cavity correctly only depends on the actual cavity recorded in the MRI data and (2) this prediction is robust to noise. Indeed, by definition of the backward mapping (Sect. 3.3), a low value of B indicates that the output will not change much when the input changes slightly.

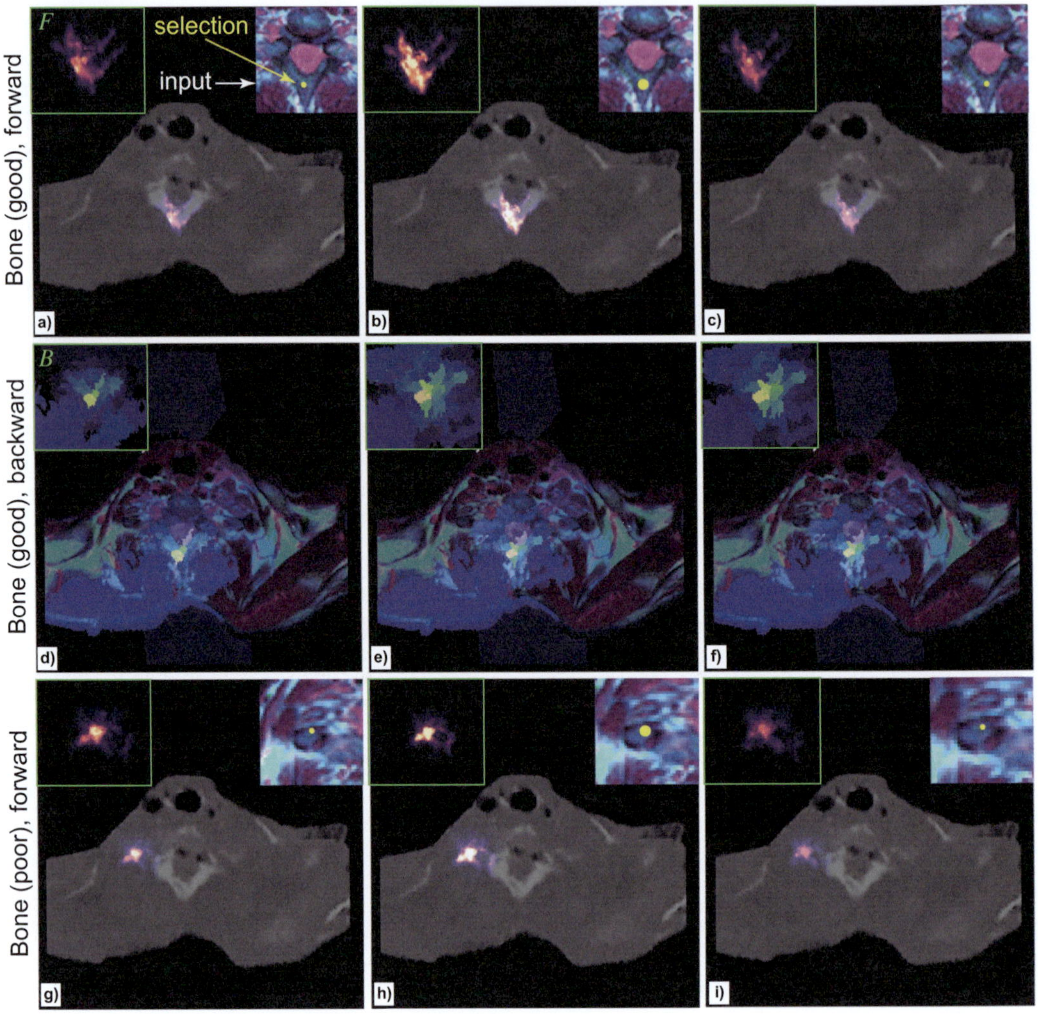

Fig. 6 Explaining MRI-to-CT generation. Forward (**a**–**c**, **g**–**i**, **m**–**o**) and backward (**d**–**f**, **j**–**l**, **p**–**r**) mappings for a well-predicted bone (**a**–**f**), poorly predicted bone (**g**–**l**), and well-predicted air cavity (**m**–**r**). Mappings are overlaid over the respective input or output images. Top-right insets show the area in the input MRI with selected pixels in yellow. Top-left insets show the mappings without overlay. See Sect. 4.2

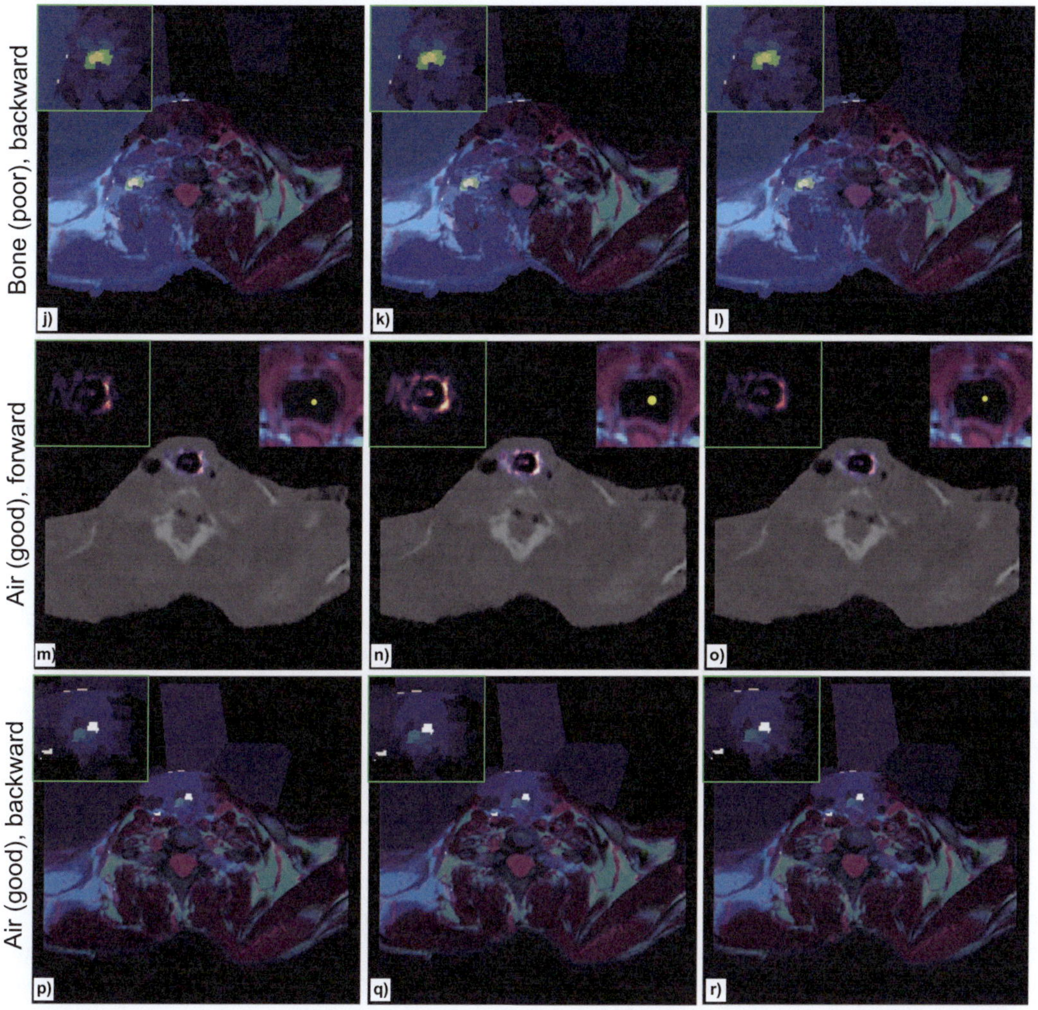

Fig. 6 (continued)

5 Discussion

We discuss next several aspects of our proposed IBIX framework.

Genericity: By construction, IBIX can handle any types of mappings f, as long as these input and output real-valued quantities. While we demonstrated IBIX only for *regressors* (which, as explained in Sect. 2, are the more complex and less covered case in the literature), our framework can handle any mapping, provided that one defines (1) ranges for the input perturbations and (2) suitable visualizations for the induced output changes. This is in stark contrast to most VA methods for XAI which work only for specific input and/or output data types [6, 48]. In the same time, IBIX is *fully* black box-compatible, needing only the ability to evaluate the model f for some given input $\mathbf{x}$, in stark contrast with many XAI techniques that need more knowledge over f [2, 48].

Ease of use: IBIX is fully automatic, requiring the use only to select a region of interest in the input ($M^{\mathbf{x}}$) or output (M^f) to explain these. The actual selection mechanism, of course, depends on the kind of input (and/or output) data.

Speed: IBIX's speed is fundamentally determined by the speed of evaluating the underlying model f.

For the forward mapping F, IBIX's cost equals the inference cost of f times the number H of jitters (Sect. 3.2). For the backward mapping B, this cost increases by a factor of K, equal to the number of blocks used to discretize the input domain. This cost can be however spread over multiple scales (Sect. 4.1.2) to generate high-resolution mappings in areas where the signal is high, thus, of interest to the user. All in all, for typical DL pipelines, F runs at interactive rates for inputs (and outputs) of dimensionality (n, respectively m) of up to one million. Computing B takes over 20 seconds for such input sizes using two scales. Using multiple scales could further reduce such costs, an investigation which is subject to future work. Note also that we currently compute our two scales using superpixels (Sect. 4.1.2), which only works for *image* inputs. However, our multiscale idea is generic—one can use any subdivision of the input domain, e.g., quadtrees, octrees or any similar multiresolution scheme.

Limitations: The arguably largest limitation of IBIX is its parameterization. That is, one should decide how many jitter levels N and jitter range size H to use (Sect. 3.2). Too conservative bounds hereof will inevitably only expose the working of the regressor f for a small part of its dynamic range. Setting N and H is, for now, application dependent, based on the expected range and dynamics of f. Separately, IBIX is designed, for now, to explain *single* input samples $\mathbf{x}$. This is on purpose, since existing VA methods do not handle this use-case well (Sect. 2). Extending IBIX to aggregate its findings for entire *datasets*, while maintaining its attractive speed, ease-of-use, and genericity, is a key direction to explore next.

IBIX can explain how the input of a regressor influences certain parts of its output, and conversely. This is aimed to help model engineers to spot problematic inference pertaining to certain input and/or output structures, such as demonstrated in Sect. 4.2. However, IBIX does not (aim to) solve such inference problems—it only exposes their presence. It is, still, the task of the model engineer to detect patterns in such problems and, based on that, devise changes to the model's training data, hyperparameters, or architecture to correct these.

6 Conclusion

We have presented Instance-Based Inference Explainers (IBIX), a framework for building visual explanations of the way multidimensional regressors infer their results for particular instances of interest. IBIX has a simple underlying operation, essentially measuring the rate of change of dimensions of an output (inferred) sample as function of change of the dimensions of the corresponding input. By relating the two changes, IBIX proposes a forward mapping explanation that highlights the output dimensions strongest affected by user-selected dimensions in an input sample; and a backward mapping explanation that, given user-selected dimensions in an output sample, highlights the input dimensions which strongest affect that selection. IBIX is simple to implement, works generically for any multidimensional regressor working on quantitative data, needs no knowledge of the regressor's internals, and is easy to use.

Several extension directions are possible. We envisage extending IBIX to explain groups of samples rather than individual ones, thereby lifting insights on the regressor's operation to a higher, more general, level. Alternatively, we consider designing specialized classes perturbations—generic but also application-specific—that users can select to 'probe' a given regressor's response to obtain finer-grained understanding of its functioning, similar to impulse-response testing in dynamical systems analysis. Separately, we aim to extend the bi-level acceleration scheme for backward mapping computation to a multilevel one, thereby bringing its operation to (near) real time without resolution trade-offs. Finally, as IBIX is fully generic in terms of the explored model, we aim to apply it to a larger class of multidimensional regressors beyond image-to-image ones or deep-learning models.

Acknowledgements We acknowledge the help of Mathijs de Boer with the implementation and evaluation of the MRI-to-pseudo-CT application. We also acknowledge the advice of dr. Matteo Maspero in developing the Pix2Pix generating network used for the same application and prof. Nico van den Berg for stimulating discussions.

References

1. Das A, Rad P. Opportunities and challenges in explainable artificial intelligence (XAI): a survey. 2020. arXiv:2006.11371
2. Ribeiro M, Singh S, Guestrin C. Why should I trust you?: explaining the predictions of any classifier. In: Proceedings of ACM SIGMOD KDD; 2016, p. 1135–44.
3. Adadi A, Berrada M, Bhateja V, Satapathy S, Satori H. Explainable AI for healthcare: from black box to interpretable models. Embedded Syst Artif Intell. 2020;1076:327–37.
4. Yang G, Ye O, Xia J. Unbox the black-box for the medical explainable AI via multi-modal and multicentre data fusion: a mini-review, two showcases and beyond. 2021. arXiv:2102.01998
5. Rodrigues F, Espadoto M, Hirata R, Telea AC. Constructing and visualizing high-quality classifier decision boundary maps. Information. 2019;10(9):280.
6. Garcia R, Telea A, da Silva B, Torresen J, Comba J. A task-and-technique centered survey on visual analytics for deep learning model engineering. Comput Graph. 2018;77:30–49.
7. van der Velden BH, Kuijf HJ, Gilhuijs KG, Viergever MA. Explainable artificial intelligence (XAI) in deep learning-based medical image analysis. 2021. arXiv:2107.10912 [eess.IV]
8. Chen L-C, Papandreou G, Kokkinos I, Murphy K, Yuille AL. Deeplab: semantic image segmentation with deep convolutional nets, atrous convolution, and fully connected crfs. IEEE Trans Pattern Anal Mach Intell. 2017;40(4):834–48.
9. Ren S, He K, Girshick R, Sun J. Faster R-CNN: towards real-time object detection with region proposal networks. 2015. arXiv:1506.01497
10. Akkus Z, Galimzianova A, Hoogi A, Rubin DL, Erickson BJ. Deep learning for brain MRI segmentation: state of the art and future directions. J Digit Imaging. 2017;30(4):449–59.
11. Spinner T, Schlegel U, Schäfer H, El-Assady M. explAiner: a visual analytics framework for interactive and explainable machine learning. IEEE Trans Vis Comput Graph. 2020;26(1):1064–74.
12. Hohman F, Kahng M, Pienta R, Chau DH. Visual analytics in deep learning: an interrogative survey for the next frontiers. IEEE Trans Vis Comput Graph. 2018;25(8):2674–93.
13. Rauber PE, Fadel SG, Falcão AX, Telea AC. Visualizing the hidden activity of artificial neural networks. IEEE Trans Vis Comput Graph. 2016;23(1):101–10.
14. Seifert C, Aamir A, Balagopalan A, Jain D, Sharma A, Grottel S, Gumhold S. Visualizations of deep neural networks in computer vision: a survey. In: Transparent data mining for big and small data. Springer; 2017, p. 123–44.
15. Ma Y, Fan A, He J, Nelakurthi AR, Maciejewski R. A visual analytics framework for explaining and diagnosing transfer learning processes. 2020. arXiv:2009.06876
16. Maaten LVD, Hinton G. Visualizing data using t-SNE. J Mach Learn Res. 2008;9:2579–605.
17. Rauber PE, Falcão AX, Telea AC. Projections as visual aids for classification system design. Inf Vis. 2018;17(4):282–305.
18. Benato BC, Telea AC, Falcão AX. Semi-supervised learning with interactive label propagation guided by feature space projections. In: Conference on graphics, patterns and images (SIBGRAPI); 2018. p. 392–99.
19. Sedlmair M, Aupetit M. Data-driven evaluation of visual quality measures. Comput Graph Forum. 2015;34(3):201–10.
20. Bernard J, Zeppelzauer M, Sedlmair M, Aigner W. VIAL: a unified process for visual interactive labeling. Vis Comput. 2018;34(9):1189–207.
21. Behrisch M, Korkmaz F, Shao L, Schreck T. Feedback-driven interactive exploration of large multidimensional data supported by visual classifier. In: IEEE conference on visual analytics science and technology (VAST); 2014. p. 43–52.
22. Tuia D, Volpi M, Copa L, Kanevski M, Munoz-Mari J. A survey of active learning algorithms for supervised remote sensing image classification. IEEE J Sel Top Signal Process. 2011;5(3):606–17.
23. Saito PTM, Suzuki CTN, Gomes JF, Rezende PJ, Falcão AX. Robust active learning for the diagnosis of parasites. Pattern Recogn. 2015;48(11):3572–83.
24. Ren M, Zeng W, Yang B, Urtasun R. Learning to reweight examples for robust deep learning. In: International conference on machine learning; 2018, p. 4334–343.
25. Harley AW, An interactive node-link visualization of convolutional neural networks. In: International symposium on visual computing; 2015, p. 867–77.
26. Bernard J, Zeppelzauer M, Lehmann M, Müller M, Sedlmair M. Towards user-centered active learning algorithms. Comput Graph Forum. 2018;37(3):121–32.
27. Zeiler MD Fergus R. Visualizing and understanding convolutional networks. In: European conference on computer vision; 2014. p. 818–33.
28. Pezzotti N, Höllt T, Van Gemert J, Lelieveldt BPF, Eisemann E, Vilanova A. Deepeyes: progressive visual analytics for designing deep neural networks. IEEE Trans Vis Comput Graph. 2017;24(1):98–108.
29. Liu M, Shi J, Li Z, Li C, Zhu J, Liu S. Towards better analysis of deep convolutional neural networks. IEEE Trans Vis Comput Graph. 2016;23(1):91–100.
30. Wongsuphasawat K, Smilkov D, Wexler J, Wilson J, Mane D, Fritz D, Krishnan D, Viégas FB, Wattenberg M. Visualizing dataflow graphs of deep learning models in tensorflow. IEEE Trans Vis Comput Graph 2017;24(1):1–12.

31. Abadi M et al. TensorFlow: large-scale machine learning on heterogeneous systems. 2015. Software available from tensorflow.org. https://www.tensorflow.org/
32. Choo J, Liu S. Visual analytics for explainable deep learning. IEEE Comput Graph Appl. 2018;38(4):84–92.
33. Yosinski J, Clune J, Nguyen A, Fuchs T, Lipson H. Understanding neural networks through deep visualization. In: Deep learning workshop, international conference on machine learning (ICML); 2015.
34. Hohman F, Park H, Robinson C, Chau DH. SUMMIT: scaling deep learning interpretability by visualizing activation and attribution summarizations. IEEE Trans Vis Comput Graph. 2019;26(1):1096–106.
35. Zeiler MD, Krishnan D, Taylor GW, Fergus R. Deconvolutional networks. In: IEEE conference on computer vision and pattern recognition; 2010. p. 2528–35.
36. Kahng M, Andrews PY, Kalro A, Chau DH. ActiVis: visual exploration of industry-scale deep neural network models. IEEE Trans Vis Comput Graph. 2017;24(1):88–97.
37. Nguyen A, Yosinski J, Clune J. Multifaceted feature visualization: Uncovering the different types of features learned by each neuron in deep neural networks. In: Visualization for deep learning workshop, international conference in machine learning; 2016. arXiv:1602.03616
38. Dosovitskiy A, Brox T. Inverting visual representations with convolutional networks. In: IEEE conference on computer vision and pattern recognition; 2016, p. 4829–37.
39. Simonyan K, Vedaldi A, Zisserman A. Deep inside convolutional networks: visualising image classification models and saliency maps. 2013. arXiv:1312.6034
40. Mahendran A, Vedaldi A. Visualizing deep convolutional neural networks using natural pre-images. Int J Comput Vis. 2016;120(3):233–55.
41. Kahng M, Thorat N, Chau DH, Viégas FB, Wattenberg M. Gan lab: understanding complex deep generative models using interactive visual experimentation. IEEE Trans Vis Comput Graph. 2018;25(1):310–20.
42. Liu M, Shi J, Cao K, Zhu J, Liu S. Analyzing the training processes of deep generative models. IEEE Trans Vis Comput Graph. 2017;24(1):77–87.
43. Wang J, Gou I, Yang H, Shen H-W. Ganviz: a visual analytics approach to understand the adversarial game. IEEE Trans Vis Comput Graph. 2018;24(6):1905–17.
44. Zhou B, Khosla A, Lapedriza A, Oliva A, Torralba A. Learning deep features for discriminative localization,. In: IEEE conference on computer vision and pattern recognition; 2016, p. 2921–29.
45. Selvaraju RR, Cogswell M, Das A, Vedantam R, Parikh D, Batra D. Grad-cam: visual explanations from deep networks via gradient-based localization. In: IEEE international conference on computer vision; 2017. p. 618–26.
46. Li H, Tian Y, Mueller K, Chen X. Beyond saliency: understanding convolutional neural networks from saliency prediction on layer-wise relevance propagation. Image Vis Comput. 2019;83:70–86.
47. Mahendran A, Vedaldi A. Salient deconvolutional networks. In: European conference on computer vision; 2016. p. 120–35.
48. Guidotti R, Monreale A, Ruggieri S, Turini F, Giannotti F, Pedreschi D. A survey of methods for explaining black box models. ACM Comput Surveys (CSUR). 2018;51(5):1–42.
49. Bazzani L, Bergamo A, Anguelov D, Torresani L. Self-taught object localization with deep networks. In: IEEE winter conference on applications of computer vision (WACV), 2016; p. 1–9.
50. Li D, Huang J-B, Li Y, Wang S, Yang M-H. Weakly supervised object localization with progressive domain adaptation. In: IEEE conference on computer vision and pattern recognition; 2016. p. 3512–520.
51. Zhang D, Han J, Cheng G, Yang M-H. Weakly supervised object localization and detection: a survey. IEEE Trans Pattern Anal Mach Intell. 2021.
52. Masci J, Meier U, Cireşan D, Schmidhuber J. Stacked convolutional auto-encoders for hierarchical feature extraction. In: International conference on artificial neural networks; 2011. p. 52–9.
53. Nair, V., Hinton GE. Rectified linear units improve restricted Boltzmann machines. In: International conference on machine learning (ICML); 2010. p. 807–14.
54. Sutskever I, Martens J, Dahl G, Hinton G. On the importance of initialization and momentum in deep learning. In: International conference on machine learning (ICML); 2013, p. 1139–147.
55. Taylor JR, Williams N, Cusack R, Auer T, Shafto MA, Dixon M, Tyler LK, Henson RN, et al. The Cambridge Centre for ageing and neuroscience (Cam-CAN) data repository: structural and functional MRI, MEG, and cognitive data from a cross-sectional adult lifespan sample. Neuroimage. 2017;144:262–9.
56. Fonov VS, Evans AC, McKinstry RC, Almli CR, Collins DL. Unbiased nonlinear average age-appropriate brain templates from birth to adulthood. Neuroimage. 2009;47:S102.
57. Sofroniew N et al.. napari/napari: 0.4.12rc2,' Oct 2021. Available https://doi.org/10.5281/zenodo.5587893
58. Achanta R, Shaji A, Smith K, Lucchi A, Fua P, Süsstrunk S. SLIC superpixels compared to state-of-the-art superpixel methods. In: IEEE Trans on Pattern Anal Mach Intell. 2012;34(11):2274–282.
59. Owrangi A, Greer P, Glide-Hurst C. MRI-only treatment planning: benefits and challenges. Phys Med Biol. 2018;63(5).
60. Spadea MF, Maspero M, Zaffino P, Seco J. Deep learning based synthetic-CT generation in radiotherapy and PET: a review. Int J Med Phys Res Pract. 2021;48(11):6537–66.
61. Low D. MRI guided radiotherapy. In: Cancer treatment and research. Springer; 2017. p. 41–67.

62. Maspero M, Savelije M, Dinkla A, Seevinck P, Intven M, Jurgenliemk-Schulz I, Kerkmeijer L, van den Berg C. Dose evaluation of fast synthetic-CT generation using a generative adversarial network for general pelvis MR-only radiotherapy. Phys Med Biol. 2018;10(63).
63. Isola P, Zhu I-Y, Zhou T, Efros AA. Image-to-image translation with conditional adversarial networks. In: IEEE conference on computer vision and pattern recognition; 2017, p. 1125–134.
64. Klein S, Staring M, Murphy K, Viergever MA, Pluim JP. Elastix: a toolbox for intensity-based medical image registration. IEEE Trans Med Imaging. 2009;29(1):196–205.
65. Shamonin DP, Bron EE, Lelieveldt BP, Smits M, Klein S, Staring M. Fast parallel image registration on CPU and GPU for diagnostic classification of Alzheimer's disease. Front Neuroinf. 2014;7:50.
66. Ronneberger O, Fischer P, Brox T. U-net: convolutional networks for biomedical image segmentation. In: Medical image computing and computer-assisted intervention (MICCAI). Springer; 2015. p. 234–41.
67. Wang Z, Bovik A, Sheikh H, Simoncelli E. Image quality assessment: from error visibility to structural similarity. IEEE Trans Imag Process. 2004;13(4):600–12.

Machine Learning—Automated Machine Learning (AutoML) for Disease Prediction

Jason H. Moore, Pedro H. Ribeiro, Nicholas Matsumoto and Anil K. Saini

Abstract

The selection and tuning of feature selection, feature engineering, and classification or regression algorithms is a major challenge in machine learning, affecting both beginners and experts. Automated machine learning (AutoML) offers a solution by automating the creation of machine learning pipelines, eliminating the guesswork associated with a manual process. This chapter reviews the challenges of building pipelines and introduces some of the most widely used AutoML methods and open-source software. We focus on TPOT, an AutoML method that utilizes genetic programming for discovery and optimization and represents pipelines as expression trees. We also explore TPOT extensions and its use in handling biomedical big data.

Keywords

Automated machine learning · Machine learning · Tree-based pipeline optimization tool · Genetic programming · AutoML · TPOT

J. H. Moore (✉) · P. H. Ribeiro · N. Matsumoto · A. K. Saini
Department of Computational Biomedicine, Cedars-Sinai Medical Center, Los Angeles, CA, USA
e-mail: jason.moore@csmc.edu

1 Introduction

Machine learning is often used for developing predictive models due to its ability to capture relationships between independent variables or features and dependent variables or outcomes that may be non-additive or heterogeneous between subjects. Machine learning algorithms adjust internal parameters and mathematical functions to reduce the gap between their predictions and target values. The modeling process consists of several stages, including feature selection, pre-processing, and engineering, followed by one or more classifier or regressor algorithms like decision trees or neural networks. The main challenge for data scientists is to find an optimal combination of algorithms and hyperparameters that strikes a balance between accuracy and interpretability, which can be a time-consuming process of trial and error. Automated machine learning (AutoML) aims to simplify this task through automation, thus removing some of the guesswork that goes into selecting and tuning algorithms. We review here some of the steps involved in creating a typical pipeline and then introduce AutoML as a powerful tool to make this modeling approach more accessible. Figure 1 provides an overview of some of the steps that go into building an analytics pipeline.

F. W. Asselbergs et al. (eds.), *Clinical Applications of Artificial Intelligence in Real-World Data*,
https://doi.org/10.1007/978-3-031-36678-9_10

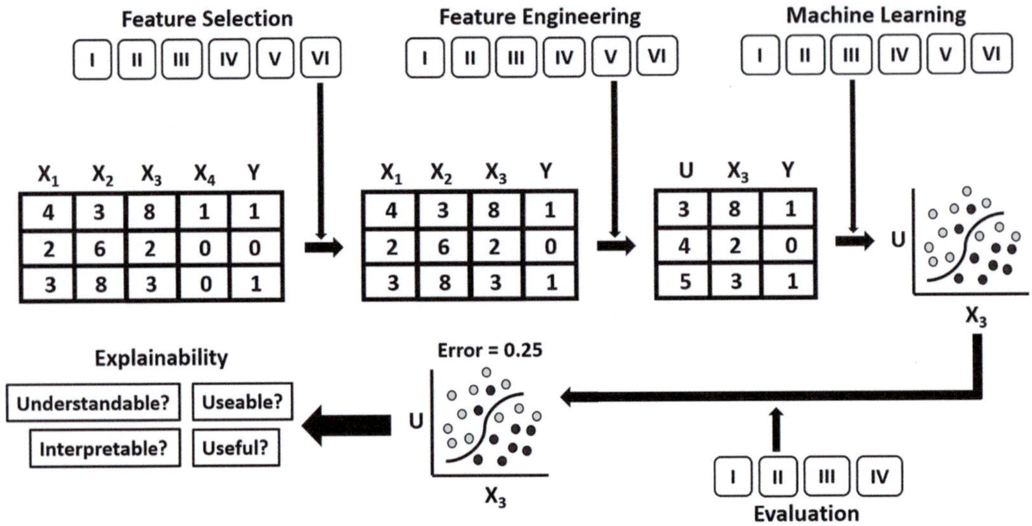

Fig. 1 Overview of the many decisions that need to be made when choosing feature selection, feature engineering, machine learning, and model evaluation algorithms. Also shown are the components of model explainability that are often necessary for clinical problem-solving and model deployment

1.1 Cleaning Data

Machine learning can be very sensitive to problems in the data such as noise, bias, missing information, outliers, and imbalanced labels. Data cleaning and quality control aim to identify and correct these issues, which may involve various algorithms and statistical methods. The outcome of these steps greatly affects the accuracy of machine learning results [1].

1.2 Feature Selection

In biomedical or clinical research studies, it is common to be faced with data with thousands or millions of features such as electronic health records or genomics, respectively. Applying machine learning algorithms to these many features can create several problems, including learning noise instead of signal (i.e., overfitting). Overfit models are much less likely to generalize to new data. Additionally, processing large number of features can be computationally expensive, which raises issues related to the carbon footprint of the analysis. A good machine learning analysis will try to balance these issues by selecting a subset of features most likely to harbor a signal. Identifying the relevant features can be done automatically through the use of algorithms that estimate feature importance scores. In some cases, expert knowledge of known interactions can be leveraged to reduce the search space. There are a wide variety of different feature selection algorithms and methods each with their own hyperparameters. And therefore, selecting the right method can be difficult.

1.3 Engineering New Features

Feature engineering involves converting raw data to a different format or encoding to make the signal in the data more accessible to modeling. Transforming the data can improve performance, interpretability, or both. While machine learning algorithms can sometimes address these issues, they often make the models more complex and less interpretable. Feature engineering offers a different solution, allowing the algorithm to concentrate on important patterns in the data for making predictions. Care must be taken, however, to avoid overfitting the data when using predicted outcomes to engineer features. As an example, the average of systolic and diastolic blood pressure could be used as an engineered feature with the hope that it captures important information missing from each feature individually. Additional examples include normalization of the values or encoding a continuous feature into a binary one using a threshold from the definition of hypertension.

1.4 Choosing Classification and Regression Algorithms

Selecting the right machine learning classifier or regressor method and setting its hyperparameters to build a model is one of the biggest challenges faced by both experts and non-experts. There are many commonly used methods, each modeling the relationship between features and outcomes differently. For instance, some methods excel at modeling linear patterns, while others are better suited for nonlinear relationships. Some methods result in more interpretable models, while others prioritize predictive performance since these are more computationally demanding. This can be especially challenging when patterns in data are unknown until after thorough analysis and evaluation. To complicate matters, each method often has multiple hyperparameters influencing how the algorithm operates. It is difficult to know beforehand what the best method is for a given dataset. This challenge has been a major motivating factor for the development of AutoML.

1.5 Assessing the Quality of a Model

Appropriately assessing the quality of a machine learning model is essential for its success. Machine learning aims to make accurate predictions as measured by a loss function. However, evaluating a model's predictive performance is not always straightforward. Overfitting, where a model memorizes the specifics of the dataset instead of general trends, is a common issue leading to poor performance on new data. Cross-validation helps estimate out-of-sample error by averaging scores on k different training/validation splits, but this metric can be overfit itself. The challenge for data scientists is to distinguish between underfit, good fit, and overfit models and choose an appropriately fit model. The ultimate value of a model is its ability make prediction in data it hasn't previously seen.

Evaluating the quality of a machine learning model goes beyond just looking at its predictive accuracy using a loss function. Other factors may include interpretability, usefulness, or interestingness. With multiple objectives, often there is a trade-off when optimizing towards the desired metrics. In particular, the trade-off between performance and interpretability should be considered when developing and evaluating models. There are several multi-objective methods like Pareto optimization that are designed to efficiently optimize towards multiple measures of quality.

1.6 Explaining a Model

The field of explainable artificial intelligence (XAI) focuses on developing machine learning models that are accurate and transparent in their decision-making. While algorithms behind machine learning algorithms can be simple, the models they generate can be highly complex and difficult to understand. Explainable artificial intelligence aims to make the reasoning behind these predictions more accessible to humans, which can lead to new insights and applications in the specific domain. Combi et al. [2] describe several components of XAI, including *interpretability*, *understandability*, *usefulness*, and *utility*. We briefly summarize each of these here.

Interpretability of machine learning models refers to the ability of a user to intuitively understand the reasoning behind a model's predictions. It is defined by understanding the basis of decisions made by the model without the need to know the exact mathematical process. For example, feature importance scores, either derived through permutation testing or the parameters of the model, can provide insight into which features the model is basing its decision on. A more interpretable model can lead to better insights, new applications, and improved decision making. As an example, a user might learn that a deep learning model used for detecting cancer from imaging data focuses only on particular regions of the image which can in turn be used to more efficiently guide the doctor towards relevant parts of the image or quickly allow them to fact check decisions.

The ability of a user to comprehend the inner workings and mathematical logic of a machine learning model is known as its *understandability*. A decision tree is an example of a model that is understandable as it is easy to read and follow its flow of logic. On the other hand, deep learning models are not as easily understood due to the abstract logic hidden in the matrix transformations. Understandability is crucial in the medical field, where incorrect decisions could lead to serious consequences. Clinicians can use their own expert knowledge to validate the reasoning of the model, providing *trust* in the model. Further, understanding the model can lead to the identification of new hypotheses and potential interventions. For example, a decision tree model that predicts disease risk from genetic data could reveal new rules that could lead to hypotheses about new drug targets for disease treatment.

Combi et al. [2] also touch on the concept of *usability* in machine learning, which refers to the practicality of implementing a solution in the clinic. A number of factors come into play when determining if a model can be practically put into use. These include the feasibility of collecting, digitizing, and inputting the necessary data, the financial cost of installing, operating, and maintaining the solution, and the ease of training users to utilize the solution and integrate it into their workflow. It is important to note that a technology's usefulness can vary depending on the context and the problems being faced, as well as the availability of alternatives.

The final component of XAI is *usefulness*. This refers to whether the technology would be used by the user if it meets their needs. In machine learning, this often refers to accuracy and *actionable* predictions. The usefulness of a model is often enhanced if it is also interpretable, understandable, and usable. Interpretability and understandability can lead to trust in the underlying predictions, leading to more efficient evaluation and decision-making and providing insights into new directions. Usability is required for people to actually use the technology in the first place. A strong usability provides incentives to use the technology as it can make workflows more efficient.

2 Automated Machine Learning

By introducing some of the components of a machine learning pipeline, we have also highlighted the many decisions that need to be made to develop a good model worthy of consideration for clinical application. For this reason, machine learning has long required computer or data scientists as collaborators because they have the knowledge and experience to make the many technical decisions required for predictive modeling. However, machine learning, like parametric statistical methods, should be accessible to all. Automated machine learning seeks to let the computer make the many decisions required to build an optimal pipeline, thus making these complex methods more accessible to those who may not be able to enlist a computational expert with the time and dedication to the project. The field of AutoML started after 2010 and has been reviewed in a recent book [3]. Some of the first AuoML methods and open-source software include Auto-WEKA [4], Auto-sklearn [5], and the tree-based pipeline optimization tool of TPOT [6, 7]. We briefly review the first two below and then present TPOT in more detail, along with some biomedical data examples. Commercial products such as DataRobot (www.datarobot.com) will not be covered since they do not provide the transparency necessary to describe their underlying algorithms.

2.1 Auto-WEKA

Auto-WEKA uses a Bayesian optimization method to search across multiple machine learning algorithms and parameter settings to select the best model for a dataset [4]. It is built on top of the popular WEKA machine learning software package [8]. Auto-WEKA has been used in the biomedical space. Examples include predicting intracerebral hemorrhage in patients with features derived from demographics, laboratory tests, and imaging [9].

2.2 Auto-sklearn

Auto-sklearn is a popular AutoML method that uses Bayesian optimization to construct machine learning pipelines [5]. It leverages the scikit-learn library [10] and was one of the first AutoML methods to incorporate meta-learning and ensemble classification. The pipelines created by Auto-sklearn consist of data pre-processing, feature selection, and machine learning classifier components. The method uses analysis results from numerous public datasets as metadata to inform the optimization of its pipelines on new data. Auto-sklearn has proven to be effective for various tasks, such as prioritizing social media posts about suicide [11] and predicting mood and anxiety disorders [12] (Fig. 2).

2.3 Tree-Based Pipeline Optimization Tool

While Auto-WEKA and Auto-sklearn use Bayesian optimization, the tree-based pipeline optimization tool (TPOT) uses genetic programming (GP) to discover and optimize machine learning pipelines represented as expression trees [6, 7]. Like Auto-sklearn, TPOT also uses the Python-based scikit-learn machine learning library [10]. We review this approach in more detail in the next section as it has been used for biomedical applications more extensively than the other methods.

3 The Tree-Based Pipeline Optimization Tool (TPOT) Algorithm

An important feature of TPOT is the representation of machine learning pipelines as expression trees. TPOT uses GP optimization algorithm [13] from evolutionary computation, an AI subfield inspired by evolution and natural selection, to evolve a population of trees towards the desired objectives. TPOT is built upon and inspired by a vast literature of GP methods and strategies for complex problems represented as expression trees. TPOT's algorithm uses a type of Pareto optimization, which enables pipelines

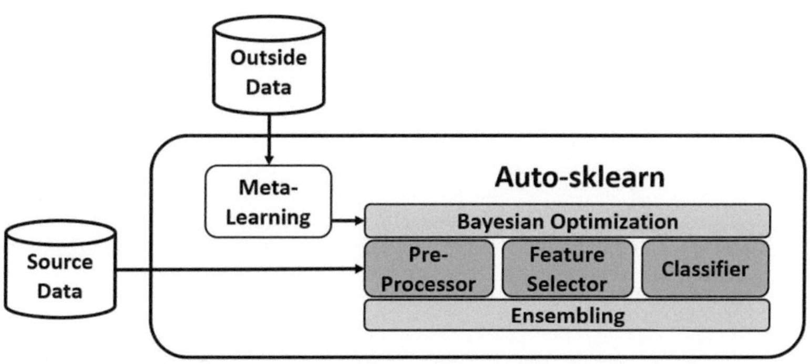

Fig. 2 Overview of the Auto-sklearn method. The included meta-learning algorithm is trained on outside data. The meta-learner informs the Bayesian optimization of a machine learning pipeline with pre-processor, feature selector, and classifier components, followed by the optimization of ensembles of built pipelines

to be evaluated based on multiple objectives like accuracy and complexity. TPOT was implemented using DEAP, an open-source Python software package for distributed evolutionary algorithms [14].

An overview of the TPOT algorithm is illustrated in Fig. 3. The algorithm starts by randomly generating *N* expression tree-based pipelines from a set of scikit-learn operators (e.g., feature selectors, classifiers, etc.) and their hyperparameters. New pipelines are generated using variation operators that mutate pipeline components and recombine branches between pipelines. The *N* old and the *N* new pipelines are evaluated, and the best *N* are selected to move forward using a selection algorithm. The variation, evaluation, selection, and iteration steps continue until a stopping criterion is reached. This is usually set to be *G* generations or iterations of the algorithm (e.g., $G = 100$ or 1000). We introduce the components of TPOT in more detail below.

3.1 Representing TPOT Pipelines

One of the key differences between TPOT and other methods is the representation of machine learning pipelines as expression trees. Tree-based data structures are ideal for this purpose, given the stepwise data processing that a pipeline performs. Here, the tree nodes are selected from feature selection, feature engineering, and machine learning algorithms from the scikit-learn library. The terminals of the tree represent the hyperparameters of the various algorithms and the data inputs. A scikit-learn pipeline is constructed by initializing models with their respective hyperparameters

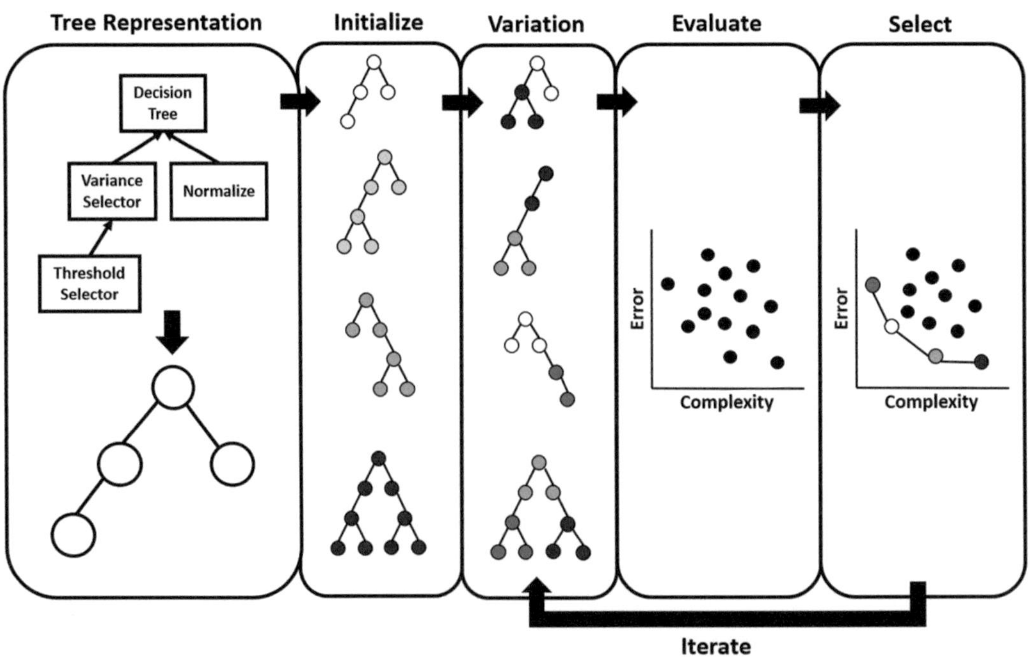

Fig. 3 An overview of the TPOT algorithm. The first step is to represent machine learning pipelines using expression trees. Pipeline trees are initialized randomly, diversified using several variation operators, evaluated, and selected using quality metrics such as an error-based loss function and the complexity of the pipelines. This process is iterated until a stopping criterion is reached

and using the feature unions to create the branching structure. To execute a tree, the data are passed into the leaves of the tree and propagated through the nodes of the tree to the root node, which serves as the final classifier or regressor.

3.2 Initializing TPOT Pipelines

The first step of the TPOT algorithm involves initializing a set of *N* pipelines (e.g., N = 100 or 1000). TPOT comes with a default set of algorithms from the scikit-learn library, which can be customized using a configuration file. Each expression tree starts with a machine learning algorithm at the root node, ensuring the pipeline's output is a set of predicted values that can be evaluated using a loss function. Child nodes are selected from a pool of allowable methods, including feature transformation, selection, engineering, and machine learning algorithms, with terminals specifying randomly selected hyperparameters. In short, the initial population of *N* expression trees is generated randomly with varying layers, drawn from a distribution of possibilities.

3.3 Generating TPOT Pipeline Variation

Each generation in TPOT starts with generating new pipelines from those in the current set or population. TPOT uses mutation and recombination operators, inspired by similar processes in natural evolution, to generate variation in the machine learning pipelines (Fig. 4). New individuals are produced through mutation of an existing tree with probability *M*, or crossover of selected subtrees or hyperparameters between two individuals with probability *R*. Mutations can insert, remove, or replace nodes. Crossover involves swapping randomly selected subtrees of two pipelines.

3.4 Evaluating TPOT Pipelines

The TPOT algorithm evaluates each expression tree based on two objectives. First, it uses a standard loss function and k-fold cross-validation to measure the predictive error of the classifier. Second, the complexity of the tree is

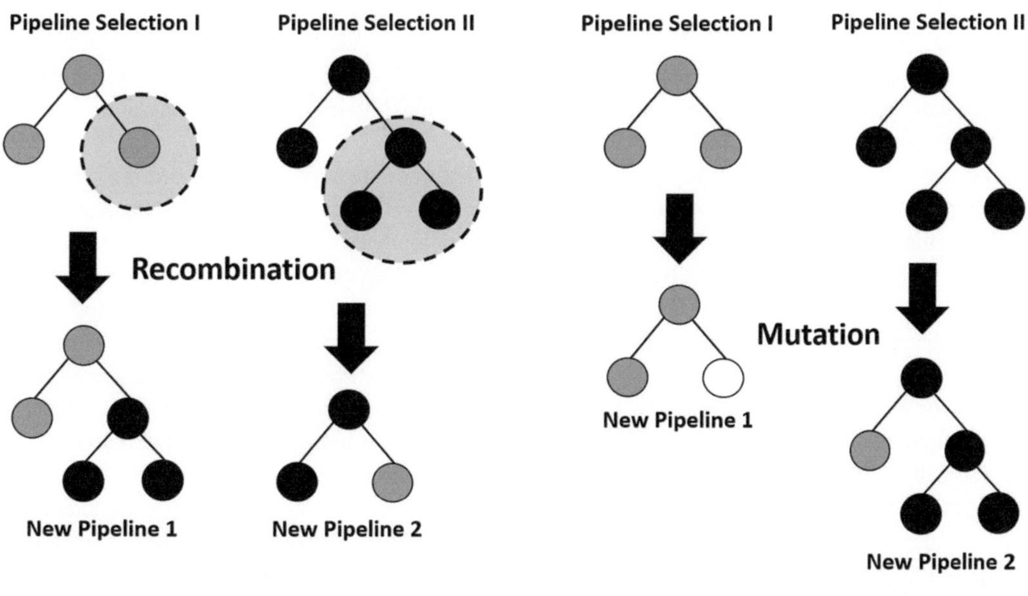

Fig. 4 Overview of the process by which variation is introduced into TPOT pipelines via recombination of subtrees (left) and mutation of nodes (right). Mutation and recombination occur separately on different trees in the same generation with some probability set by the user

estimated by counting the number of nodes. Other complexity measures could be used that take into account the complexity of the individual algorithms and their hyperparameters. For instance, machine learning methods, such as XGBoost that have higher complexity and are less interpretable than simpler methods such as decision trees or logistic regression, could be given different weights. Assessing complexity allows TPOT to prioritize simpler pipelines that are more interpretable, less prone to overfitting, and better suited for generalization to new data. TPOT can be customized for multi-objective optimization with the development of different or additional criteria.

3.5 Selecting TPOT Pipelines

An important component of TPOT is the method used to pick the best trees or pipelines from the current population to move forward. An optimal model should have low complexity and high performance as measured by the loss function. In reality, there is often a compromise between interpretability and performance, with simpler models compromising some performance. Also, there is a trade-off between generalizability and overfitting, where cross-validation addresses this to some extent but is not foolproof. TPOT models can become too complex and overfit the cross-validation score. This is a particular concern when evaluating many pipelines. If unrestricted, TPOT may form overly complex pipelines that significantly overfit the data, and if too limited, TPOT might not discover better solutions.

To balance interpretability and performance, TPOT optimizes a Pareto front of non-dominated models defined by both the loss function and pipeline complexity (usually measured by the number of ML operators used in the pipeline). During training, TPOT selects the set of non-dominated models from a Pareto front using the non-dominated sorting genetic algorithm II or NSGA-II [15]. These models will then be mutated or recombined in the next generation. Other methods, such as lexicase selection [16], may also be explored.

3.6 Picking the Final TPOT Pipeline

There are several approaches to selecting the best TPOT model once the algorithm has completed its run. The simplest method is to return the pipeline from the final iteration with the best predictive accuracy determined by cross-validation. Another approach is to identify the Pareto optimal models and select the one that balances accuracy and complexity according to the wishes of the user. The best approach may depend on the goals of the user.

4 Scaling TPOT to Big Data

Le et al. [17] tackled the challenge of computational complexity in AutoML by making two key modifications to TPOT. First, they introduced a template option that allows the user to specify a fixed linear pipeline structure. This feature was designed to help speed up execution time, as using a template reduces the complexity of generating and evaluating pipelines. For example, the template option can be used to limit TPOT to a simple feature selector and classifier, making it run faster than more complex trees.

Second, the authors introduced the feature set selector (FSS) operator, which functions as an expert-knowledge-based feature selector. This operator uses pre-defined groupings of features into S subsets, allowing the user to apply their domain knowledge to the pipeline generation process. The FSS operator includes a hyperparameter that points to one of the feature subsets, which is then used to generate the data set to be used for the next step in the tree.

The combination of a simple template tree structure and smaller feature sets can significantly improve the execution time of TPOT, making it a more efficient solution for working with big data. By reducing the computational

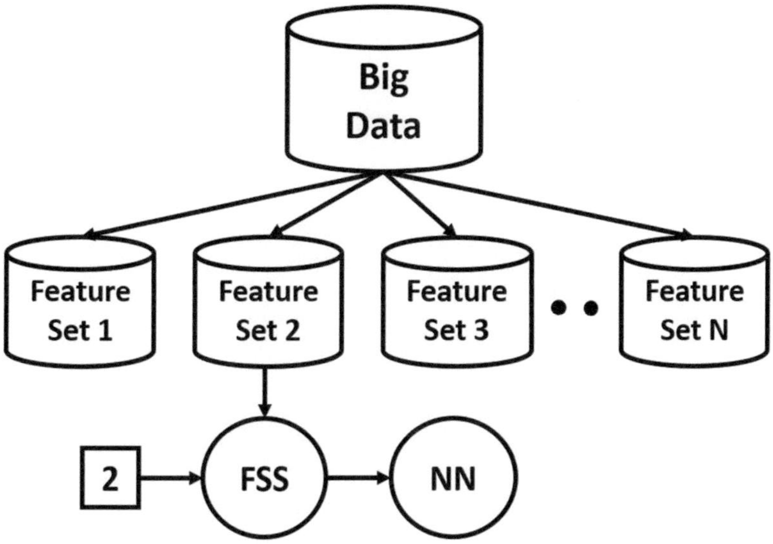

Fig. 5 Including a Feature Set Selector (FSS) allows TPOT to select a subset of features for analysis in a pipeline. In the example pipeline shown, the FSS operator has a hyperparameter set to 2, which in turn selects data subset 2. This subset of the data is then passed to the Neural Network (NN) algorithm to develop a predictive model

load, TPOT can also minimize its carbon footprint, making it a more sustainable option for machine learning practitioners (Fig. 5).

5 Using TPOT to Automate Neural Networks

An advantage of deep learning neural networks over other machine learning algorithms is that they can perform feature selection and feature engineering in the early layers of the network prior to classification or regression in later layers. An important question is whether AutoML pipelines are able to approximate the performance of a deep learning algorithm by piecing together feature selection and feature engineering algorithms with simpler feed-forward neural networks. The value of this approach is that it might be more computationally efficient (i.e., greener) and yield models that are more explainable.

To address this question, Romano et al. [18] investigated the performance of TPOT, NNs, and TPOT with shallow NN classifiers (referred to as TPOT-NN) on several publicly available data sets (see Fig. 6 for an overview of TPOT-NN). The results showed that TPOT-NN performed better on several data sets compared to standard TPOT and NNs, without performing worse on others. The study raises the possibility of using TPOT-NN to approximate complex deep learning models by combining simple NN operators with feature selection and engineering algorithms. It will be interesting to explore the potential for TPOT-NN to generate high-performing and easily interpretable pipelines.

6 Biomedical Applications of TPOT

There have been a number of biomedical applications of TPOT with an emphasis on genetics and genomics [19]. These include predicting depression using genomic data [17], coronary artery disease using metabolomics data [20], schizophrenia using genomics data [21], predicting renal cell carcinoma grade using radiologic images [22], childhood dental carries using metabolomics data [23], and coronary artery disease using genetics data [24]. We focus here

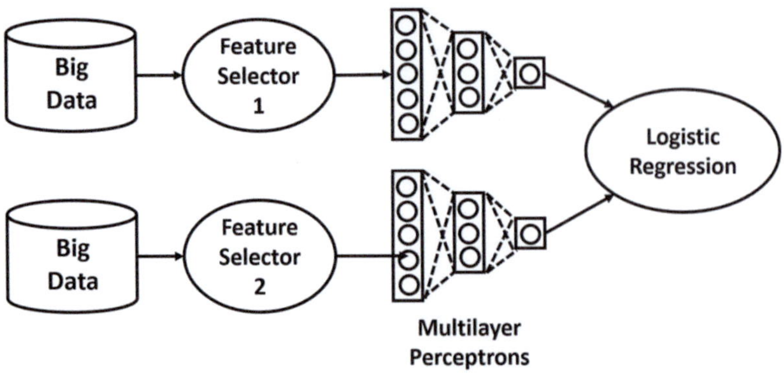

Fig. 6 A hypothetical TPOT-NN pipeline. Here, two different Feature Selector operators select different subsets of features that are then passed to multilayer perceptron neural networks. The predictions made by these feed-forward neural networks are passed to logistic regression that makes the final prediction

on the latter study by Manduchi et al. that illustrates several of abovementioned concepts.

Manduchi et al. [24] conducted a study to predict the presence of coronary artery disease (CAD) in over 340,000 subjects using data from the UK Biobank resource, which included more than one million genetic features. This posed several machine learning challenges, including a severely imbalanced class distribution and a large feature set that presented computational difficulties for AutoML. To overcome these challenges, the authors randomly downsampled the larger class to balance the dataset and used expert knowledge to focus on a smaller set of promising genetic features for CAD. In this case, features were selected based on whether genes were valid drug targets based on the biochemistry and structure of their corresponding protein products [25]. The final models were evaluated using fivefold cross-validation and holdout datasets to assess their generalizability and predictive accuracy.

The pipeline described in Fig. 7 was generated using TPOT to predict CAD. The TPOT algorithm selected a pipeline of feature selection and feature engineering methods, including percentile feature selection, variance thresholding, and a stacking estimator, with a stochastic gradient descent classifier. The final pipeline used an extra trees classifier to classify subjects

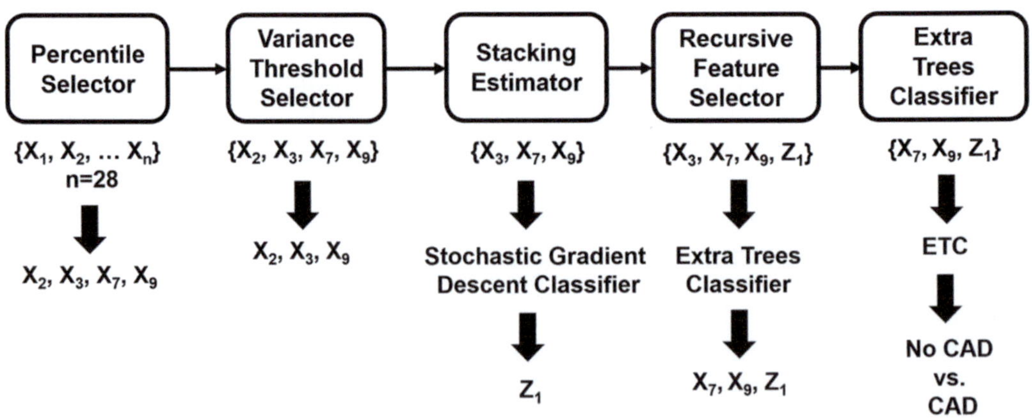

Fig. 7 A TPOT-generated machine learning pipeline for predicting risk of CAD. This pipeline contains a combination of feature selector (first, second, and fourth), feature engineering (third), and classification (fifth) algorithms

as having or not having CAD. The pipeline was statistically significant and had a testing accuracy of 0.55, comparable to other predictive studies using genetic data. The use of TPOT allowed for the automatic identification of a complex pipeline, which would have been difficult for a human user to construct manually.

The study used Shapley values, a game theoretic approach, to interpret the predictive model. The results showed that different features contributed differently to the prediction of different subsets of subjects, indicating the presence of genetic heterogeneity. Machine learning methods, such as the one used by TPOT, have an advantage over linear methods, such as regression, as they can detect and model complex relationships between features and outcomes, including this heterogeneity pattern. TPOT was able to automatically find a pipeline that could model these complex relationships.

7 Future Directions

Automated machine learning or AutoML shows tremendous promise in biomedical and clinical research because it can reduce pipeline development time and thus make these analytical techniques much more accessible to those without in-depth knowledge and experience with the algorithms being used. This accessibility should accelerate their use and help users become comfortable with advanced machine learning methods similar to how the user-friendly statistical analysis software packages brought the t-test, analysis of variance, and linear regression to the masses decades ago. Before AutoML becomes mainstream in medicine, several challenges still need to be addressed.

First, it will be important to more thoroughly explore how to integrate existing biological and clinical knowledge in the processes of feature selection, model selection, and explainability. Machine learning algorithms are often agnostic to the problem being studied. However, biologists and clinicians sometimes have detailed knowledge from which the algorithm can benefit. For example, expert knowledge could be used as a quality metric for multiobjective optimization via Pareto optimization. The Manduchi example [24] used the druggability of genes [25] as a pre-processing step prior to analysis with TPOT. An alternative approach could have been to develop a druggability score for each gene and then add an additional objective function to maximize the enrichment of druggable genes selected by a TPOT pipeline for modeling.

Second, the potential of AutoML for democratizing machine learning is only realized when it is accessible to non-experts. TPOT, while effective in constructing pipelines, lacks a user-friendly graphic-user interface (GUI) which can be a hindrance for widespread adoption. A GUI designed specifically for those who are not machine learning experts can help to reduce barriers and make advanced technology more accessible to everyone. A great example of this is Aliro AI, which provides a simple, intuitive interface for AutoML [26] and could be extended to support TPOT. Auto-WEKA also includes a GUI as part of the WEKA software [8].

Third, it is currently not known whether AutoML tools like TPOT and Auto-sklearn are more susceptible to issues with the fairness and bias of the models generated than more traditional machine learning approaches. Does optimizing a complex machine learning algorithm amplify biases in the data that might further discriminate against certain classes of patients? Building operators and checks into AutoML pipelines that can detect and self-correct bias to yield fair models will be an important topic for future studies.

Fourth, natural language processing (NLP) is an important AI methodology for extracting structured data and meaning from clinical notes and other text-based sources. NLP has been used for tasks such as text classification and sentiment analysis. AutoML has not been fully explored as a tool to assist with NLP-related goals.

Fifth, the ease of deployment of models derived from AutoML will need to be explored and evaluated. For example, it is important for clinicians to trust and feel comfortable with models generated by AutoML methods. This means that they need to understand how AutoML algorithms work, where the models come from, the biases of the models, and what their predictions mean.

Finally, one can imagine taking AutoML algorithms a step or two further to produce persistent and self-updating models that receive feedback from users and improve over time in an autonomous manner. This is especially important for clinical applications where data is being continuously collected. Additionally, smoothly transitioning models to new data sources as the technology used for lab tests, imaging, etc. changes would allow clinicians to stay continuously updated rather than waiting for major updates which can be hard to implement. This approach might be also appealing for complex problems where the search space is effectively infinite, and best model can't be found in a short period of time.

Automated machine learning is a relatively new field of AI. These methods show tremendous promise for accelerating discovery using machine learning pipelines by democratizing access. As machine learning continues to be used across biomedical and clinical disciplines, it will be important to assess the impact of AutoML for moving from discovery to deployment. Do automated methods speed up the biomedical data science process? Do they yield better predictive models that generalize across health systems and patient populations? Are models generated by AutoML more explainable to clinicians? Are they fairer and more unbiased? Do they allow more clinicians without specific computational training to enter the applied AI field? Do they yield better biological discoveries and clinical outcomes? As with any new technology, there are currently more questions than answers.

References

1. Chicco D, Oneto L, Tavazzi E. Eleven quick tips for data cleaning and feature engineering. PLOS Comput Biol. 2022;18: e1010718.
2. Combi C, Amico B, Bellazzi R, Holzinger A, Moore JH, Zitnik M, et al. A manifesto on explainability for artificial intelligence in medicine. Artif Intell Med. 2022;133: 102423.
3. Hutter F, Kotthoff L, Vanschoren J, editors. Automated machine learning: methods, systems, challenges. Springer; 2019.
4. Thornton C, Hutter F, Hoos HH, Leyton-Brown K. Auto-WEKA: combined selection and hyperparameter optimization of classification algorithms. In: Proceedings of the 19th ACM SIGKDD international conference on knowledge discovery and data mining. New York, NY, USA: ACM; 2013. p. 847–55.
5. Feurer M, Klein A, Eggensperger K, Springenberg J, Blum M, Hutter F. Efficient and Robust automated machine learning. In: Cortes C, Lawrence ND, Lee DD, Sugiyama M, Garnett R, editors. Advances in neural information processing systems 28. Curran Associates Inc; 2015. p. 2962–70.
6. Olson RS, Bartley N, Urbanowicz RJ, Moore JH. Evaluation of a tree-based pipeline optimization tool for automating data science. In: Proceedings of the genetic and evolutionary computation conference 2016. New York, NY, USA: ACM; 2016. p. 485–92.
7. Olson RS, Urbanowicz RJ, Andrews PC, Lavender NA, Kidd LC, Moore JH. Automating biomedical data science through tree-based pipeline optimization. In: Squillero G, Burelli P, editors. Applications of Evolutionary Computation. Cham: Springer; 2016. p. 123–37.
8. Kotthoff L, Thornton C, Hoos HH, Hutter F, Leyton-Brown K. Auto-WEKA 2.0: automatic model selection and hyperparameter optimization in WEKA. J Mach Learn Res. 2017;18:826–30.
9. Wang H-L, Hsu W-Y, Lee M-H, Weng H-H, Chang S-W, Yang J-T, et al. Automatic machine-learning-based outcome prediction in patients with primary intracerebral hemorrhage. Front Neurol. 2019;10:910.
10. Pedregosa F, Varoquaux G, Gramfort A, Michel V, Thirion B, Grisel O, et al. Scikit-learn: machine learning in python. J Mach Learn Res. 2011;12:2825–30.
11. Howard D, Maslej MM, Lee J, Ritchie J, Woollard G, French L. Transfer learning for risk classification of social media posts: model evaluation study. J Med Internet Res. 2020;22: e15371.
12. van Eeden WA, Luo C, van Hemert AM, Carlier IVE, Penninx BW, Wardenaar KJ, et al. Predicting the 9-year course of mood and anxiety disorders with automated machine learning: a comparison between auto-sklearn, naïve Bayes classifier, and traditional logistic regression. Psychiatry Res. 2021;299: 113823.
13. Koza JR. Genetic programming: on the programming of computers by means of natural selection. Cambridge, MA, USA: MIT Press; 1992.
14. Fortin F-A, Rainville F-MD, Gardner M-A, Parizeau M, Gagné C. DEAP: evolutionary algorithms made easy. J Mach Learn Res. 2012;13:2171−2175.

15. Deb K, Pratap A, Agarwal S, Meyarivan T. A fast and elitist multiobjective genetic algorithm: NSGA-II. IEEE Trans Evol Comput. 2002;6:182–97.
16. Helmuth T, McPhee NF, Spector L. Lexicase selection for program synthesis: a diversity analysis. In: Riolo R, Worzel WP, Kotanchek M, Kordon A, editors. Genetic programming theory and practice XIII. Cham: Springer; 2016. p. 151–67.
17. Le TT, Fu W, Moore JH. Scaling tree-based automated machine learning to biomedical big data with a feature set selector. Bioinforma Oxf Engl. 2020;36:250–6.
18. Romano J, Le T, Fu W, Moore J. TPOT-NN: augmenting tree-based automated machine learning with neural network estimators. Genet Program Evolvable Mach. 2021;1–21.
19. Manduchi E, Romano JD, Moore JH. The promise of automated machine learning for the genetic analysis of complex traits. Hum Genet. 2022;141:1529–44.
20. Orlenko A, Kofink D, Lyytikäinen L-P, Nikus K, Mishra P, Kuukasjärvi P, et al. Model selection for metabolomics: predicting diagnosis of coronary artery disease using automated machine learning. Bioinforma Oxf Engl. 2020;36:1772–8.
21. Manduchi E, Fu W, Romano JD, Ruberto S, Moore JH. Embedding covariate adjustments in tree-based automated machine learning for biomedical big data analyses. BMC Bioinf. 2020;21:430.
22. Purkayastha S, Zhao Y, Wu J, Hu R, McGirr A, Singh S, et al. Differentiation of low and high grade renal cell carcinoma on routine MRI with an externally validated automatic machine learning algorithm. Sci Rep. 2020;10:19503.
23. Heimisdottir LH, Lin BM, Cho H, Orlenko A, Ribeiro AA, Simon-Soro A, et al. Metabolomics insights in early childhood caries. J Dent Res. 2021;100:615–22.
24. Manduchi E, Le TT, Fu W, Moore JH. Genetic analysis of coronary artery disease using tree-based automated machine learning informed by biology-based feature selection. IEEE/ACM Trans Comput Biol Bioinform. 2022;19:1379–86.
25. Tragante V, Hemerich D, Alshabeeb M, Brænne I, Lempiäinen H, Patel RS, et al. Druggability of coronary artery disease risk loci. Circ Genomic Precis Med. 2018;11: e001977.
26. La Cava W, Williams H, Fu W, Vitale S, Srivatsan D, Moore JH. Evaluating recommender systems for AI-driven biomedical informatics. Bioinforma Oxf Engl. 2021;37:250–6.

Machine Learning—Evaluation (Cross-validation, Metrics, Importance Scores...)

Abdulhakim Qahtan

Abstract

The high performance of machine learning (ML) techniques when handling different data analytics tasks resulted in developing a large number of models. Although these models can provide multiple options for performing the task at hand, selecting the right model becomes more challenging. As the ML models perform differently based on the nature of the data and the application, designing a good evaluation process would help in selecting the appropriate ML model. Considering the nature of the ML model and the user's interest, different evaluation experiments can be designed to get better insights about the performance of the model. In this chapter, we discuss different evaluation techniques that suit both supervised and unsupervised models including cross-validation and bootstrap. Moreover, we present a set of performance measures that can be used as an indication on how the model would perform in real applications. For each of the performance measures, we discuss the optimal values that can be achieved by a given model and what should be considered as acceptable. We also show the relationship between the different measures, which can give more insights when interpreting the results of a given ML model.

Keywords

Machine learning · Training · Testing · Regression · Classification · Clustering

Before discussing how to evaluate the Machine Learning (ML) models, we give a brief summary about the different models and how they work. Depending on the nature of the data and the task at hand, different machine learning models can be selected. These models are usually parameterized to automatically adjust their performance according to the data and the performance criteria through a set of tunable parameters. The values of the different parameters are learned and automatically adjusted during a training (fitting) stage of the model development. Learning the models' parameters can be achieved using one of three main approaches.

- **Supervised learning**: When the training set consists of labeled examples (exemplars), the algorithms use the labeled examples to learn how to generalize to the set of all possible inputs. Examples of techniques that belong to supervised learning category include logistic regression [3], support vector machines [6], neural networks [11] decision trees [22], random forest [6], etc.

A. Qahtan (✉)
Department of Information and Computing Sciences, Utrecht University, Utrecht, The Netherlands
e-mail: a.a.a.qahtan@uu.nl

F. W. Asselbergs et al. (eds.), *Clinical Applications of Artificial Intelligence in Real-World Data*,
https://doi.org/10.1007/978-3-031-36678-9_11

- **Unsupervised learning**: Refers to the set of algorithms that learn from a set of unlabeled examples. These algorithms learn the patterns that exist in the data according to a specific criterion that could be statistical, geometric or similarity criterion. Examples of unsupervised learning include k-means clustering [5] and kernel density estimation [17].
- **Reinforcement learning**: In this set of algorithms, learning is achieved by iterative exploring the solution space and receiving a feedback on the quality of the solution. The exploration is repeated until a satisfactory performance measure value is reached.

The decision on using supervised/unsupervised learning technique will depend mainly on the availability of the labeled examples in the training set. In this chapter, we focus on the evaluation of the different machine learning techniques.

1 Background

Evaluation is a key and challenging task when selecting a Machine Learning (ML) model for a specific problem. There are lots of models that can be used, but which one will perform better than the others. This requires a systematic way for evaluating the different models. In this chapter, we will discuss the different measures for evaluating the ML models. We will restrict our discussion on the predictive models that include the regression models, the classifiers and the clustering algorithms.

Selecting the performance measure to evaluate a ML model should consider the problem at hand. Evaluating a supervised model should be based on comparing the value of the target variable that has been predicted by the model with the actual value. However, evaluating the unsupervised learning techniques is more challenging and is based on computing a set of statistical measures such as Silhouette score [13] in measuring the quality of a clustering algorithm. Moreover, in case of supervised learning, the evaluation measures that are used to evaluate the regression models are different from those that are used to evaluate the classifiers. Deciding whether to use a regression model or a classifier depends on the target variable that should be predicted. If the variable contains continuous values, a regression model should be used. Otherwise (when the variable contains a few distinct values that represent class labels of the data records), a classifier is trained for this purpose. Evaluating the regression models is carried out by measuring the difference between the actual and the predicted values. This difference is used as an indicator of the performance of the regression model. For classifiers, matching the predicted class label with the actual label of the record is used as an indicator of the performance of the classifier.

Example 1 Considering the diabetes dataset,[1] a classifier should be trained and used to predict if a person is diabetic or not based on the existing information. However, predicting the person's *weight* based on the *waist circumference*, which could be useful for validating the recorded data, requires building a regression model.

However, the main idea of building supervised ML models is to train the models on a training set that contains the data records and their corresponding target variable (the variable that should be predicted for new unseen records). When using the ML model to predict the value of the target variable for an unseen record, we should have a certain level of confidence on the correctness of the predicted value. Using the proper evaluation method helps in building such confidence. Moreover, when comparing the performance of different ML models, it is important to ensure that the apparent differences in the performance is not caused by chance.

To build a supervised ML model, a labeled set that contains records with values for the independent variables and their corresponding responses (values of the target variable) is required. A typical question that could be asked is: why we do not select the model that best fits the labeled data? To answer this question, we extract a set of ten values from the feature *waist circumference* and their corresponding values from the *weight* feature for training regression models. After that, we train three different regression models to fit the

[1] https://github.com/semerj/NHANES-diabetes.

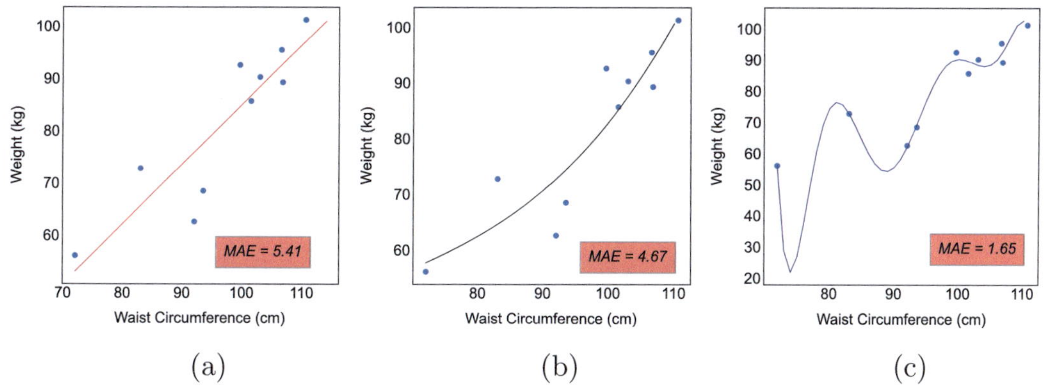

Fig. 1 Training three regression models **a** linear regression model, **b** polynomial regression model with degree 3 and **c** polynomial regression model with degree 7. In each subfigure, the mean absolute error between the actual values and the predicted ones is calculated and displayed in the red box inside the subfigure. Polynomial regression with degree 7 shows the smallest error

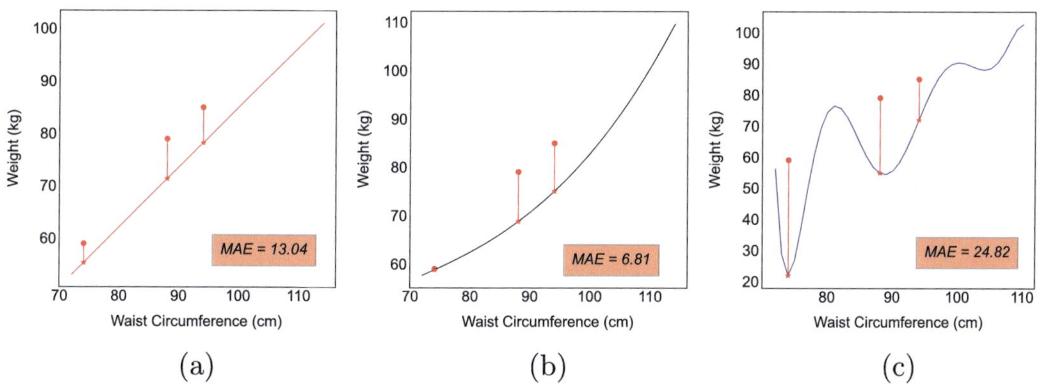

Fig. 2 Testing the three regression models on unseen data samples. In each subfigure, the mean absolute error between the actual values and the predicted ones is calculated and displayed in the red box in the subfigure. Polynomial regression with degree 3 shows the smallest error. The red vertical lines represent the difference between the actual test value (red circle) and the predicted values (red star on the regression curve)

training data as shown in Fig. 1. The Mean Absolute Error (MAE) [16] between the actual readings and the predicted ones is used as an indicator of the accuracy of the different models (MAE will be discussed later in the chapter). Comparing the MAE values in Fig. 1 (on the training data) with Fig. 2 (on the test data), it can be concluded that the model, which fits the training data the best is not necessarily the best model to be used for predicting new unseen values. This problem is a well-known problem and is called model over-fitting.

Based on the earlier discussion, the labeled data should be split into two parts (sometimes three parts) when building a supervised ML model. The first part is used for training the model and the second part is used to evaluate the model on data samples that have not been used during the training step. In some cases, a third subset of the data is used for parameter tuning of the model and is called the validation set. Evaluating the different ML models on values that have not been used during the training step is very important for comparing the different models and deciding which model to use. There are a lot of techniques that can be used to split the data into training and testing.

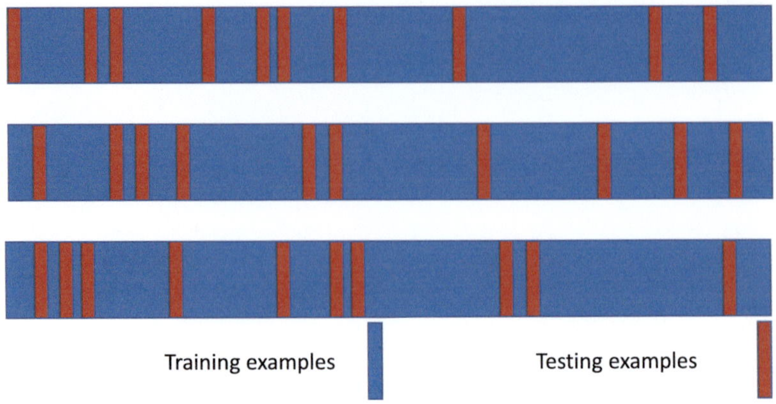

Fig. 3 Selecting random samples for training and testing from the labeled data

2 Train-Test Split

In this section, we discuss the different techniques that can be used to split the labeled data into training and testing in order to accurately estimate the performance of the ML models. The main idea is to split the labeled data into $x\%$ for training and $(100 - x)\%$ for testing (usually x is taken from the set $\{70, 75, 80\}$). The training subset is used to train (build) the ML model and the test subset is used to evaluate the performance of the model. In order to have a good estimation of the model's performance, this process is repeated multiple times and the average of the performance measure estimates is used as an indicator of the model's performance.

2.1 Random Split

For random sampling with $x\%$ for training and $(100 - x)\%$ for testing, a data example (record) from the labeled data is selected to be in the training set with probability $p = x/100$. Practically, this can be achieved by generating a random permutation for the index (sequence numbers of the records) and selecting the records with the first $x\%$ index values in the permutation. The rest of the records are assigned to the test set.

Alternatively, a random number generator can be used to generate random numbers between 0 and 100. For each record, the number r that is generated by the random number generator is compared to x and the record is selected to be in the training set if $r < x$; otherwise, the record is added to the test set. Figure 3, shows examples of splitting the labeled dataset into train and test substes randomly.

2.2 Split with Stratification

In a set of classification problems with imbalanced classes, splitting the labeled dataset into training and testing randomly may result with a training/testing dataset that contains records from only one class. For example, consider a data set of X-ray images, where the records are labeled as 0 if the person does not have cancer and 1 if the person has cancer. In such data set, the number of records that are labeled 1 is significantly smaller than those with label 0. If the training set contains only records with label 0, the trained model will not be able to recognize the records with label 1. Moreover, if test set contains records with label 0 only, the values of performance measures will be misleading.

To overcome such problem, train-test split with stratification [2] is introduced. This technique recognizes the different categories in the labeled data and generates the required ratio from each category. For example, to split the labeled data with $x\%$ for training, the labeled data is divided into a number of subsets equal to the number of classes and the records that belong to the same class fall in the same subset. After that, for each subset, an $x\%$ of the records in that subset are selected for training and the rest are held out to be used for testing.

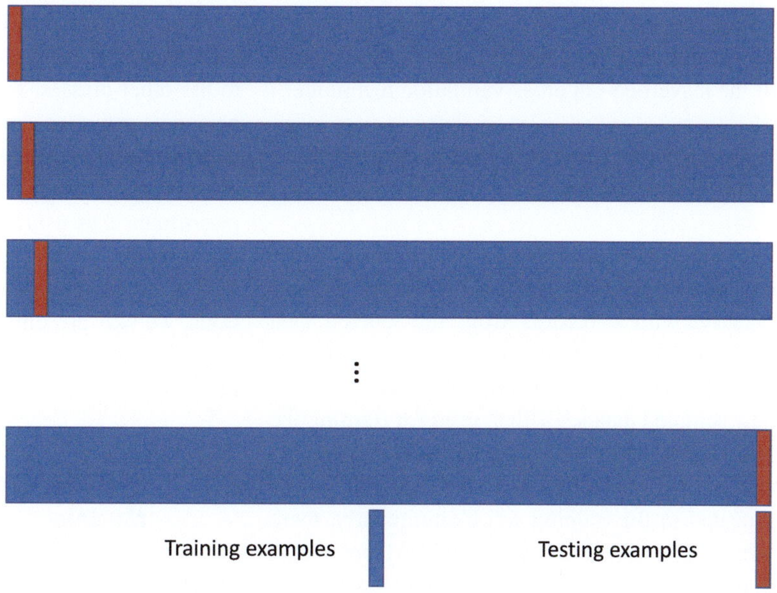

Fig. 4 Leave-one-out cross-validation for splitting the labeled dataset into training and testing

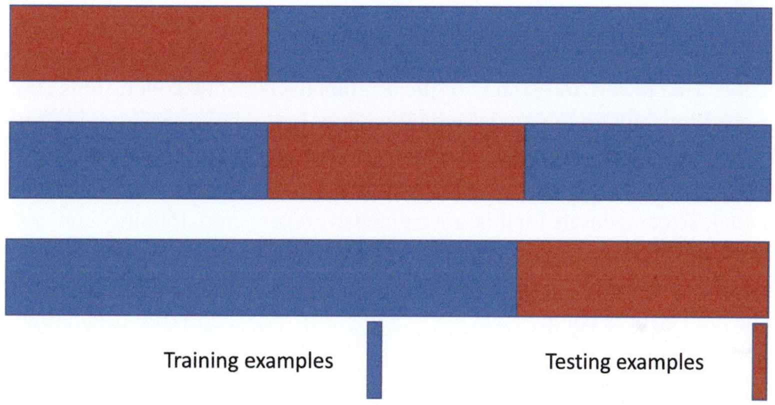

Fig. 5 Three fold cross-validation for splitting the labeled dataset into training and testing

2.3 Cross-validation

Cross validation [14] is one of the most popular techniques for train-test split. Such technique is based on performing the evaluation step multiple times where each single record in the labeled data is assigned at least once to the test set. In cross-validation, the user decides on a fixed number of folds or partitions of the data. The labeled data is then partitioned into that number of partitions. For example, if the user chose five folds, the labeled data is partitioned into five (approximately equal) partitions and each partition is used once for testing and the rest of the partitions are used for training. Figure 5, shows an example for a threefold cross-validation. A stratified 10-fold cross-validation is becoming a standard way of train-test split of the labeled data for the purpose of evaluating the ML models.

Another variation of the cross-validation is called leave-one-out cross-validation [15]. This technique is simply n-fold cross-validation when the labeled data set has n records. In this technique, each record is left out exactly once and the ML model is trained on the rest of the records. The record that is left out is used to test the model and the process is repeated n times to use each record for testing the model exactly once. This technique is preferred by the researchers, in many cases, as it maximizes the number of records that are used for training the model and the error estimation process is deterministic. Figure 4 shows an example of the leave-one-out cross-validation technique.

2.4 Bootstrap

Given a labeled data set with n records (examples), the idea of bootstrap [18] is to sample another data set with n records from the labeled data with replacement. That means, a record from the labeled data can be selected more than once. The new sampled data set is then used for training the ML model. Since sampling the new training set is done with replacement, a set of records will be repeated in the training set. Consequently, there will be a set of records in the original labeled data that have not been selected. These records are used for testing the model.

It can be shown that the probability of a record in the labeled data to be picked more than once is 0.368. That means, only 0.632 of the original data is used for training the model which is quite low compared to the 10-fold cross-validation where 90% of the labeled data is used for training the model. To compensate for this, a weighted average of the error on the training and the testing sets is used as an indicator of the model's performance. The final error is computed as

$$e = 0.632 \times e_{te} + 0.368 \times e_{tr},$$

where e_{te} is the error on the test set and e_{tr} is the error on the training set.

3 Evaluation Measures

As mentioned earlier, the evaluation measure that can be used to determine the performance of a given ML model depends on the nature of the data (labeled/unlabeled), the used ML model and the application. When the data is labeled, a supervised ML model can be used and the selection of the evaluation measure will depend on the nature of the predicted variable if it is continuous or categorical. Moreover, in many classification tasks, we might be interested in predicting the labels of a set of records that belong to a specific class more than the labels of the records that belong to the other classes. For example, predicting if a person is going to develop cancer accurately is more important than predicting if the person is not going to develop cancer. In such case, the performance measure should give more weight for correctly predicting the labels of the records from the desirable class. In the upcoming subsections, we will present and discuss different measures that can be used to evaluate the different ML models.

3.1 Evaluating the Supervised Models

In supervised learning, the ML model is trained to predict the value of the target variable using labeled data. We assume that the labels for the evaluation (test) set are also available so we can draw conclusions about the model's performance before using it in production applications for predicting the values of unseen examples (objects). As mentioned earlier, the labeled data is split into training and testing (sometime validation) sets. Comparing the predicted value with the actual value of the target variable is the logical step when evaluating the supervised ML models. Consequently, the selection of the performance measures that can be used to evaluate the supervised ML model depend on the nature of the target variable.

Evaluating the Regression Models Regression models are used to predict the values of continuous target variables. For example, predicting the blood pressure based on the lab results of a patient requires using a regression model. Let us consider that $y = \{y_1, y_2, \ldots, y_n\}$ represent the set of actual values of the target variable in the test set and $\hat{y} = \{\hat{y}_1, \hat{y}_2, \ldots, \hat{y}_n\}$ represent the set of predicted values. We compute the difference between the actual values and their corresponding predicted values $e_i = |y_i - \hat{y}_i|, \quad 1 \leq i \leq n$. We define a set of performance measures based on the values of e_i. The most common measures are the mean absolute error (MAE), sum/mean of squared error (SSE/MSE), the l_∞ and the coefficient of determination R^2.

The mean absolute error is defined as $MAE = \frac{1}{n}\sum_{i=1}^{n}|y_i - \hat{y}_i|$. It represents the arithmetic average of the absolute error between the actual and the predicted values. This measure is usually used for computing the forecast error in time series analysis. However, it is used in a lot of applications as an indicator of the regression models' performance. The optimal value for MAE is 0; However, when comparing different regression models, the regression with smallest value for the MAE is considered better than the other models.

The sum/mean squared error are computed as $SSE = \sum_{i=1}^{n}\left(y_i - \hat{y}_i\right)^2$ and $MSE = \frac{1}{n}\sum_{i=1}^{n}\left(y_i - \hat{y}_i\right)^2$. It is clear that SSE/MSE are the arithmetic summation/average of the squared difference (absolute error) between the actual and the predicted values. Similar to MAE, a value close to 0 means that the model is accurate. However, this measure reduces the contribution of the error values that are close to 0 and gives more weight to the error values that are greater than 1.

In order to make sure that the regression model provides accurate predictions for all examples in the test set, a measure called l_∞ is proposed. The $l_\infty = \max\limits_{1\le i\le n}|y_i - \hat{y}_i|$ error is computed as the maximum value of the absolute error e_i, $1 \le i \le n$. This measure is used to highlight the worst performance of the model.

The coefficient of determination is denoted by R^2 [10] and represents the proportion of the variance in the target variable that is predictable from the independent (determinant or exploratory) variables. It is a measure of how the regression equation accounts for the variation in the dependent variable. It is well-known that the closer the regression curve to the points, the better the models fits the data. The main idea behind R^2 is to determine if a regression model can utilize the knowledge from the independent variables to predict the dependent (target) variable accurately. To compute the R^2 value, we start by considering the average value of the target variable as our baseline predictor. After that, we compute the deviation of the predicted values of the regression model from the mean value and from the actual values, i.e, we compute three quantities

$$\begin{aligned} TSS &= \sum_{i=1}^{n}(y_i - \bar{y})^2 \\ RSS &= \sum_{i=1}^{n}\left(\hat{y}_i - \bar{y}\right)^2 \\ ESS &= \sum_{i=1}^{n}\left(y_i - \hat{y}_i\right)^2 \end{aligned} \tag{1}$$

where $\bar{y}$ is the mean of the target variable y in the test set, TSS refers to the sum of squared deviation and RSS refers to the sum of squared deviation between the predicted values using the regression model and the mean of the target variable. Moreover, ESS is the sum of squared deviation between the actual and the values that predicted using the regression model. From Eq. (1), we can see that $TSS = RSS + ESS$. The coefficient of determination R^2 is then computed as

$$R^2 = \frac{RSS}{TSS} = \frac{TSS - ESS}{TSS} = 1 - \frac{ESS}{TSS}. \tag{2}$$

The optimal score for R^2 is 1.0, which can be achieved when the value of the term $ESS \to 0$. Smaller values for R^2 means that the model is not accurate.

In Table 1, we summarize the measures that can be used to evaluate the regression models. It is clear that the main term in each measure is the difference between the actual and the predicted value. Usually, we need to compare two different learning models to see which one performs better on a specific problem. To have a better indication on the performance of the different models, we need to apply the techniques that we mentioned earlier such as cross validation and repeat the tests multiple times to choose the model that

Table 1 Summary of regression evaluation measures

Measure	Formula
MAE	$\frac{1}{n}\sum_{i=1}^{n}\lvert y_i - \hat{y}_i\rvert$
MSE	$\frac{1}{n}\sum_{i=1}^{n}\left(y_i - \hat{y}_i\right)^2$
SSE	$\sum_{i=1}^{n}\left(y_i - \hat{y}_i\right)^2$
l_∞	$\max_{1\le i\le n}\lvert y_i - \hat{y}_i\rvert$
R^2	$1 - \frac{\sum_{i=1}^{n}(y_i - \hat{y}_i)^2}{\sum_{i=1}^{n}(y_i - \bar{y})^2}$

gives the lower estimated error. However, we need also to check if the difference in the error is not happening by chance due to the randomness in the process. We leave this issue as it is out of the scope of this chapter.

Evaluating the Classifiers Classifiers predict a categorical value for each data example that represents the class label for that example. Based on this property, evaluating the classification models can be done by matching the predicted class label with the actual one and counting the number of examples that have the same value for the predicted and the actual labels. The large number of correct predictions indicates high performance of the classification model.

In the case of two class problem, we can consider the labels for the classes to be positive and negative or 0 and 1. The possible outcomes for matching a predicted class label with the actual one can be one of the the following:

- True positive (TP): the actual and the predicted labels are positive.
- False positive (FP): the actual label is negative while the predicted label is positive.
- False negative (FN): the actual label is positive while the predicted label is negative.
- True negative (TN): both (actual and predicted) labels are negative.

These different outcomes are usually summarized in matrix form, which is called the *confusion matrix* [21] (see Table 2). In Table 2, we see the confusion matrix for two classes with entries labeled as TP, FP, FN, and TN. From the confusion matrix, a set of performance measures can be defined. The basic performance measure for a classifier is its accuracy, which can be defined as follows

Table 2 The confusion matrix

		Prediction	
		Positive	Negative
Actual	Positive	TP	FN
	Negative	FP	TN

$$\text{Accuracy (acc)} = \frac{\text{number of correct prediction}}{\text{size of the test set}} \tag{3}$$

In terms of the confusion matrix entries, the accuracy can be written as

$$\begin{aligned}\text{Accuracy (acc)} &= \frac{TP+TN}{TP+FP+FN+TN}\\ &= \frac{TP+TN}{n},\end{aligned} \tag{4}$$

where n is the number of examples in the test set. As we can see, all misclassification errors are given the same weight. However, optimizing the classifiers to have better accuracy values is usually misleading. This is a well-known problem when the class distribution of the samples (examples) is imbalanced [1]. By imbalanced data, we refer to the situation when the representative samples of the classes are unevenly distributed [19]. Let us consider the example in [4], where a set of images are labeled as either cancerous or noncancerous. The annotation resulted in labeling 10,923 images as noncancerous (majority class) and 260 as cancerous (minority class). When optimizing the ML model for accuracy, the model will tend to classify more examples to be noncancerous. If the ML model classifies every sample to be from the noncancerous (majority) class, it will achieve 99.98 % accuracy. However, in many applications, it is more costly to misclassify the examples from the minority class. For this reason, a set of measures have been proposed to tackle the imbalanced data problem and give better indications about the classifiers' performance.

In the information retrieval community, the *precision (P)* and *recall (R)* [20] are used to evaluate the performance of the information retrieval systems. When the user sends a query to retrieve a set of documents that are related to a specific topic, the precision represents the ratio of the correctly retrieved documents that are related to the topic in the set of the retrieved documents, whereas the recall represents the ratio of correctly retrieved documents in the set of he related documents in the whole dataset. In terms of the confusion matrix entries, we can consider:

- TP = the number of relevant retrieved documents
- FP = the number of irrelevant retrieved documents
- FN = the number of relevant unretrieved documents
- TN = the number of irrelevant unretrieved documents

Using this analogy, the precision and recall can be defined as:

$$\text{Precision (P)} = \frac{TP}{TP + FP}$$

$$\text{Recall (R)} = \frac{TP}{TP + FN}$$

Since, the precision and the recall can be expressed in terms of the entries in the confusion matrix, they have been used for measuring the performance of the classifiers. Moreover, a measure that combines the values of precision and recall is called the *F-Measure* or *F-Score* [7] is also used for measuring the classifiers' performance. In its generic form, the F-Score is defined as:

$$F_\beta = (1 + \beta^2)\frac{P \times R}{(\beta^2 \times P) + R},$$

where P, R are the precision and recall and β is a parameter that controls the importance of the recall compared to the precision when computing the F-Score. When $\beta > 1$, the recall has more weight than the precision and vice versa. The balance between precision and recall is achieved when $\beta = 1$. In this case, F-Score represents the harmonic mean between P and R and is written as:

$$F_1 = 2\frac{P \times R}{P + R}.$$

Usually, the discussion of the precision, recall and F-Score focuses on measuring the performance of the ML models with respect to the positive class (+ve). However, they can be used to measure the performance with respect to the negative class (−ve). We can write:

$$P(+ve) = \frac{TP}{TP + FP} \text{ and } P(-ve) = \frac{TN}{TN + FN}.$$

Similarly:

$$R(+ve) = \frac{TP}{TP + FN} \text{ and}$$
$$R(-ve) = \frac{TN}{TN + FP}.$$

In general, if we have k classes, we can compute k different values for each of the precision, recall and F-Score as they are associated with the class labels.

In the data mining community, the $R(+ve)$ is also known as the *sensitivity* of the ML model while the $R(-ve)$ is known as the *specificity*. The sensitivity and the specificity are used to define another performance measure that is more suitable for evaluating the ML models on biased data, which is called *the balanced accuracy* and is defined as follows:

$$\text{Balanced Accuracy (BA)} = \frac{\text{sensitivity} + \text{specificity}}{2} = \frac{R(+ve) + R(-ve)}{2}$$

The balanced accuracy provides a better measure for the performance of the ML models when the dataset is biased (there is a significant difference between the number of representative examples from each class in the dataset).

Example 2 Consider the case of training an ML model for classifying an input record to be cancerous or not using the dataset in [4]. We have 10,923 examples from noncancerous (U) and 260 examples from the cancerous class (C). If we split the dataset using the 70-30 rule (70% for training and 30% for testing) with stratification then we will have the number of records in each subset as in Table 3. We train an ML model (M) using the training set and test it on the test set. We present the output of the ML model in Table 4.

Table 3 Train-test split of the cancer dataset with stratification

	Cancerous (C)	Noncancerous (U)
Training	182	7646
Testing	78	3277

Table 4 The confusion matrix that represents the results of testing M using the test set of the cancer dataset

		Prediction	
		C	U
Actual	C	47	31
	U	327	2950

Table 5 Performance measures of the ML model on the cancer dataset

Acc.	$P(C)$	$P(U)$	$R(C)$	$R(U)$	$F_1(C)$	$F_1(U)$	BA
89.33	12.57	98.96	60.26	90.02	20.80	94.28	75.14

The reported values are out of 100, where 100 is the optimal value

The values for the different performance measures that are used to evaluate the ML model (M) are presented in Table 5. As we can see in the results, considering the values of the measures that are computed for the class (C) are lower than those for the class (U). Moreover, small changes in the classification outcomes would lead to significant changes in the values of the performance measures when considering the class (C) as it has a few examples. The accuracy is an exception.To show that, assume that your ML model is able to classify all the examples from the class (C) correctly. In this case, the value of the accuracy will be $acc. = 90.25\%$ whereas the balanced accuracy will be $BA = 95\%$. As we can see, the balanced accuracy increased by 20% while the accuracy increased by less than 1%. Hence, the balanced accuracy can be considered as a better classification performance measure when the data is biased as it gives more weight for correctly classifying an example from the minority class.

It is worth noting that these measures are easily extendable for the cases when we have more than two classes. To show that, let us consider a dataset that contains k classes $C = \{C_1, C_2, \ldots, C_k\}$. In this case, the confusion matrix can be constructed

Table 6 The confusion matrix for the case of k classes

		Prediction			
		C_1	C_2	$\ldots$	C_4
Actual	C_1	C_{11}	C_{12}	$\ldots$	C_{1k}
	C_2	C_{21}	C_{22}	$\ldots$	C_{2k}
	$\ldots$	$\ldots$	$\ldots$	$\ldots$	$\ldots$
	C_k	C_{k1}	C_{k2}	$\ldots$	C_{kk}

as in Table 6 and the accuracy can be computed as the summation of the values in the main diagonal over the summation of all entries in the confusion matrix. That is

$$acc. = \frac{\sum_{i=1}^{k} C_{ii}}{\sum_{i=1}^{k}\sum_{j=1}^{k} C_{ij}}$$

Moreover, the precision and recall can be expressed as

$$P(C_i) = \frac{C_i}{\sum_{j=1}^{k} C_{ij}} \quad \text{and} \quad R(C_i) = \frac{C_i}{\sum_{j=1}^{k} C_{ji}},$$

where $P(C_i)$ is the precision and $R(C_i)$ is the recall with respect to (w.r.t) class C_i. The other measures can be expressed in a similar way.

3.2 Evaluating the Unsupervised Models

In unsupervised learning, the training data is not labeled. In this case, there is no error or reward that can help in optimizing the ML model. Instead, the ML techniques learn the patterns that exist in the data in order to categorize the examples (objects) according to a specific geometric or statistical criteria. The ML models are trained to summarize the key features or structures of the data by optimizing for the specified criteria. For example, clustering is an unsupervised technique that tends to increase the intra-cluster similarity and reduce the inter-cluster similarity. The different clustering techniques (algorithms) try to satisfy this criteria using different optimization functions. In this section we will focus on evaluating the clustering techniques since they are the most widely used unsupervised learning techniques.

As the clustering techniques tend to group similar items (objects) together, a similarity measure should be introduced that can determine how two objects are similar to each other. For numerical attributes, the *Minkowski distance* is a well-known similarity measure between the objects. The Minkowski distance is defined as

$$d(\mathbf{x}, \mathbf{y}) = \left(\sum_{i=1}^{d} |x_i - y_i|^p \right)^{1/p},$$

where $d(\mathbf{x}, \mathbf{y})$ is the distance between two objects $\mathbf{x}, \mathbf{y} \in \mathbb{R}^d$, d is the data dimensionality and $\mathbb{R}$ is the set of real numbers. For categorical data, a match/mismatch or string dissimilarity functions can be used as dissimilarity (distance) measures. These dissimilarity measures are also used to define similarity measures to determine the membership level of an object to a given cluster. We use the similarity measures to compute *Silhouette coefficient* [13], which is used to measure the quality of a given clustering technique.

When evaluating the different clustering techniques, it is important to define a measure that can check if two clustering techniques (algorithms) produce similar groups (clusters) of the objects in the data. For this purpose, a measure called *Rand Index* is proposed in [12]. To explain how rand index can be used to compare two clustering algorithms, assume that we have a set $\mathbf{X} = \{\mathbf{x_1}, \mathbf{x_2}, \ldots, \mathbf{x_n}\}$ of objects (examples) that needs to be clustered (grouped). We use two different clustering algorithms $\mathcal{A}_1, \mathcal{A}_2$ to cluster the data into $\mathcal{A}_1(\mathbf{X}) = \{A_{11}, A_{12}, \ldots, A_{1r}\}$ and $\mathcal{A}_2(\mathbf{X}) = \{A_{21}, A_{22}, \ldots, A_{2s}\}$. There are four different types of relations that can be found between any pair of elements in the set $\mathbf{X} \times \mathbf{X}$ (Cartesian product of $\mathbf{X}$ with itself)

$$\begin{aligned}
\Gamma_1 &= \{(\mathbf{x_i}, \mathbf{x_j}) \ : (\exists p, \exists q),\ \mathbf{x_i}, \mathbf{x_j} \in A_{1p} \ \wedge\ \mathbf{x_i}, \mathbf{x_j} \in A_{2q}\} \\
\Gamma_2 &= \{(\mathbf{x_i}, \mathbf{x_j}) \ : (\exists p, \forall q),\ \mathbf{x_i}, \mathbf{x_j} \in A_{1p} \ \wedge\ \mathbf{x_i}, \mathbf{x_j} \notin A_{2q}\} \\
\Gamma_3 &= \{(\mathbf{x_i}, \mathbf{x_j}) \ : (\forall p, \exists q),\ \mathbf{x_i}, \mathbf{x_j} \notin A_{1p} \ \wedge\ \mathbf{x_i}, \mathbf{x_j} \in A_{2q}\} \\
\Gamma_4 &= \{(\mathbf{x_i}, \mathbf{x_j}) \ : (\forall p, \forall q),\ \mathbf{x_i}, \mathbf{x_j} \notin A_{1p} \ \wedge\ \mathbf{x_i}, \mathbf{x_j} \notin A_{2q}\},
\end{aligned}$$

where $p \in \{1, 2, \ldots, r\}$ and $q \in \{1, 2, \ldots, s\}$. Let $\gamma_l = |\Gamma_l|,\ 1 \le l \le 4$, then the values for $\gamma_l,\ 1 \le l \le 4$ can be interpreted as follows: i) γ_1 represents the cardinality of the set that contains the pairs of objects which fall in the same cluster using both algorithms $\mathcal{A}_1, \mathcal{A}_2$; ii) γ_2 is the number of pairs of objects in $\mathbf{X}$ that are in the same cluster according to algorithm $\mathcal{A}_1$, but in different clusters according to algorithm $\mathcal{A}_2$; iii) γ_3 is the number of pairs of elements in $\mathbf{X}$ that are in different clusters according to algorithm $\mathcal{A}_1$, but in the same cluster according to algorithm $\mathcal{A}_2$; and iv) γ_4 is the number of pairs of objects in $\mathbf{X}$ that fall in different clusters according to both algorithms $\mathcal{A}_1$ and $\mathcal{A}_2$. Based on these quantities, the rand index is computed as

$$RI = \frac{\gamma_1 + \gamma_4}{\gamma_1 + \gamma_2 + \gamma_3 + \gamma_4}.$$

The RI takes values in the interval [0, 1], where 1 represents the optimal value and means that both algorithms divided the original dataset $\mathbf{X}$ into the same set of clusters. When $RI = 0$, then the two algorithms are completely different. However, when assigning the objects in $\mathbf{X}$ into clusters randomly, the value of RI will not be 0, which requires correction-for-chance that has been proposed in [8] to define the adjusted random index (ARI). The ARI can be written as [9]

$$ARI = \frac{\binom{n}{2}(\gamma_1 + \gamma_3) - [(\gamma_1 + \gamma_4)(\gamma_1 + \gamma_2) + (\gamma_2 + \gamma_3)(\gamma_3 + \gamma_4)]}{\binom{n}{2}^2 [(\gamma_1 + \gamma_4)(\gamma_2 + \gamma_3) + (\gamma_2 + \gamma_3)(\gamma_3 + \gamma_4)]},$$

where $n = |\mathbf{X}|$ and $\binom{n}{2}$ is the total number of pairs. We consider that the pairs $(\mathbf{x_i}, \mathbf{x_j})$ and $(\mathbf{x_j}, \mathbf{x_i})$ are equal so they are counted only once.

When the dataset $\mathbf{X}$ is labeled, we can select algorithm $\mathcal{A}_1$ as the dummy clustering algorithm that assigns each object in $\mathbf{X}$ to its class and creates a number of clusters that is equivalent to the number of the classes in the dataset. In this case, the value of RI that is used to compare a given clustering algorithm $\mathcal{A}_2$ with the dummy algorithm $\mathcal{A}_1$ is exactly the accuracy that we discussed when evaluating the classification techniques earlier. Based on this observation, the other performance measures that we defined to evaluate the classification techniques, can be used to evaluate the clustering algorithms when the labels of the object are available. However, the performance measures have been given different names when they are used to evaluate the clustering algorithms. For example, the precision is called *purity* or *homogeneity*, the recall is called the *completeness* and the F-Score is called the *V-measure*.

When the labels of the objects in the dataset are available, we count the number of objects that belong to each class in a given cluster and associate that cluster with the class which includes the majority of the objects. A cluster is said to satisfy the purity (homogeneity) criterion if all the values in that cluster belong to the same class. Moreover, a cluster is said to satisfy the completeness criterion if all examples that belong to the class associated with that cluster are included in the cluster. To compute the purity and completeness of cluster $\mathbb{C}_i$, we assume that $\mathbb{C}_i$ is associated with class C_j.[2] In this case, the purity of $\mathbb{C}_i$ is defined as $purity(\mathbb{C}_i) = \frac{|\{\mathbf{x}:\mathbf{x}\in\mathbb{C}_i \wedge \mathbf{x}\in C_j\}|}{|\mathbb{C}_i|}$ and the completeness is defined as $completeness(\mathbb{C}_i) = \frac{|\{\mathbf{x}:\mathbf{x}\in\mathbb{C}_i \wedge \mathbf{x}\in C_j\}|}{|C_j|}$. The V-measure is defined similar to the F_1-Score as follows

$$\text{V-measure} = \frac{2 \times purity \times completeness}{purity + completeness}.$$

The purity, completeness and V-measure take values in the interval [0, 1] where 1 represents the optimal outcome of the clustering algorithm. Obviously, these measures will not take the value of 0 in case of random clustering. Instead, their values will increase as the number of clusters increases, which could give misleading indication about the goodness of the clustering algorithm. However, this problem can be overcome when the number of the objects in the dataset $\mathbf{X}$ is large and the number of clusters is small.

Another measure that can be used to evaluate the goodness of the clustering algorithm is the *Silhouette coefficient* [13]. This measure determines how similar an example is to the examples in its own cluster compared to the examples in the other clusters without using the labels in the dataset. To compute the Silhouette coefficient for a given object (example $\mathbf{x_i}$) in the dataset, we compute two quantities $a(\mathbf{x_i})$ and $b(\mathbf{x_i})$ as follows:

$$a(\mathbf{x_i}) = \frac{1}{|\mathbb{C}_k| - 1} \sum_{\mathbf{x_j}\in\mathbb{C}_k \wedge \mathbf{x_j}\neq\mathbf{x_i}} d(\mathbf{x_i}, \mathbf{x_j}),$$

where $\mathbb{C}_k$ is the cluster that contains the object $\mathbf{x_i}$ and $d(\mathbf{x_i}, \mathbf{x_j})$ is a dissimilarity (distance) measure. The quantity $a(\mathbf{x_i})$ represents the average distance between $\mathbf{x_i}$ and all other objects in the same cluster. We define $\alpha_{im}(\mathbf{x_i}, \mathbb{C}_m)$ to be the average dissimilarity between the object $\mathbf{x_i}$ and all other objects in the cluster $\mathbb{C}_m$. That is

$$\alpha_{im}(\mathbf{x_i}, \mathbb{C}_m) = \frac{1}{|\mathbb{C}_m|} \sum_{\mathbf{x_j}\in\mathbb{C}_m} d(\mathbf{x_i}, \mathbf{x_j}).$$

Assuming that we have λ clusters, we select $b(\mathbf{x_i})$ to be the minimum value of $\alpha_{it}(\mathbf{x_i}, \mathbb{C}_t),\ 1 \le t \le \lambda \wedge t \neq k$. Using the quantities $a(\mathbf{x_i})$ and $b(\mathbf{x_i})$, we define the Silhouette coefficient for $\mathbf{x_i}$ as:

$$Sil(\mathbf{x_i}) = \frac{b(\mathbf{x_i}) - a(\mathbf{x_i})}{\max(b(\mathbf{x_i}), a(\mathbf{x_i}))}.$$

The Silhouette coefficient takes values in the interval $[-1, 1]$, where a value of 0 means that the object is in the border between two clusters, a negative value means that the object is more similar to objects in the nearest cluster than the objects in its own cluster. The average Silhouette coefficient over all objects in a given cluster determines the goodness of the cluster where a value close to 1 would mean a compact cluster. The average Silhouette coefficient over all clusters defines the quality of the clustering algorithm.

4 Conclusion

In this chapter, we provided a brief summary about the different machine learning approaches including the supervised, unsupervised and reinforcement learning. We introduced different performance measures that can be used to evaluate the ML models. Our main focus was on the regression, classification and clustering as these are the most widely used ML techniques. We showed that the values of some measures can be misleading when the dataset has specific characteristics. For example, the accuracy is not a good measure for

[2] We use the symbol $\mathbb{C}$ to represent a cluster while the regular C is used to represent a class.

the classification performance when the dataset is biased (the majority of the examples in the dataset belong to one class). Consequently, selecting the performance measure should consider the ML technique, the characteristics of the dataset and the task at hand. A good performance measure would lead to better optimization of the ML model to produce high quality results especially in fields where ML models have high impact people's lives such as in the health domain.

References

1. A comprehensive data level analysis for cancer diagnosis on imbalanced data. J Biomed Inf. 2019;90.
2. César CC, Carvalho MS. Stratified sampling design and loss to follow-up in survival models: evaluation of efficiency and bias. BMC Med Res Methodol. 2011;11(1):1–9.
3. Cox DR. The regression analysis of binary sequences. J Roy Stat Soc: Seri B (Methodol). 1958;20(2):215–32.
4. Fotouhi S, Asadi S, Kattan MW. A comprehensive data level analysis for cancer diagnosis on imbalanced data. J Biomed Inf. 2019;90.
5. Hartigan JA, Wong MA. A k-means clustering algorithm. JSTOR: Appl Stat. 1979;28(1):100–108.
6. Ho TK. Random decision forests. In: Proceedings of 3rd international conference on document analysis and recognition. vol. 1. IEEE; 1995. p. 278–282.
7. Hripcsak G, Rothschild AS. Agreement, the f-measure, and reliability in information retrieval. J Ame Med Inf Assoc. 2005;12:296–8.
8. Hubert L, Arabie P. Comparing partitions. J Classif. 1985;2(1):193–218.
9. Igual L, Seguí S. Introduction to data science. 2017.
10. Lewis-Beck C, Lewis-Beck M. Applied regression: an introduction, vol. 22. Sage Publications; 2015.
11. McCulloch WS, Pitts W. A logical calculus of the ideas immanent in nervous activity. Bull Math Biophys. 1943;5(4):115–33.
12. Rand WM. Objective criteria for the evaluation of clustering methods. J Am Stat Assoc. 1971;66(336):846–50.
13. Rousseeuw PJ. Silhouettes: a graphical aid to the interpretation and validation of cluster analysis. J Comput Appl Math. 1987;20:53–65.
14. Sammut C, Webb GI, editors. Cross-validation. Boston, MA, USA: Springer; 2010.
15. Sammut C, Webb GI editors. Leave-one-out cross-validation. 2010. p. 600–601.
16. Sammut C, Webb GI editors. Mean absolute error. 2010.
17. Scott DW. Multivariate density estimation: theory, practice, and visualization. Wiley; 1992.
18. Stine R. An introduction to bootstrap methods: examples and ideas. Soc Methods Res. 1989;18(2–3):243–91.
19. Sun Y, Wong AK, Kamel MS. Classification of imbalanced data: a review. Int J Pattern Recognit Artif Intell. 2009;23(04):687–719.
20. Ting KM. Precision and recall. 2010.
21. Ting KM. Confusion matrix. Boston, MA, USA: Springer; 2017.
22. Wu X, Kumar V, Quinlan JR, Ghosh J, Yang Q, Motoda H, McLachlan GJ, Ng A, Liu B, Philip SY, et al. Top 10 algorithms in data mining. Knowl Inf Syst. 2008;14(1):1–37.

Deep Learning—Prediction

Chris Al Gerges, Melle B. Vessies, Rutger R. van de Leur and René van Es

Abstract

Deep learning is a subfield of artificial intelligence (AI) that is concerned with developing large and complex neural networks for various tasks. As of today, there exists a wide variety of DL models yielding promising results in many subfields of AI, such as computer vision (CV) and natural language processing (NLP). In this chapter, we provide an overview of deep learning, elaborating on some common model architectures. Furthermore, we describe the advantages and disadvantages of deep learning compared to machine learning. Afterwards, we discuss the application of deep learning models in various clinical tasks, focusing on clinical imaging, electronic health records and genomics. We also provide a brief overview of prediction tasks in deep learning. The final section of this chapter discusses the limitations and challenges of deploying deep learning models in healthcare and medicine, focusing on the lack of explainability in deep learning models.

C. Al Gerges (✉) · M. B. Vessies ·
R. R. van de Leur · R. van Es
UMCU, Utrecht, Netherlands
e-mail: chrisalgerges@hotmail.com

Keywords

Deep learning · Machine learning · Regression · Classification · Segmentation · Clinical imaging · Electronic health records · Explainable AI (XAI)

1 Introduction

This chapter describes the field of deep learning (DL) and its application in the medical field for the purpose of prediction, both for diagnosis and prognosis. First, we will provide a theoretical overview of DL, focusing on some common models and their components. Furthermore, we will discuss the process of training these models on data, and the benefits and limitations of DL concerning the field of machine learning (ML). Second, we will describe several prediction tasks that DL models perform, focusing on classification, regression, survival analysis, and segmentation. Third, we provide several examples that illustrate the potential real-world application of DL models in healthcare and medicine, focusing on clinical imaging, electronic health records (EHRs), and genomics. Finally, we discuss the possible implications of deploying DL models in medicine and healthcare. We conclude this chapter by describing several limitations of DL within the medical domain, focusing on explainability and its necessity in DL models.

F. W. Asselbergs et al. (eds.), *Clinical Applications of Artificial Intelligence in Real-World Data*,
https://doi.org/10.1007/978-3-031-36678-9_12

2 Deep Learning: A Theoretical Overview

DL is a subfield of artificial intelligence (AI) that is concerned with developing large and complex neural networks for various tasks. It emerged from the field of ML when more research was done on artificial neural networks (ANNs), models that have been inspired by the biological neural networks of animal brains [1]. A DL model is simply an ANN with many hidden layers. Each DL model is trained with the *backpropagation algorithm* [2] (Fig. 1). It consists of two parts: the forward pass and the backward pass. In the forward pass, the DL model is fed a *batch* of input data x, transforming it to an output y'. Here, a batch is simply a small subset of randomly sampled datapoints from a dataset. The size of this subset is called the *batch size*. After the forward pass, an error measure between the model output y' and the ground truth y is calculated with a *loss function*, which depends on the task of the DL model. This error is then propagated through the DL model in the backward pass by calculating the gradient of each hidden layer. Finally, these gradients are used to update the parameters of the DL model. The exact method that performs this update is called the *optimizer* of the DL model. In general, an optimizer iteratively minimizes (or maximizes) the value of the loss function. The rate at which this optimization takes place is called the *learning rate*. One of the first optimizers used in DL is stochastic gradient descent (SGD). Currently, there exist many other optimizers, including AdaGrad [3], RMSProp [4], and Adam [5], the latter of which is one of the most popular optimizers in DL. After the parameters have been updated, the backpropagation algorithm is repeated for a different batch of input data until all datapoints have been fed to the DL model. When that is the case, we say that the DL model has finished an *epoch*. Training of the DL model ends when it has completed a specified number of epochs, depending on the task of the model.

Compared to ML, one of the main advantages of DL is that no feature extraction step is required when building a predictive model for a dataset (Fig. 2). Here, a feature is a property derived from the raw data input with the purpose of providing a suitable representation [6]. In ML systems, such as support vector machines (SVMs), the raw data needs to be transformed into useful features before it can be fed to a learning algorithm for detecting patterns. Historically, constructing feature extractors required domain knowledge and human engineering. Conversely, in DL the feature extraction is done automatically, as a DL model learns its own representations needed for pattern recognition. This occurs in each layer of the DL model, where the lower layers contain more primitive and data specific features, while the higher layers contain rather abstract and complex features. This framework allows for DL models to directly work with the raw data and to extract useful features from multiple data sources [7]. Another advantage that DL has over ML is that DL models can handle noisy and unstructured data better than ML models, due to the aforementioned automated feature learning of DL models [6]. Finally, DL models continue to

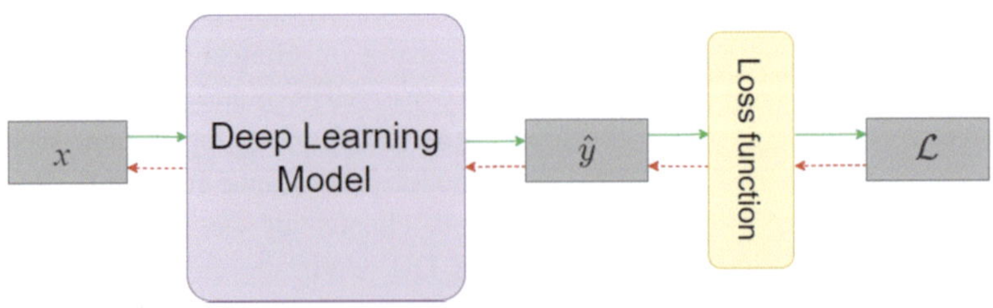

Fig. 1 Schematic overview of the backpropagation algorithm. The green solid arrows represent the forward pass, while the dashed red arrows represent the backward pass

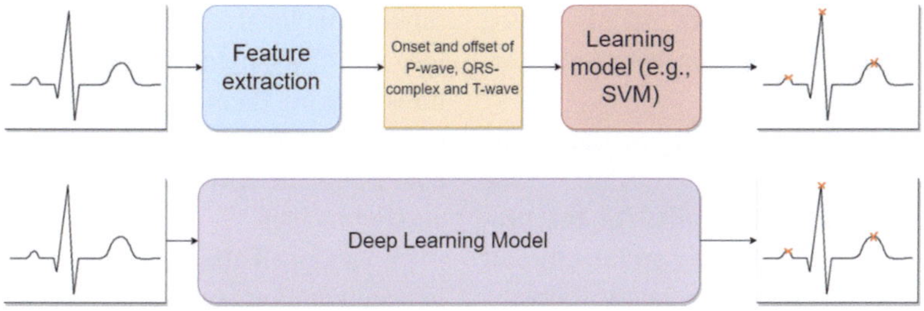

Fig. 2 Schematic overview of a ML approach (top) and a DL approach (bottom) for the task of peak detection in electrocardiograms (ECGs). In an ML approach, features are extracted from the raw ECG signal and fed into a learning model. In a DL approach on the other hand, the raw ECG signal can be directly fed to the model, as it automatically learns the features from the data

improve with more data, enabling them to outperform many classical ML approaches [7].

Despite the rise in popularity of DL in AI research, there are also disadvantages of DL compared to ML. One of the main disadvantages of DL is that most DL models are *black-box models*. This means that the decision-making process of DL models is not transparent. In other words, end users of such models have no indication how the input corresponded to the model's output. As such, when a DL model makes a prediction, it may not be possible to explain why the model has made that prediction. This lack of transparency forms one of the main reasons why DL models are not prevalent in healthcare and medicine, because many clinicians feel uncomfortable to apply DL models in medicine, even when these models achieve impressive results in clinical tasks [8]. This feeling of discomfort is likely due to the fact that healthcare and medicine contain many high-stake scenarios (e.g., surgery, diagnosis), where decisions could greatly impact people's lives. As such, physicians would like to explain these decisions to their patients [9]. Another limitation is that DL models require a large amount of processing power and memory due to their complexity and size, which limits the use of DL models in small industries. Finally, DL models need a large amount of data in order to obtain state-of-the-art results. For some tasks, such as the diagnosis of rare diseases, such large datasets are not always available, limiting the application of DL in certain fields. We will elaborate more on the shortcomings of DL in the final section of this chapter.

3 Deep Learning: Model Architectures

As of today, there exists a wide variety of DL models yielding promising results in many subfields of AI, such as computer vision (CV) and natural language processing (NLP). The simplest type of DL model is the multilayer perceptron (MLP). MLPs are ANNs that contain fully connected layers, meaning that each node in the previous layer is connected to every other node in the next layer. Within a fully connected layer, a matrix multiplication between the input matrix X and a weight matrix W is performed. Afterwards, a bias vector b is added to the result. Because of the aforementioned calculation, a fully connected layer is also referred to as a *linear layer* in literature. Usually, linear layers are followed by an activation layer, applying an activation function f to the output of the linear layer. Generally, an MLP comprises of an input layer, followed by multiple consecutive hidden layers and ending with an output layer. The input layer is responsible for receiving the data. The hidden layers are composed of many fully connected layers, extracting features from the input data. Finally, the output layer produces the final prediction result [10]. MLPs are often present at the end of large DL architectures, integrating high-level features to produce a task-dependent prediction. However, MLPs are mainly suited for processing rather simple data structures, particularly tabular data [10].

A more complex type of DL model is the convolutional neural network (CNN). These models are a very popular choice for the processing of image data. The basic architecture of CNNs consists of a convolution layer, followed by an activation layer. The convolution layer extracts features from the input data by performing a convolution with a fixed size convolution filter, after which an activation function f is applied. Usually, a pooling (subsampling) layer follows the activation layer, performing a subsampling operation in each region covered by the convolution filter. This extracts more representative features and makes them more robust to noise [10]. Common subsampling operations include taking the average (i.e., mean pooling) or taking the maximum (i.e., max pooling) in each region. If the features need to be aggregated for prediction tasks, a linear layer could be added at the end of the CNN [10, 11]. By relying on local connections and weight sharing, the CNN obtains translation invariant features, making them especially suitable to encode spatial dependencies of the input data [11]. This could explain why CNNs are effective in processing images.

A variant of the CNN that is primarily used in segmentation tasks is the U-Net [12] (Fig. 3). A U-Net contains two parts: the contractive path and the expansive path. The contractive path is the typical CNN, each step containing successive convolution layers with rectifier linear unit (ReLU) activation, followed by a max pooling operation. This decreases the spatial resolution of the image and increases the resolution of the feature map. Thus, the contractive path learns features at multiple resolution levels, capturing context information of the image. In the symmetric expansive path, each step contains a transposed convolution as upsampling operation, followed by the same amount of convolution layers as in the contractive path. This increases the spatial resolution of the image at each step.

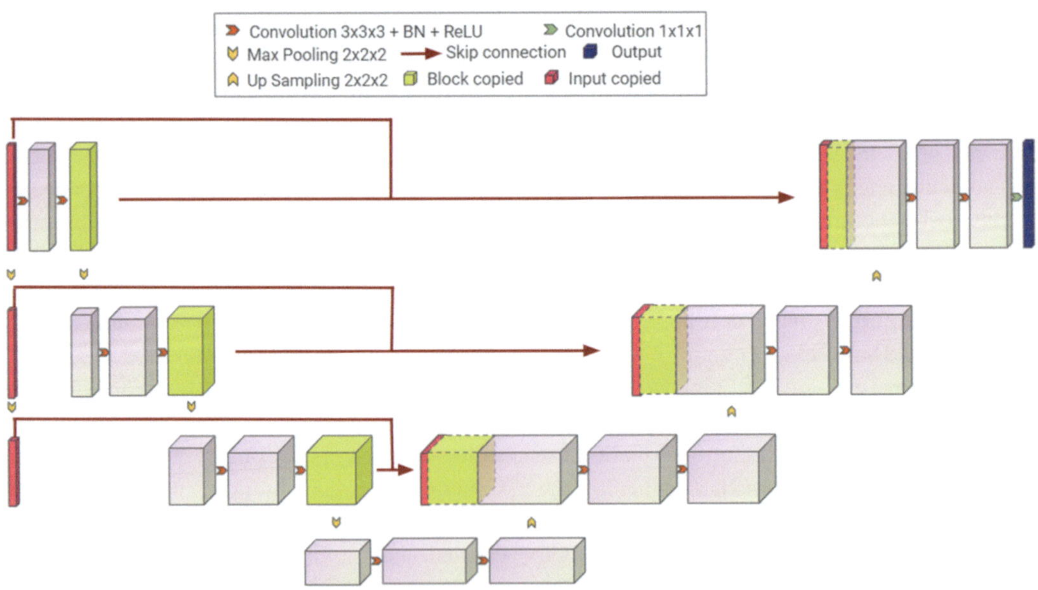

Fig. 3 Architecture of a U-net model. The contractive path starts at the top left and ends at the bottom. Each step consists of successive convolutions with ReLU activation, followed by a max pooling layer, increasing the resolution of the features. The expansive path of the U-net is symmetric to the contractive path, starting from the bottom and ending at the top right. Each step performs an upsampling operation, followed by the same convolutions as in the contractive path. The skip connections concatenate the high-resolution features from the contractive path to the expansive path. Optionally, the input could be subsampled in the contractive path and concatenated in the expansive path

Furthermore, at each step there is a skip connection that concatenates the high-resolution features from the contractive path to the input of the expansive path. Therefore, the expansive path combines spatial information of the image with high-resolution features from the contractive path, enabling precise localization of the segments.

Another important type of DL model is the recurrent neural network (RNN). RNNs are ANNs where nodes in the hidden layers have a connection with themselves. This allows the RNN to use the internal state (or 'memory') of the hidden layer to model sequential data of arbitrary length. Specifically, the output value of each element in the sequence of inputs is dependent on the calculations of previous elements [11]. This makes RNNs suitable for processing text data and time series, as these data types contain sequential dependencies [10]. In the original formulation, RNNs could not properly process long-term dependencies within the input sequence due to vanishing and exploding gradients [11]. The long short-term memory (LSTM) and gated recurrent unit (GRU) networks address this issue by modelling the hidden state with a gating mechanism that determines how much of the information flow is kept given the previous state, the current memory, and the input value. LSTMs and GRUs have been capable of capturing long-term dependencies effectively, yielding impressive results in various NLP tasks.

4 Prediction Tasks for Deep Learning in Healthcare

In the context of healthcare and medicine, the goal of each DL model is to improve the care that patients need for his/her disorder by making accurate predictions for the specific task that the model is trained for. When the DL model needs to predict a continuous value, then we perform a *regression* task [13]. Principally, the term regression refers to a technique where the relationship between independent variables and a dependant variable is modelled. The independent variables could be each dimension of the input data, while the dependant variable is the value of interest that the model needs to predict. The relationship between the independent variables and the dependant variable is then characterized by the parameters of the DL model. Since ANNs are considered as universal function approximators [14], a regression task could be seen as fitting an extremely complex function to the input data, quantifying the relationship between the input data and the predicted output value. What the predicted value represents is heavily dependent on the prediction task. Examples include predicting the age [15] or blood pressure [16] of patients from electrocardiograms (ECGs), the absorbed dose of radiation after administering patients with radiopharmaceuticals [17], or the tolerable dose of chemotherapy [18].

For many tasks in medicine, however, a DL model is required to distinguish between discrete categories. In this case, the model performs a *classification* task [13]. Depending on the specific task, we can further distinguish classification tasks into three subtypes. When there are only two possible classes in the classification task, then the DL model performs *binary* classification. If there are more than two possible classes, and these classes are mutually exclusive, then we perform *multiclass* classification. Finally, when there are more than two possible classes, but they are not necessarily mutually exclusive, then we perform *multilabel* classification. In this case, a datapoint can belong to two or more classes. In each classification task, the DL model predicts the probability of a datapoint belonging to a particular class. For binary and multilabel classification, this class probability is calculated by applying the *sigmoid* function on the output of the final layer of the model. For multiclass classification, a *softmax* function is applied instead. Examples of classification tasks include predicting the mortality of COVID-19 patients from ECGs [19], or performing a triage on 12-lead ECGs [20].

In healthcare, some tasks not only require DL models to predict a particular event, but also the time until that event occurs. In this case, the DL model performs a *survival analysis*. In general, survival data are modelled with two probabilities. The first is the *survival probability* (or survival function), conventionally denoted as $S(t)$, representing the probability that an individual survives from the time origin (e.g., the diagnosis of an illness) to a specified time t in the future. The second probability is the *hazard probability*, conventionally denoted as $h(t)$ or $\lambda(t)$, which represents the probability that an individual observed in time t has an event at that time [21]. Usually, these two probabilities are estimated through statistical methods. As such, a DL model could estimate the necessary parameters of a survival model based on survival data. An example is the proportional hazards model, or Cox regression method [22], which estimates a survival curve of a patient by estimating the effect parameters (e.g., age, gender, disease of patient) of the Cox model. The effect parameters could then be estimated by a DL model [23]. In one study, Sammani et al. used a Cox regression model to predict life-threatening ventricular arrhythmias from 21 ECG factors [24]. These factors were generated by a variational autoencoder (VAE) that encoded the raw ECG into a fixed-sized vector.

When DL models are applied to clinical image data (e.g., ECGs or magnetic resonance imaging (MRI) scans), some tasks require the model to *localize* certain parts of the input image and distinguish those into semantic categories. In this case, the DL model performs a *segmentation* task, producing as output the input image with highlighted regions. As such, segmentation tasks could be considered as a classification task since we are essentially classifying each pixel of the input image into the desired categories. Segmentation tasks are often used as intermediate steps for a subsequent classification or regression task, where the highlighted segments of the input data could be used as input for such a task. Examples of segmentation tasks include the segmentation of heart chambers (i.e., atria and ventricles) from MRI scans [25], or predicting the onset and offset values of P and T-waves and QRS-complexes from ECGs [26].

5 Applications: Medical Imaging

Since some of the greatest opportunities for DL have been found in CV tasks, such as object detection, classification, and segmentation, the first applications of DL models to clinical data were on processing medical image data [11], including X-ray, computed tomography (CT) and MRI scans, ultrasounds, and ECGs. Concretely, DL models can assist physicians in tasks that are labour-intensive and prone to errors, such as analysing and processing pathology images [7]. Furthermore, DL models performing object detection and segmentation tasks can supplement physicians on urgent and easily missed cases [27]. Moreover, the patterns discovered by DL models in clinical images could provide more information about the patient's survival probability [28] or receptiveness to types of drugs [29].

Many studies in clinical imaging have shown remarkable results, sometimes achieving physician-level accuracy, in a wide variety of diagnostic tasks, categorizing the image into classes (e.g., diseases or degrees of urgency). For example, DL models have been applied to analyse brain MRI scans to predict Alzheimer disease and its variants, outperforming state-of-the-art ML techniques [30]. Furthermore, CNNs have been used to classify skin lesions directly from medical images, which is impressive given the great variety of the appearance of skin lesions [31]. In other studies, CNNs have been applied for identifying diabetic retinopathy and cardiovascular risks from retinal fundus images [32, 33], detecting breast lesions from mammograms [34], performing automated triage of 12-lead ECGs [20], analysing MRI scans of the spine [35], and distinguishing between benign and malignant breast nodules from ultrasounds [36].

Besides diagnostics, DL has also been successfully applied in segmentation and detection tasks, identifying specific parts of the image that belongs to a particular object. In one study, a CNN has been used to segment large-artery occlusions in the brain from computed tomography angiographies (CTAs) [27]. Moreover, CNNs have been applied to detect mitotic cells and metastatic tumours in pathology images [37, 38]. In other studies, DL models have been utilized for segmenting multiple sclerosis lesions in multi-channel 3D MRI scans [39], segmenting heart chambers from foetal ultrasound images [40], and segmenting waves and intervals of ECGs [41].

Segmentation models are not limited to detecting and categorizing objects from images. They could also be used for predicting complex patterns. In one study, Mahmud et al. [42] developed NABNet, a DL model that predicts arterial blood pressure (ABP) waveforms by segmenting ECG and photoplethysmogram (PPG) signals. The architecture of NABNet is based on a U-net model, with the addition of attention-guided bi-convolutional LSTM blocks instead of direct skip connections between the contractive path and the expansive path. The final ABP estimation is then obtained by linearly transforming the ABP prediction of NABNet with predicted blood pressure values. These blood pressure values were obtained with the method described in [16]. Figure 4 shows the results of the NABNet procedure.

6 Applications: Electronic Health Records Data

Electronic health records (EHRs) are digital repositories of patients containing medical records about the patients and their treatment [43]. The main purpose of EHRs is to support continuing, efficient, and quality health care for patients. EHRs contain both structured and unstructured data. Structured data in EHRs are stored in a table, where the rows denote the patients while the columns represent the content of the patient's information, such as demographics, diagnosis, vital signals, and laboratory results. Unstructured data on the other hand

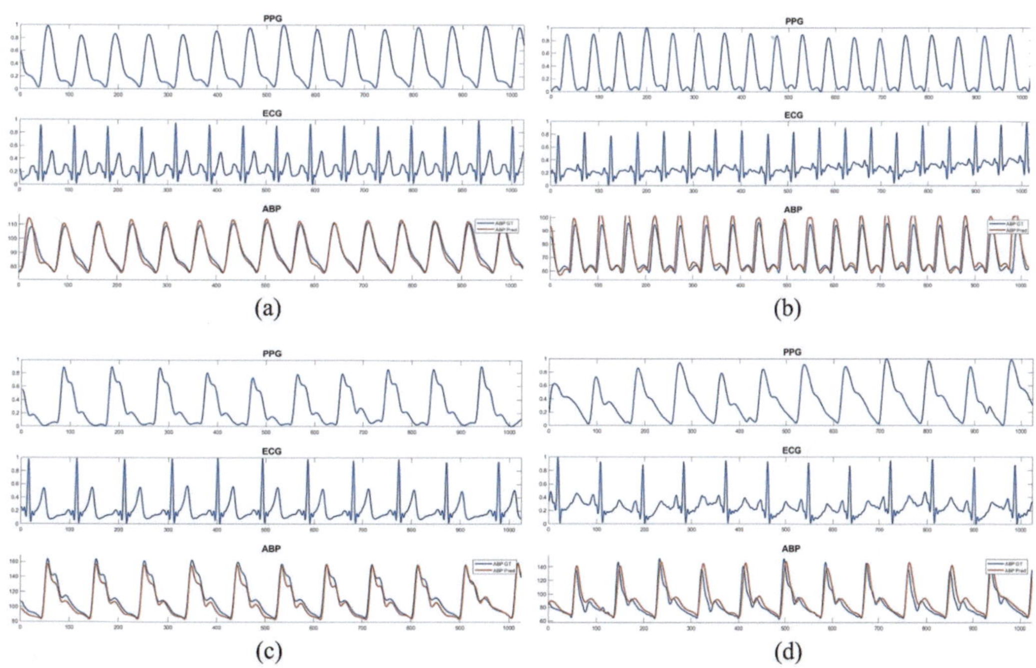

Fig. 4 Results of the NABNet procedure as described by Mahmud et al. [42] on four datapoints from the test set. In each subfigure, the top subplot is the PPG signal, the middle subplot is the ECG signal, and the bottom subplot shows the predicted ABP waveforms (orange) and the ground-truth ABP waveforms (blue). Image obtained and modified from https://github.com/Sakib1263/NABNet/blob/main/Documents/1-s2.0-S1746809422007017-gr7.png in accordance with MIT license

are usually text files containing clinical notes [10, 11]. Currently, the data contained in EHRs have increased considerably in volume. To illustrate, the EHR of a large medical organization contains medical records of roughly 10 million patients within a decade, covering a plethora of rare conditions and illnesses [7]. Analysing this vast amount of medical knowledge can significantly benefit the efficiency and efficacy of healthcare. Since DL models are suitable to process such large amounts of data, they have been increasingly applied to EHRs.

In most studies, DL models have been utilized on structured EHR data to predict future medical events, regularly surpassing traditional ML techniques with hand-engineered features. For such tasks, the DL model is required to capture the temporal relationships between structural events occurring in a patient's records. As such, RNNs are ubiquitous in these studies, since they are well suited for processing sequential data, including time series. However, CNNs and other DL models have been studied as well. In one study, a GRU model was trained to predict diagnoses and medications of subsequent visits based on patient history, achieving a higher recall than shallow baselines [44]. In another study, LSTMs were used on EHRs of diabetes and mental health patients to model the disease progression and future risk [45]. A decay effect was added to the LSTM model to handle irregular timed events, which are common in longitudinal EHRs. Differently, a deep CNN was used to predict unplanned readmissions after discharge, outperforming traditional methods and detecting meaningful patterns about the patient's disease and intervention records [46]. Other studies of DL models applied to structured EHR data include predicting disease onsets from longitudinal laboratory records [47], classifying 128 diagnoses from multivariate time series of clinical measurements [48], and predicting clinical interventions from EHRs of intensive care units [49]. On unstructured EHR data (e.g., clinical notes), deep language models have been applied to learn embedded representations of medical concepts such as diagnoses and medications. These embeddings could be useful for other analysis and prediction tasks such as patient summarization and cohort selection [50]. In another study, deep language models have also been used to remove protected information from EHRs in order to protect the confidentiality of patients [51].

7 Applications: Genomics

Because of their ability to learn complex high-end features, DL models have been increasingly applied on biological data to capture their inner structure. DL has especially been studied on biological data describing genetic structures (e.g., DNA sequencing, RNA measurements) [11]. Initially, DL was mainly used to replace conventional ML techniques with simple DL models. A feature extraction step was still necessary. For instance, an MLP was used on input features extracted from exons and adjacent introns to predict the splicing activity of individual exons, surpassing the simpler ML approaches [52].

With the rise in popularity of CNNs, the raw DNA sequence could be directly fed into the model. Since they are excellent at capturing spatial dependencies from the input data, CNNs could directly capture the inner structure of the DNA sequence, improving the detection of relevant patterns compared to ML approaches and MLPs. This is because CNNs could process a larger window of DNAs, which in turn is due to the fact that CNNs perform convolutions on small windows of the input data and that the parameters are shared across these regions [11]. Therefore, CNNs form the bulk of the DL models used to extract feature from DNA sequences. For example, CNNs were used to predict specificities of DNA- and RNA-binding, uncovering interesting patterns such as known and novel sequence motifs and identify functional single nucleotide variations (SNVs) [53]. In another study, CNNs were used to annotate and interpret the noncoding genome of eukaryote cells. Concretely, it was used to predict DNase I hypersensitivity across multiple cell types and to quantify the effect of SNVs on chromatin accessibility [54]. In other studies, CNNs have been used for predicting chromatin marks from DNA sequences [55], predicting methylation states in single-cell bisulfite sequencing studies [56], and classifying gene expressions from histone modification data [57].

8 Shortcomings and Challenges of Deep Learning in Healthcare

Despite the impressive results that DL models achieve in various prediction tasks, there still remain some shortcomings and challenges that prevents DL to be widely applied in healthcare and medicine. As mentioned in the first paragraph, one of the main shortcomings of DL models is that they are black-box models. In this case, the DL model is considered to be not *explainable*. Before discussing the importance of explainable DL models in the medical field, it is important to define the notion of *explainability*. There exist numerous definitions of explainability in the context of DL models. In this chapter, we follow the definitions from Markus et al. [58], stating that an AI model is explainable if it is intrinsically *interpretable*. For interpretability, we will use the definition of Doshi-Velez and Kim [59], arguing that interpretability is the degree in which the inner logic of an AI model can be explained in human understandable terms. In principle, explainability requires DL models to explain how the relationships between the input and output are established. A consequence of the lack of explainability in DL models is that end-users do not know what parts of the input data contribute to the predictions of the model, which could have negative consequences in case the model makes an incorrect prediction. As an example, if an AI model that predicts atrial fibrillation (AF) from ECG data makes an incorrect diagnosis, cardiologists would have serious suspicions about the trustworthiness of the AI model, since AF can be easily detected from ECGs. This leads to a lack of confidence in applying DL models in healthcare by physicians. Furthermore, since diagnoses can be impactful events in people's lives, physicians would like to explain the reason behind a (false) diagnosis from DL models [9]. If such an explanation could not be given due to the lack of explainability of the DL model, then physicians may lose trust in deploying such DL models for clinical decision making. Therefore, enhancing the explainability of DL models is a necessary requirement for applying them in healthcare and medicine.

Possible solutions to resolve the black-box issue of DL models are provided by the field of explainable AI (XAI), which is concerned with highlighting the inner mechanisms of DL models. The bulk of the studies in XAI is focused on *post-hoc* explanation methods that explain pre-trained DL models [60]. Post-hoc methods form a popular direction of research in XAI, because they can be applied on any type of DL model. One way in which post-hoc methods explain DL models is to calculate *attribute scores*, where their value indicates how much (parts of) the input contributed to the output. This highlights the importance of input features for certain predictions, indirectly explaining the DL model itself. This relationship can sometimes be visualized more qualitatively by highlighting regions of the input that contributed the most to the output (see Fig. 5). Although attribution scores can give an indication of the model's inner logic, they may not always be accurate or physiologically sensible, showing that enhancing explainability remains a key challenge to overcome [61].

Instead of generating post-hoc explanations for a pre-trained DL model, we could also make use of interpretable features to enhance explainability of the DL approach. One technique that could be used for this is called *disentanglement learning* [62]. This technique is concerned with learning *disentangled representations*, where each dimension or subset of dimensions stands for a generative factor of the input data that is independent of other generative factors. VAEs could be used for learning disentangled representations. Here, an encoder compresses the input data into a fixed-sized vector. A decoder is then used to reconstruct the original input from the fixed-sized vector. After training time,

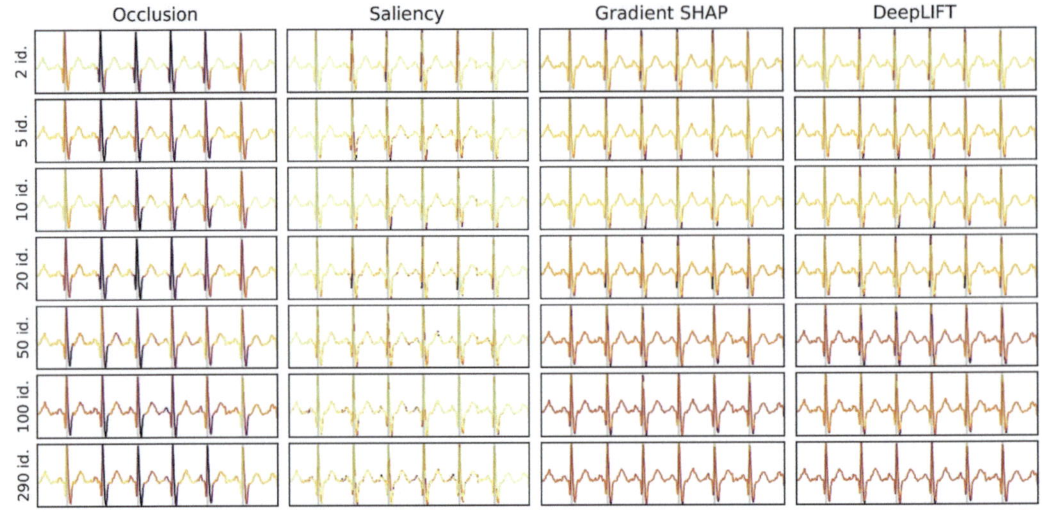

Fig. 5 Explanations of a 5 s ECG sample. These explanations were obtained with four different post-hoc explanation methods (columns), highlighting which time samples of the ECG signal contribute the most to the identification of human patients [65, 66]. Lighter yellow colours represent less relevant time samples, while darker purple colours represent more relevant time samples. The rows in this figure represents the population size in which the human identification task is performed (e.g., 100 id. means that 100 unique patients were used for the task). Image obtained from https://github.com/jtrpinto/xECG/blob/master/plots/ptb_segment16_id0.pdf in accordance with MIT license

the disentangled representations could be used as input for other models to perform prediction tasks. By modifying and decoding the disentangled representation, the influence of each factor on the original data could be visualised. This allows disentangled representations to improve explainability of both an individual prediction of the model (i.e., local explanation) and the model itself (i.e., global explanation) [63]. As an example, Sammani et al. used disentangled representations and a Cox regression model to predict life-threatening ventricular arrhythmia (LTVA) [24]. The disentangled representations were generated by a VAE that encodes raw ECGs into fixed-sized vectors of 32 independent elements [64]. The collection of these vectors is called *FactorECG*. From the 32 elements 21 of those were identified to represent a certain generative factor (e.g., PR-interval, Ventricular rate) of the raw ECG data. As such, these were fed to the Cox regression model for prediction. By modifying and decoding the disentangled representations, the influence of each factor on the ECG morphology could be visualised. This highlights the relationships between ECG morphology and the risk in LTVA found by the model on a global scale.

Besides the black-box problem, there are other technical shortcomings of DL models. One such shortcoming is that DL models require an enormous amount of data to achieve state-of-the-art performance on their prediction task. The great success of DL in CV and NLP tasks is due to the accessibility of large volumes of data in those fields. However, this is not always the case in healthcare, as the data may not always be available in great quantities, or difficult to access. As such, medical data is limited compared to data from other domains [10, 11]. A related shortcoming of DL models is that they not only need large volumes of data, but also clean and well-structured data. Unfortunately, medical data are relatively unstructured compared to other domains, being heterogeneous, ambiguous, incomplete, and noisy. As such, medical data needs to be carefully pre-processed before it can be fed to the DL model, unlike in other domains (e.g., CV) where for some tasks little pre-processing is required [10, 11]. Finally, tasks from healthcare (e.g., modelling diseases, genome structure) are much more complicated than tasks from other domains (e.g., CV, NLP). This is because diseases are highly heterogeneous and there is still no complete knowledge about their cause and their progression [11]. As a result, much more medical data is needed to obtain good performance compared to tasks from other domains. Another reason for the complexity of the medical domain is that biological processes change over time in a non-deterministic way. However, most existing DL models assume a static and vectorized input. Therefore, the temporal factor behind biological processes is not properly modelled by DL models [11].

In addition to technical shortcomings, the application of DL models in healthcare also brings some ethical issues. One such issue involves the principle of fairness, which evaluates the predictions of DL models in terms of discrimination [60]. Generally, predictions of DL models are considered *fair* if they are not based on *sensitive* factors [67], such as race, gender, or the type of insurance policy. These sensitive factors could be present in the training data [60] or could be learned by the DL model during training time [68]. If this bias is not taken into account, it could lead to discrimination, lack of equity, lack of diversity inclusion and lack of just provision of care [68]. As a consequence, it may lead to unfair care of patients in clinical decision making [69]. A number of techniques to enhance the fairness of DL models involves removing bias from training data [70–72] or forcing DL models to make fair predictions [73, 74].

Another ethical issue of DL models in healthcare involves the privacy of patients. The consent of patients to share their medical data is crucial for the successful application of DL models in healthcare [68]. Patients provide this consent on the condition that their privacy is protected by the hospital. If the privacy of the patients is broken, their willingness to share medical data would decrease considerably, hindering the progress of DL models in healthcare. Therefore, privacy is an important issue to address if DL models will be widely deployed in healthcare. In fact, Tramèr et al. [75] shows that model parameters or training data could be inferred from AI models deployed for commercial use, breaking the model and personal privacy. Solutions that addresses the privacy risks includes differential privacy methods to protect the model parameters [76–78] or homomorphic encryption for encrypting the model gradients [79].

References

1. Artificial neural network—An overview. ScienceDirect topics. https://www.sciencedirect.com/topics/neuroscience/artificial-neural-network. Accessed 17 Sept 2022.
2. Hecht-Nielsen. Theory of the backpropagation neural network. In: International 1989 joint conference on neural networks, vol 1; 1989. p. 593–605. https://doi.org/10.1109/IJCNN.1989.118638
3. Duchi J, Hazan E, Singer Y. 2011. Adaptive subgradient methods for online learning and stochastic optimization. p. 39.
4. Tieleman T, Hinton G. Lecture 6.5-rmsprop: divide the gradient by a running average of its recent magnitude. In: Presented at the COURSERA: neural networks for machine learning; 2012.
5. Kingma DP, Ba J. Adam: a method for stochastic optimization. 29 Jan 2017. Accessed 04 Oct 2022. Available http://arxiv.org/abs/1412.6980
6. Janiesch C, Zschech P, Heinrich K. Machine learning and deep learning. Electron Mark. 2021;31(3):685–95. https://doi.org/10.1007/s12525-021-00475-2.
7. Esteva A, et al. A guide to deep learning in healthcare. Nat Med. 2019;25(1):24–9. https://doi.org/10.1038/s41591-018-0316-z.
8. Wang F, Kaushal R, Khullar D. Should health care demand interpretable artificial intelligence or accept 'black box' medicine? Ann Intern Med. 2020;172(1):59–60. https://doi.org/10.7326/M19-2548.
9. Ahmad MA, Eckert C, Teredesai A. Interpretable machine learning in healthcare. In: Proceedings of the 2018 ACM international conference on bioinformatics, computational biology, and health informatics. New York, NY, USA, Aug 2018. p. 559–60. https://doi.org/10.1145/3233547.3233667
10. Yang S, Zhu F, Ling X, Liu Q, Zhao P. Intelligent health care: applications of deep learning in computational medicine. Front Genet. 2021;12: 607471. https://doi.org/10.3389/fgene.2021.607471.
11. Miotto R, Wang F, Wang S, Jiang X, Dudley JT. Deep learning for healthcare: review, opportunities and challenges. Brief Bioinform. 2018;19(6):1236–46. https://doi.org/10.1093/bib/bbx044.
12. Ronneberger O, Fischer P, Brox T (2015) U-Net: convolutional networks for biomedical

image segmentation. 18 May 2015. https://doi.org/10.48550/arXiv.1505.04597
13. Sidey-Gibbons JAM, Sidey-Gibbons CJ. Machine learning in medicine: a practical introduction. BMC Med Res Methodol. 2019;19(1):64. https://doi.org/10.1186/s12874-019-0681-4.
14. Hornik K, Stinchcombe M, White H. Multilayer feedforward networks are universal approximators. Neural Netw. 1989;2(5):359–66. https://doi.org/10.1016/0893-6080(89)90020-8.
15. Attia ZI, et al. Age and sex estimation using artificial intelligence from standard 12-lead ECGs. Circ Arrhythm Electrophysiol. 2019;12(9): e007284. https://doi.org/10.1161/CIRCEP.119.007284.
16. Mahmud S et al. A shallow U-Net architecture for reliably predicting blood pressure (BP) from photoplethysmogram (PPG) and electrocardiogram (ECG) signals. Sensors. 2022;22(3):Art no 3. https://doi.org/10.3390/s22030919
17. Götz TI, Schmidkonz C, Chen S, Al-Baddai S, Kuwert T, Lang EW. A deep learning approach to radiation dose estimation. Phys Med Ampmathsemicolon Biol. 2020;65(3): 035007. https://doi.org/10.1088/1361-6560/ab65dc.
18. Lou B, et al. An image-based deep learning framework for individualising radiotherapy dose: a retrospective analysis of outcome prediction. Lancet Digit Health. 2019;1(3):e136–47. https://doi.org/10.1016/S2589-7500(19)30058-5.
19. van de Leur R et al. Electrocardiogram-based mortality prediction in patients with COVID-19 using machine learning. Neth Heart J Mon J Neth Soc Cardiol Neth Heart Found. 2022; 30(6): 312–18. https://doi.org/10.1007/s12471-022-01670-2
20. van de Leur RR, et al. Automatic triage of 12-lead ECGs using deep convolutional neural networks. J Am Heart Assoc. 2020;9(10): e015138. https://doi.org/10.1161/JAHA.119.015138.
21. Clark TG, Bradburn MJ, Love SB, Altman DG. Survival analysis Part I: basic concepts and first analyses. Br J Cancer. 2003;89(2):Art no 2. https://doi.org/10.1038/sj.bjc.6601118
22. Cox DR. Regression models and life-tables. J R Stat Soc Ser B Methodol. 1972;34(2):187–202. https://doi.org/10.1111/j.2517-6161.1972.tb00899.x.
23. Nagpal C, Yadlowsky S, Rostamzadeh N, Heller K. Deep cox mixtures for survival regression. In: Proceedings of the 6th machine learning for healthcare conference, Oct 2021p. 674–708. Accessed 06 Oct 2022. Available https://proceedings.mlr.press/v149/nagpal21a.html
24. Sammani A et al. Life-threatening ventricular arrhythmia prediction in patients with dilated cardiomyopathy using explainable electrocardiogram-based deep neural networks. Eur Eur Pacing Arrhythm Card Electrophysiol J Work Groups Card Pacing Arrhythm Card Cell Electrophysiol Eur Soc Cardiol. 2022;24(10):1645–54. https://doi.org/10.1093/europace/euac054
25. Avendi M, Kheradvar A, Jafarkhani H. Fully automatic segmentation of heart chambers in cardiac MRI using deep learning. J Cardiovasc Magn Reson. 2016;18(1):P351. https://doi.org/10.1186/1532-429X-18-S1-P351.
26. Moskalenko V, Zolotykh N, Osipov G. Deep learning for ECG segmentation. In: Advances in neural computation, machine learning, and cognitive research III. Cham. 2020. p. 246–54. https://doi.org/10.1007/978-3-030-30425-6_29
27. Rodrigues G, et al. Automated large artery occlusion detection in stroke: a single-center validation study of an artificial intelligence algorithm. Cerebrovasc Dis. 2022;51(2):259–64. https://doi.org/10.1159/000519125.
28. Beck AH et al. Systematic analysis of breast cancer morphology uncovers stromal features associated with survival. Sci Transl Med. 2011;3(108):108ra113–108ra113. https://doi.org/10.1126/scitranslmed.3002564.
29. Charoentong P, et al. Pan-cancer immunogenomic analyses reveal genotype-immunophenotype relationships and predictors of response to checkpoint blockade. Cell Rep. 2017;18(1):248–62. https://doi.org/10.1016/j.celrep.2016.12.019.
30. Liu S, Liu S, Cai W, Pujol S, Kikinis R, Feng D. Early diagnosis of Alzheimer's disease with deep learning. In: 2014 IEEE 11th international symposium on biomedical imaging (ISBI), Apr 2014. p. 1015–18. https://doi.org/10.1109/ISBI.2014.6868045
31. Esteva A et al. Dermatologist-level classification of skin cancer with deep neural networks. Nature. 2017;542(7639):Art no 7639. https://doi.org/10.1038/nature21056
32. Gulshan V, et al. Development and validation of a deep learning algorithm for detection of diabetic retinopathy in retinal fundus photographs. JAMA. 2016;316(22):2402–10. https://doi.org/10.1001/jama.2016.17216.
33. Poplin R et al. Prediction of cardiovascular risk factors from retinal fundus photographs via deep learning. Nat Biomed Eng. 2018; 2(3):Art no 3. https://doi.org/10.1038/s41551-018-0195-0
34. Kooi T, et al. Large scale deep learning for computer aided detection of mammographic lesions. Med Image Anal. 2017;35:303–12. https://doi.org/10.1016/j.media.2016.07.007.
35. Jamaludin A, Kadir T, Zisserman A. SpineNet: automatically pinpointing classification evidence in spinal MRIs. In: Medical image computing and computer-assisted intervention—MICCAI 2016, Cham; 2016. p. 166–75. https://doi.org/10.1007/978-3-319-46723-8_20
36. Cheng J-Z et al. Computer-aided diagnosis with deep learning architecture: applications to breast lesions in us images and pulmonary nodules in CT scans. Sci Rep. 2016;6(1):Art no 1. https://doi.org/10.1038/srep24454
37. Liu Y et al. Detecting cancer metastases on gigapixel pathology images. 07 Mar 2017. https://doi.org/10.48550/arXiv.1703.02442

38. Cireşan DC, Giusti A, Gambardella LM, Schmidhuber J. Mitosis detection in breast cancer histology images with deep neural networks. In: Medical image computing and computer-assisted intervention—MICCAI 2013, Berlin, Heidelberg; 2013, p. 411–18. https://doi.org/10.1007/978-3-642-40763-5_51
39. Yoo Y, Brosch T, Traboulsee A, Li DKB, Tam R. Deep learning of image features from unlabeled data for multiple sclerosis lesion segmentation. In: Machine learning in medical imaging, Cham; 2014, p. 117–24. https://doi.org/10.1007/978-3-319-10581-9_15
40. Pu B et al. MobileUNet-FPN: a semantic segmentation model for fetal ultrasound four-chamber segmentation in edge computing environments. IEEE J Biomed Health Inform. 2022;1–11. https://doi.org/10.1109/JBHI.2022.3182722
41. Malali A, Hiriyannaiah S, Siddesh GM, Srinivasa KG, Sanjay NT. Supervised ECG wave segmentation using convolutional LSTM. ICT Express. 2020; 6(3):166–69. https://doi.org/10.1016/j.icte.2020.04.004
42. Mahmud S, et al. NABNet: a nested attention-guided BiConvLSTM network for a robust prediction of blood pressure components from reconstructed arterial blood pressure waveforms using PPG and ECG signals. Biomed Signal Process Control. 2023;79: 104247. https://doi.org/10.1016/j.bspc.2022.104247.
43. Häyrinen K, Saranto K, Nykänen P. Definition, structure, content, use and impacts of electronic health records: a review of the research literature. Int J Med Inf. 2008;77(5):291–304. https://doi.org/10.1016/j.ijmedinf.2007.09.001.
44. Choi E, Bahadori MT, Schuetz A, Stewart WF, Sun J. Doctor AI: predicting clinical events via recurrent neural networks. In: Proceedings of the 1st machine learning for healthcare conference, Dec 2016. p. 301–18. Accessed 26 Sep 2022. Available https://proceedings.mlr.press/v56/Choi16.html
45. Pham T, Tran T, Phung D, Venkatesh S. DeepCare: a deep dynamic memory model for predictive medicine. Advances in knowledge discovery and data mining, Cham; 2016. p. 30–41. https://doi.org/10.1007/978-3-319-31750-2_3
46. Nguyen P, Tran T, Wickramasinghe N, Venkatesh S. Deepr: a convolutional net for medical records. IEEE J Biomed Health Inform. 2017;21(1):22–30. https://doi.org/10.1109/JBHI.2016.2633963.
47. Razavian N, Marcus J, Sontag D. Multi-task prediction of disease onsets from longitudinal laboratory tests. In: Proceedings of the 1st machine learning for healthcare conference, Dec 2016. p. 73–100. Accessed 27 Sep 27 2022. Available https://proceedings.mlr.press/v56/Razavian16.html
48. Lipton ZC, Kale DC, Elkan C, Wetzel R. Learning to diagnose with LSTM recurrent neural networks. 21 Mar 2017. https://doi.org/10.48550/arXiv.1511.03677
49. Suresh H, Hunt N, Johnson A, Celi LA, Szolovits P, Ghassemi M. Clinical intervention prediction and understanding with deep neural networks. In: Proceedings of the 2nd machine learning for healthcare conference, Nov 2017, p. 322–37. Accessed 27 Sep 2022. Available https://proceedings.mlr.press/v68/suresh17a.html
50. Choi Y, Chiu CY-I, Sontag D. Learning low-dimensional representations of medical concepts. AMIA Summits Transl Sci Proc. 2016;2016:41–50.
51. Dernoncourt F, Lee JY, Uzuner O, Szolovits P. De-identification of patient notes with recurrent neural networks. J Am Med Inform Assoc. 2017;24(3):596–606. https://doi.org/10.1093/jamia/ocw156.
52. Xiong HY, et al. The human splicing code reveals new insights into the genetic determinants of disease. Science. 2015;347(6218):1254806. https://doi.org/10.1126/science.1254806.
53. Alipanahi B, Delong A, Weirauch MT, Frey BJ. Predicting the sequence specificities of DNA- and RNA-binding proteins by deep learning. Nat Biotechnol. 2015;33(8):Art no 8. . https://doi.org/10.1038/nbt.3300
54. Kelley DR, Snoek J, Rinn JL. Basset: learning the regulatory code of the accessible genome with deep convolutional neural networks. Genome Res. 2016;26(7):990–9. https://doi.org/10.1101/gr.200535.115.
55. Zhou J, Troyanskaya OG. Predicting effects of noncoding variants with deep learning–based sequence model. Nat Methods. 2015;12(10):Art no 10. https://doi.org/10.1038/nmeth.3547
56. Angermueller C, Lee HJ, Reik W, Stegle O. DeepCpG: accurate prediction of single-cell DNA methylation states using deep learning. Genome Biol. 2017;18(1):67. https://doi.org/10.1186/s13059-017-1189-z.
57. Singh R, Lanchantin J, Robins G, Qi Y. DeepChrome: deep-learning for predicting gene expression from histone modifications. Bioinformatics. 2016;32(17):i639–48. https://doi.org/10.1093/bioinformatics/btw427.
58. Markus AF, Kors JA, Rijnbeek PR. The role of explainability in creating trustworthy artificial intelligence for health care: A comprehensive survey of the terminology, design choices, and evaluation strategies. J Biomed Inform. 2021;113: 103655. https://doi.org/10.1016/j.jbi.2020.103655.
59. Doshi-Velez F, Kim B. Towards a rigorous science of interpretable machine learning. 02 Mar 2017. https://doi.org/10.48550/arXiv.1702.08608
60. Linardatos P, Papastefanopoulos V, Kotsiantis S. Entropy, and undefined 2021, Explainable AI: a review of machine learning interpretability methods. mdpi.com. 2020. https://doi.org/10.3390/e23010018
61. Ghassemi M, Vector, Beam AL, Ghassemi M, Oakden-Rayner L, The false hope of current approaches to explainable artificial intelligence in health care. Lancet Digit Health.

2021;3(11):e745–e750. https://doi.org/10.1016/S2589-7500(21)00208-9
62. Liu X, Sanchez P, Thermos S, O'Neil AQ, Tsaftaris SA. Learning disentangled representations in the imaging domain. Med Image Anal. 2022;80: 102516. https://doi.org/10.1016/j.media.2022.102516.
63. van de Leur RR, et al. Improving explainability of deep neural network-based electrocardiogram interpretation using variational auto-encoders. Eur Heart J Digit Health. 2022;3(3):390–404. https://doi.org/10.1093/ehjdh/ztac038.
64. van de Leur RR et al. Inherently explainable deep neural network-based interpretation of electrocardiograms using variational auto-encoders. Cardiovasc Med. Preprint, 2022. https://doi.org/10.1101/2022.01.04.22268759
65. Pinto JR, Cardoso JS. Explaining ECG biometrics: is it all in the QRS? p. 12.
66. Pinto JR, Cardoso JS, Lourenço A. Deep neural networks for biometric identification based on non-intrusive ECG acquisitions. In: Arya KV, editors. The biometric computing, 1st ed. Chapman and Hall/CRC; 2019. p. 217–34. https://doi.org/10.1201/9781351013437-11
67. Barocas S, Hardt M, Narayanan A. Fairness and machine learning. p 300.
68. Karimian G, Petelos E, Evers SMAA. The ethical issues of the application of artificial intelligence in healthcare: a systematic scoping review. AI Ethics. 2022. https://doi.org/10.1007/s43681-021-00131-7.
69. Petkus H, Hoogewerf J, Wyatt JC. What do senior physicians think about AI and clinical decision support systems: quantitative and qualitative analysis of data from specialty societies. Clin Med. 2020;20(3):324. https://doi.org/10.7861/clinmed.2019-0317.
70. Kamiran F, Calders T. Data preprocessing techniques for classification without discrimination. Knowl Inf Syst. 2012;33(1):1–33. https://doi.org/10.1007/s10115-011-0463-8.
71. Kamiran F, Calders T. Classifying without discriminating. In: Control and communication 2009 2nd international conference on computer, Feb 2009. pp 1–6. https://doi.org/10.1109/IC4.2009.4909197
72. Calders T, Kamiran F, Pechenizkiy M. Building classifiers with independency constraints. In: 2009 IEEE international conference on data mining workshops, Dec 2009. p. 13–18. https://doi.org/10.1109/ICDMW.2009.83
73. Kamiran F, Karim A, Zhang X. Decision theory for discrimination-aware classification. In: 2012 IEEE 12th international conference on data mining, Dec 2012. p. 924–29. https://doi.org/10.1109/ICDM.2012.45
74. Dwork C, Hardt M, Pitassi T, Reingold O, Zemel R. Fairness through awareness. In: Proceedings of the 3rd innovations in theoretical computer science conference, New York, NY, USA, Jan 2012. p. 214–26. https://doi.org/10.1145/2090236.2090255
75. Tramèr F, Zhang F, Juels A, Reiter MK, Ristenpart T. Stealing machine learning models via prediction {APIs}. In: Presented at the 25th USENIX security symposium (USENIX security 16); 2016, p. 601–18. Accessed 07 Nov 2022. Available https://www.usenix.org/conference/usenixsecurity16/technical-sessions/presentation/tramer
76. Abadi M et al. Deep learning with differential privacy. In: Proceedings of the 2016 ACM SIGSAC conference on computer and communications security, New York, NY, USA, Oct 2016, p. 308–18. https://doi.org/10.1145/2976749.2978318
77. Phan N, Wang Y, Wu X, Dou D. Differential privacy preservation for deep auto-encoders: an application of human behavior prediction. In: Thirtieth AAAI conference on artificial intelligence, Feb 2016. Accessed 07 Nov 2022. Available https://www.aaai.org/ocs/index.php/AAAI/AAAI16/paper/view/12174
78. Shokri R, Shmatikov V. Privacy-preserving deep learning. In: Proceedings of the 22nd ACM SIGSAC conference on computer and communications security, New York, NY, USA, Oct 2015, p. 1310–21. https://doi.org/10.1145/2810103.2813687
79. Phong LT, Aono Y, Hayashi T, Wang L, Moriai S. Privacy-preserving deep learning via additively homomorphic encryption. IEEE Trans Inf Forensics Secur. 2018;13(5):1333–45. https://doi.org/10.1109/TIFS.2017.2787987.

Deep Learning—Autoencoders

Melle Vessies, Rutger van de Leur, Philippe Wouters and René van Es

Abstract

Auto-encoders and their variational counterparts form a family of (deep) neural networks that serve a wide range of applications in medical research and clinical practice. In this chapter we provide a comprehensive overview of how auto-encoders work and how they can be used to improve medical research. We elaborate on various topics such as dimension reduction, denoising auto-encoders, auto-encoders used for anomaly detection and the applications of representations of data created using auto-encoders. Secondly, we touch upon the subject of variational auto-encoders, explaining their design and training process. We end the chapter with small scale examples of auto-encoders applied to the MNIST dataset and a recent example of an application of a (disentangled) variational auto-encoder applied to ECG-data.

Keywords

Auto-encoder · Variational auto-encoder · Deep learning · Dimension reduction · Denoising · Anomaly detection · Disentanglement · Explainable AI · ECG

1 Introduction

In this chapter the workings of auto-encoders are explained in a way that is understandable for medical researchers and clinicians who have little or no prior training in the field of artificial intelligence (AI). For the more experienced reader we provide several technical intermezzos that contain a more in depth and mathematical explanation of the subject. Furthermore, we provide several examples that show potential use cases of auto-encoders for medical research, whilst also giving a broad set of guidelines on how auto-encoders can be implemented and used by other researchers in medical AI applications.

Auto-encoders and their variational counterparts form a family of (deep) neural networks that serve a wide range of applications in medical research and clinical practice. Auto-encoders were first contemplated in the late 80s, and their popularity grew with the increase in computing power [1]. Their use cases range anywhere from

M. Vessies · R. van de Leur · P. Wouters · R. van Es (✉)
University Medical Center Utrecht, Utrecht, Netherlands
e-mail: R.vanEs@umcutrecht.nl

F. W. Asselbergs et al. (eds.), *Clinical Applications of Artificial Intelligence in Real-World Data*,
https://doi.org/10.1007/978-3-031-36678-9_13

signal/image denoising and anomaly detection tasks to advanced dimension reduction and complex data generation [2, 3].

Unlike most types of deep neural networks, auto-encoders are generally trained in an 'unsupervised' manor, meaning that only raw data, without any labels, are required to train the models. This unsupervised nature and the broad set of possible applications make auto-encoders a popular choice in various fields of medical AI research.

2 The Intuition Behind Auto-encoders

Auto-encoders can be considered a dimension reduction or compression technique. Dimension reduction techniques aim to retain as much information from a raw data input as possible into a compressed vector representation (i.e. a set of numbers). The numbers in this vector, which are often referred to as 'latent variables', contain (as much as possible) information about the raw data input. If a dimension reduction technique is for example applied to images of written digits (e.g. the MNIST dataset), the reduced vector form of the images may contain information about what digits the image contained, the orientation of the digit and the stroke width of the drawn digit [4]. The amount of reduction applied to the input data is usually inversely related to the amount of information that is retained in the compressed vector form. For example, if an image is reduced to only 3 numbers, a lot of information is lost, and the original cannot be accurately reconstructed. In contrast, if an image that contained 28×28 ($= 784$) pixels is reduced to a vector of 392 digits, much more information is left, albeit in a reduced form. In this context, "information" is a rather abstract concept, and depends on the goal of the user of the dimension reduction technique. For auto-encoders, the main objective is typically to enable both compression and decompression, or in other words reduce the data to such a form that the original data can be reconstructed from this compressed form. Auto-encoders therefore aim to learn the optimal (de) compression functions.

3 Principal Component Analysis

The general idea of auto-encoders has been around for decades. Traditionally the use of auto-encoders has been centered around dimensionality reduction and feature learning. For these purposes, auto-encoders are closely related to Principal Component Analysis (PCA), a technique commonly used in medical research. Both PCA and auto-encoders transform data into a lower dimensional representation, while retaining the original information as much as possible. PCA is a purely mathematical approach to dimension reduction that involves calculating the Singular Value Decomposition (SVD), and is limited to linear transformations. Conversely, (deep) auto-encoders can learn non-linear transformations. For complex data linear transformations are often insufficient for tasks such as classification and dimension reduction. Because of this (deep) auto-encoders often achieve better results than PCA. In fact, when an auto-encoder without any non-linear activations is used, the auto-encoder is likely to approximate PCA [5].

4 Methodology Behind Auto-encoders

Auto-encoders can reconstruct raw input data from extracted latent variables. We therefore make a distinction between the extraction step (i.e. *encoding*) and the reconstruction step (i.e. *decoding*). During the training of the auto-encoder, both these steps are performed in sequence. First the raw data is encoded into a set of latent variables, and then the latent variables are decoded back into the raw data form. This approach is what enables the unsupervised learning of auto-encoders, as the output of the model is effectively an approximation of the input. Meanwhile, the latent representation or compressed form of the input data, can be extracted from the middle of the network (after the encoding step). To train the model, a loss or error function is defined, which captures how well the model is doing in terms of reconstructing the original input. The model is then progressively optimized to reduce this reconstruction error.

While the exact architecture of the model may vary depending on the task and data at hand, all auto-encoder models contain a distinctive 'bottleneck' or funnel structure. Here the dimensionality of the data is reduced during the encoding step, and increased again during the decoding step. This bottleneck structure ensures the model is unable to simply copy information from the input to the output. Instead it has to compress the data and reconstruct it. By forcing compression of the data through the bottleneck structure and optimizing the model for accurate reconstructions, auto-encoders learn to perform complex steps that allow it to create a latent representation of the data that contains as much important information as possible. We provide a more formal explanation of this process in the technical intermezzo below.

Technical Intermezzo 1

The auto-encoder neural network is trained to ensure that its output data are the same as the input data, which is done through a funnel represented by the latent space (Fig. 1). Even though an auto-encoder is technically a single model; it is common to define the encoder step and the decoder step separately. The encoder $\boldsymbol{E}$ takes the raw data $\boldsymbol{x}$ as input and outputs a latent representation z (Eq. 1). Subsequently, decoder $\mathbf{D}$ takes the latent representation z as input and outputs a reconstruction of $\boldsymbol{x}$, now called $\hat{\boldsymbol{x}}$ (Eq. 2). The so-called latent vector z has a lower dimensionality (is smaller) than the input $\boldsymbol{x}$ and output $\hat{\boldsymbol{x}}$, that both have the same dimensions. As per the MNIST example above, $\boldsymbol{x}$ and $\hat{\boldsymbol{x}}$ would both be of size 28×28 pixels, while z is a vector of arbitrary size that is determined by the design and purpose of the auto-encoder (e.g. 1×2 for compression to 2 latent variables per sample or 1×32 for 32 latent variables per sample).

$$z = E(x) \tag{1}$$

Equation 1 Function that represents the encoder part of an auto-encoder. The latent vector (z) is calculated by the encoder (E) based on the input data x.

$$\hat{x} = D(z) \tag{2}$$

Equation 2 Function that represents the decoder part of an auto-encoder. The output (x̂) is calculated by the decoder (D) based on the latent vector (z) that was previously calculated by the encoder.

Using this formalization, we can thus define the auto-encoder as two functions as shown above. The objective of the model is to output a reconstruction $\hat{\boldsymbol{x}}$ that is as similar as possible to the original input $\boldsymbol{x}$ while also generating a latent representation (z) of the data after the encoding step. To enforce this similarity, a so-called loss term (or error term) is used during training of the auto-encoder. This loss term is a measure for the difference between input $\boldsymbol{x}$ and output $\hat{\boldsymbol{x}}$. A relatively simple and commonly used function to calculate the loss is the mean squared error (MSE). The loss calculation of the model can then be represented by the following function:

$$\text{Loss} = \text{MSE}(x, \hat{x}) = \frac{1}{N}\sum_{i=0}^{N}(x_i - \hat{x}_i)^2 \tag{3}$$

Equation 3 Function to calculate the mean squared error (MSE) loss of the input data x and output data x̄. N = total number of data point in data, i = ith data point in the dataset.

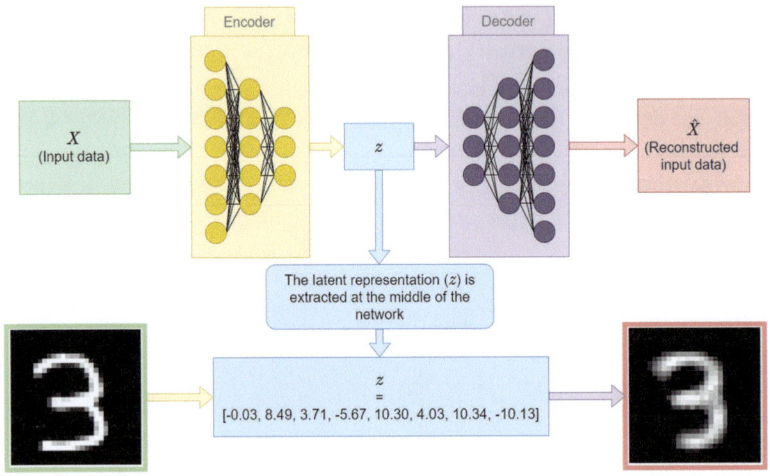

Fig. 1 General schematic layout of an Auto-encoder neural network. The network input $\boldsymbol{x}$ can be any form of data (e.g. images, signals or other measurements). The network learns to reconstruct the input by minimizing the mean squared error (MSE) between the input and the output of the network

5 Auto-encoders for Denoising and Anomaly Detection

In this section we will provide some use cases for auto-encoders. The first example of a potential use-case is that of denoising data. In the field of medical imaging, the presence of noise in images may limit resolution or decrease interpretability, thereby hampering it's use for evaluation or further analysis. Therefore, removing noise (i.e. denoising) is commonly performed as a first step. Conventional methods for denoising (medical) images ranges from spatial filters, such as Gaussian or convolutional filters to wavelet based techniques [6]. As described before, auto-encoders can also be used for denoising images. Recent studies have shown that auto-encoder based denoising methods often outperform conventional methods. Gondara showed that using convolutional layers in an auto-encoder led to efficient denoising of medical images, and maybe more importantly, can be used on smaller datasets [7].

Auto-encoders extract information from the input and reconstruct the input data as good as possible. We can use this characteristic to create an auto-encoder that extracts information from a noisy input and reconstructs the input but without the noise. We do this under the assumption that a noisy image is composed of a clean image with noise added to it. We thus want to train the auto-encoder such that it extracts the important information of the clean image but ignores the noise. In order to do so we start with a, non-noisy, input $\boldsymbol{x}$ and add some random noise $\boldsymbol{\lambda}$ to it. We thus have a new input for the model, which we will call $\boldsymbol{x}^*$, that is the sum of $\boldsymbol{x}$ and $\boldsymbol{\lambda}$ (e.g. $\boldsymbol{x}^*$ (noisy image) $= \boldsymbol{x}$ (image) $+ \boldsymbol{\lambda}$ (noise)). We pass this noisy input through the network and obtain $\hat{\boldsymbol{x}}$, the reconstructed image, as we did before. Meanwhile, we keep the original MSE loss calculation fixed, so it is still the difference between $\boldsymbol{x}$ and $\hat{\boldsymbol{x}}$, however, $\hat{\boldsymbol{x}}$ is now based on the noisy input $\boldsymbol{x}^*$ rather than $\boldsymbol{x}$. The network will thus have to learn how to remove the noise from $\hat{\boldsymbol{x}}$ in order to make it as similar as possible to $\boldsymbol{x}$.

Denoising auto-encoders can be a useful tool to clean data that stems from real world observations that tend to be very noisy. Lu et al., for example, use denoising auto-encoders to enhance speech recordings [8]. Jifara et al.

take a slightly different approach and design their auto-encoder in such a way that it outputs the estimated noise, instead of a reconstruction of the input image (the noise can be subtracted from the noisy image to create a clean image) [9]. They show that this approach improves upon standard denoising auto-encoders on images obtained using chest radiography. Nawarathne et al. use denoising auto-encoders on spectral images extracted from accelerometric data measured on pregnant mothers' abdomen, in order to improve the analysis of fetal motion during pregnancy [10].

Auto-encoders can also be used as a fully unsupervised method of anomaly detection. For these applications, it is important to understand that auto-encoders only learn to reconstruct data that they have seen during the training of the network. While a network may learn to handle slight differences, it likely performs worse on samples that are very different from the training data. To illustrate this using the MNIST (a dataset containing images of hand drawn digits) example; if a network is only trained on images of the digit 3, it will fail to properly reconstruct the digit 7. Interestingly, we can use this property to detect anomalies or outliers in the dataset, by purposefully training the network on a dataset of which we are certain does not contain any anomalous samples. If we then apply the network to another dataset that does contain outliers, the outliers are likely to have a significantly larger reconstruction error than the non-anomalous samples. It must be kept in mind that all data that is different from that in the training set is considered anomalous. It may therefore be very hard to distinguish between expected anomalous data, and noise in the observations.

Shvetsova et al. show that this approach can be used to detect tissue with metastases in H&E-stained lymph nodes and abnormal chest x-rays [11]. Wei et al. use a similar method to detect suspicious areas in mammograms showing how auto-encoders can also be used to detect the position of the anomaly in an image while only requiring a set of images obtained from healthy 'normal' patients [12].

6 Auto-encoders for Latent Vector and Feature Learning

Perhaps the most interesting applications of auto-encoders are based on the latent vector extracted after the encoding step. The latent vectors contain a condensed form, or a summary, of all the important information in the input data. Exactly what that information is however, is unknown. We only know that the latent vector contains information that the decoder can use to reconstruct the original data. An important aspect of auto-encoders is that they do not guarantee that the latent space is normally distributed. What this means is that we may get unexpected results when we reconstruct samples after manipulating latent representations or when we calculate relationships between latent representations of different samples. For instance, one might expect that two similar looking images yield similar latent vectors when passed through the encoder. However, it is entirely possible that two very different images have a very similar latent vector, while two very similar images have very different latent vectors. An example of this is given in Fig. 4 where we can see that if we look at some MNIST images that are similar in terms of their latent representation, that some of the original non-compressed images are in fact very different. The fact that the latent space of the auto-encoder is not normally distributed also hampers us from directly linking the values in the latent representations to underlying features of the data. In the case of the MNIST example we may for example observe an increase in line-width if we increase the first latent variable of a latent representation by +2 and reconstruct the image. It is however possible that a step of +5 yields a reconstruction in which the digit is rotated instead of a reconstruction where the linewidth is increased further. Variational auto-encoders, discussed later in this chapter, try to enforce a normally distributed latent space which enables a wide range of additional applications.

While the latent representations of auto-encoder are limited by the non-linearity of the latent space they can still be used for a number of applications. The created latent vectors may for example serve as input to other models [13]. If a user has a very large dataset, of which only a small fraction is labeled, it may be beneficial to first train an auto-encoder on the full dataset, and then train a separate classifier on the latent representations of the previously labelled dataset. This approach ensures that sufficient information is extracted from the input data, with less risk of overfitting and unwanted biases.

It is also possible to use the latent vectors as input for another dimension reduction technique that is better at preserving the relationship between samples, but worse at handling large/complex data [14]. It is for example not uncommon to reduce image data to 32 or 64 dimensions using an auto-encoder and then apply t-SNE (or similar dimension reduction techniques) to further reduce the dimension to 2 or 3, so that the data can easily be visualized in a graph [15]. This approach generally performs better than only using an auto-encoder or t-SNE.

7 Variational Auto-encoders

Variational auto-encoders (VAE) are closely related to auto-encoders in terms of their network structure and purposes [16]. The main goal with which they were proposed is however very different from the original 'vanilla' auto-encoders. VAEs are a type of generative model, meaning that they can generate (new) data, instead of just compressing and reconstructing existing data. In order to do so, VAEs attempt to learn the distribution (or process) that generated the data on which the model is trained, opposed to simply finding the optimal solution that minimizes reconstruction loss. The latent space variables of regular auto-encoders may have large gaps in their distribution and may be centered around an arbitrary value, while those of VAEs are all normally distributed with a mean of 0 and standard deviation of 1 (stochastic normal distribution). In the case of the latent space of an auto-encoder, there is little relation between values in the latent space and its reconstruction, slightly changing z might lead to completely different reconstructions. With the VAE, there is a very direct relation between the two and slightly changing z will slightly alter the reconstruction while changing z in the opposite direction will have the opposite result. By inserting a latent vector z (with values around zero, and within a few standard deviations) into the decoder of a VAE, one can create 'new' data that can usually be considered comparable to the data the VAE was trained on, where a latent vector z containing all zeros approximates the mean of the training data. The general structure of a VAE is visualized in Fig. 2.

The training of VAEs is more complex than that of normal auto-encoders, and is described in more detail in the technical intermezzo. It is important to know that VAEs are trained with an additional loss term: the Kullback-Leiber Divergence (KL Divergence). The KL-divergence loss term encourages the latent space of the VAE to have the desired properties described above by enforcing that each individual latent variable follows a unit normal gaussian distribution (with mean = 0 and standard deviation = 1).

Technical Intermezzo 2

VAEs are based on the assumption that all data in the dataset used to train the model was generated from a process involving some unobserved random variable. The data generation process then consists of 2 steps: (1) a value z is generated from some prior distribution $\boldsymbol{P_\theta}$ (z); ; (2) a value $\boldsymbol{x}$ is generated from a conditional distribution $\boldsymbol{P_\theta}$ $(\boldsymbol{x}|z)$. In this process the optimal values of $\boldsymbol{\theta}(\boldsymbol{\theta}^*)$ and z are unknown, and thus need to be calculated from the known values in $\boldsymbol{x}$. VAEs aim to approximate $\boldsymbol{\theta}*$ and $\mathbf{z}$ even if calculation of the marginal likelihood and true posterior density are intractable. To do so, VAEs use a recognition

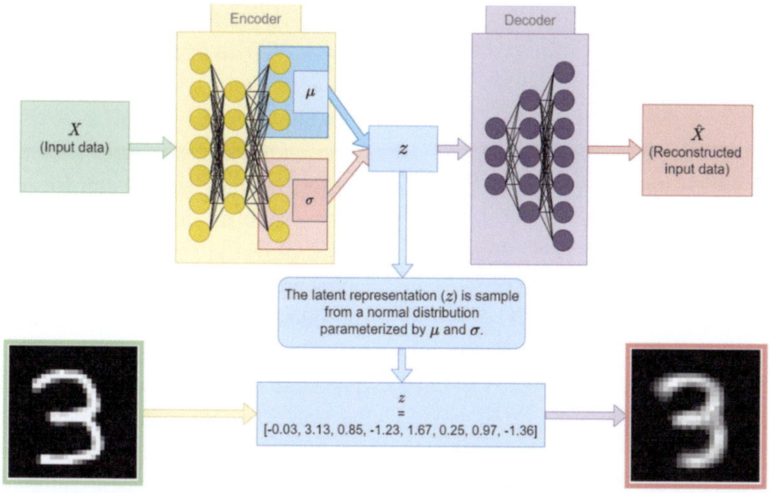

Fig. 2 General schematic layout of a Variational Autoencoder neural network. During the training the network latent vector z is sampled from a gaussian distribution parameterized by the outputs of the encoder. These outputs are also used for the calculation of the KL-divergence, which is then combined with the MSE loss (calculated from the original input and the reconstruction) to form the VAE loss function

model $\boldsymbol{q_\varphi(z|x)}$ that approximates the true posterior $\boldsymbol{P_\theta}$ $\boldsymbol{(x|z)}$ and jointly learn the recognition parameter $\boldsymbol{\varphi}$ together with the generative parameter $\boldsymbol{\theta}$. Using this formalization, we can distinguish between learning a probabilistic encoder $\boldsymbol{q_\varphi(z|x)}$, from which we can sample z when given $\boldsymbol{x}$ and a probabilistic decoder $\boldsymbol{P_\theta(x|z)}$, from which we can sample $\boldsymbol{x}$ when given z. In practice both the probabilistic encoder and decoder are neural networks of which the appropriate architecture can be picked based on the nature of the data in $\boldsymbol{x}$.

The VAE training objective

To ensure that the approximate distribution $\boldsymbol{q_\varphi(z|x)}$, is close to the real distribution $\boldsymbol{P_\theta(x|z)}$, , we can use the Kullback-Leiber Divergence (KL Divergence) which quantifies the deference between 2 distributions. In the case of VAEs the goal is to minimize this KL Divergence which can be written as follows:

$$D_{KL}\left(q_\varphi(z|x), p_\theta(z|x)\right) = p_\theta(x) + D_{KL}(q_\varphi(z|x), p_\theta(z)) - E_{z\sim q_\varphi}(z|x)\log p_\theta(x|z) \tag{4}$$

Equation 4. The Kullback-Leiber Divergence.

Equation 4 can then be rearranged to Eq. 5.

$$p_\theta(x) - D_{KL}\left(q_\varphi(z|x), p_\theta(z|x)\right) = E_{z\sim q_\varphi}(z|x)\log p_\theta(x|z) - D_{KL}\left(q_\varphi(z|x), p_\theta(z)\right) \tag{5}$$

The left-hand side of Eq. 5 exactly fits the objective of the VAE: we want to maximize the probability of $\boldsymbol{x}$ from distribution $\boldsymbol{p_\theta(x)}$ and minimize the difference between the estimated distribution $\boldsymbol{q_\varphi(z|x)}$ and real distribution $\boldsymbol{p_\theta(z|x)}$. The negation of the right-hand side of the equation gives us the loss which we minimize to find the optimal values for $\boldsymbol{\varphi}$ and $\boldsymbol{\theta}$.

$$L_{VAE} = E_{z\sim q_\varphi}(z|x)\log p_\theta(x|z) + D_{KL}\left(q_\varphi(z|x), p_\theta(z)\right)$$
$$\theta^*, \varphi^* = argmin_{\theta,\varphi} L_{VAE} \tag{6}$$

Equation 6. The training objective function of the variational auto-encoder.

Equation 6 is known as the Evidence Lower Bound (ELBO) because the KL-divergence is always positive. This means that $-L_{VAE}$ is the lowest value $p_\theta(x)$ can take, minimizing L_{VAE} thus equates to maximizing $p_\theta(x)$. Even tough Eq. 6 gives a clear definition of a loss term, it cannot directly be used to train a VAE. The expectation term in the loss has to be approximated using a sampling operation, which prevents the flow of gradients during training. To solve this issue, VAEs use the 'reparameterization trick' which relies on the assumption that $p(z|x)$ follows a known distribution. This distribution is usually assumed to be a multivariate Gaussian with a diagonal covariance structure (even though the trick works for other distributions as well). Using the parameters of $q_\varphi(x|z)$ and the assumption $q_\varphi(x|z)$ is Gaussian, z can be expressed as a deterministic variable that is produced by some function $\tau_\varphi(x, \varepsilon)$ where ε is sampled form an independent unit normal Gaussian distribution.

$$z = \tau_\varphi(x, \varepsilon) = \mu + \sigma \odot \varepsilon \tag{7}$$

Equation 7. The 'reparameterization trick' used to enable the training of variational auto-encoders through backpropagation.

In practice the encoder model of the VAE is constructed so that is outputs a mean (μ) and standard deviation (σ) that parameterize the Gaussian distribution $q_\varphi(x|z)$. Using this set up, the reparameterization trick equates to Eq. 7.

In this chapter we often refer to the embedding or latent representation of data which means the mean μ output of the encoder of the VAE was used and the standard deviation σ was ignored. This can be considered standard practice if a latent representation of input data is desired.

8 Disentanglement and Posterior Collapse

The latent variables of a VAE often encode some underlying characteristics of the data. For images, latent variables can for example encode factors such as the width, height or angle of a shown object [17]. However, different latent variables are often entangled, meaning that multiple variables influence the same characteristic of the data. To improve the explainability of the latent space and better control the generative process of the VAE [18–21] it can be desirable to disentangle the latent space. Higgins et al. proposed the β-VAE, which adds an additional weight β to the KL-term of the VAE loss, as a very simple but effective way to improve disentanglement [17]. The value of β can be picked based on the desired amount of disentanglement of the latent space. A higher β generally corresponds to better disentanglement. There is however a trade-off between the amount of disentanglement and the reconstruction quality of the VAE, where more disentanglement results in worse reconstructions [22]. VAEs also suffer from a phenomenon called posterior collapse (or KL-vanishing), which causes the model to ignore a subset of the latent variables. Posterior collapse occurs when the uninformative prior distribution matches the variational distribution too closely for a subset of latent variables. This is likely caused by the KL-divergence loss term which encourages the two distributions to be similar [23]. During training, posterior collapse can often be observed when the KL-loss term decreases to (near) zero, which is even more prevalent in VAE variants that add additional weight to the KL-term such as β-VAE [17]. To prevent posterior collapse and improve reconstruction quality of disentangled VAEs, Shao et al. propose the Control-VAE [24]. This method requires a 'target value' for the KL-divergence and tunes the weight of the KL-divergence such that it stays close the target value during training.

9 Use Cases for VAEs and Latent Traversals

The generative capabilities and their (disentangled) latent spaces allow for a large number of use-cases of VAEs. VAEs (and VAE based models) can for example be used to improve anomaly detection compared to normal auto-encoders, to create interpretable latent representations that can serve as input for conventional classification models such as logistic regressions, or to perform further analysis of the learned latent variables using techniques such as latent traversals [25, 26].

A latent traversal is a method in which we change one or more latent variables from a sample encoded using the encoder of a VAE, and reconstruct the input sample from these changed latent variables using the decoder. By comparing the original sample and the sample reconstructed from the changed variables one can see which aspects of the data are encoded by these variables. Especially when the latent space is sufficiently disentangled, it is often possible to relate individual latent variables to underlying physiological characteristics of the data.

Latent traversals can be combined with logistic regressions (or other classical statistical models) to infer and visualize relationships between latent variables and the use case (e.g. classification, prediction etc.). We do this by analyzing the weights/coefficients of the logistic regression to see which latent variables have a positive predictive value for a certain class. We can then perform a latent traversal by increasing and decreasing these important latent variables and examining how the reconstructed sample changes. This whole process thus allows us to visualize which features are important for a class. We elaborate on this approach in a practical example applied to electrocardiogram (ECG) data later in this chapter.

10 Auto-encoders Versus Variational Auto-encoders (Summary)

Now that we have discussed both auto-encoders and variational auto-encoders, we can summarize the pros and cons of both model types. An overview of these is given in Table 1. In general, VAEs provide a wider range of applications, while auto-encoders generally produce better reconstructions. We have discussed a similar trade-of regarding the disentanglement of VAEs, where the reconstruction quality of VAEs is inversely related to the amount of disentanglement. These trade-offs lead to the conclusion that it is desirable to use a (disentangled) VAE if a normal auto-encoder is insufficient for the desired use-case.

11 Designing an Auto-encoder and Common Pitfalls

The first step in training an auto-encoder (or any other model) is collecting a representative dataset that can ensure the validity of any findings or insights [27]. As discussed before, auto-encoders only learn to reconstruct data that is similar to the data used during the preceding training

Table 1 Use cases, pros and cons of using (variational) auto-encoders

Use-case	Auto-encoder	Variational quto-encoder
Denoising	+	+
Anomaly detection	+	+
Representation learning	+	+
Data generation	−	+
Latent traversals	−	+
Possibility to disentangle latent variables	−	+
Optimal reconstruction quality	+	−

phase. It is thus important to collect a heterogeneous dataset that spans the full range of sample variation that will be used for further analysis. The actual type of data can range anywhere from images, to signals to any arbitrary measurement. There is, to the best of our knowledge, no datatype that can inherently not be used to train an auto-encoder. It is however important to remember that more complex data may require a more complex network architecture, or more training data. It is also possible that the standard MSE loss term may not be adequate for certain datatypes where it is important to accurately reconstruct small features, because the MSE loss will deem large features to be more important than small features. An example of this is in the use-case of ECGs, where minor variations in the P-wave can be overshadowed by larger variations in the larger T-wave, and are thus not adequately captured by the auto-encoder.

Both the encoder and decoder part of the auto-encoder consist of a more elaborate neural network. The choice for the network architecture is generally dependent on the data to which the auto-encoder is applied. For simpler data it may be sufficient to use a small number of fully connected linear layers, in combination with non-linear activation functions [28]. For more complex data, such as for example medical images, the encoder network is often composed of several convolutional layers (connected by non-linear activation functions) [7, 9–11]. Convolutions are currently the most popular architecture type because they show optimal performance on various types of different data. For signal or timeseries data, 1-dimsional convolutions are a popular choice; for images it is common to use 2-dimensional convolutions [8]. Depending on the number of chosen layers it may also be beneficial to add skip connections (residual connections) to improve the flow of gradients through the network during backpropagation [29]. Various regularization techniques like batch normalization and dropout may also improve performance. It is however generally better to first design a simple network and be certain that these additional tricks improve performance before using them.

In essence, the decoder of the network is often designed to be a mirrored version of the encoder network. Hence, if convolutional layers are used in the encoder, transposed convolutions are used in the decoder [30]. The usage of pooling layers (e.g. min/max-pool, average pool) in the encoder may pose a problem, as no sufficient inverse of these functions exist. In this case it is possible to simply up sample the data in the decoder under the assumption that the model will be expressive enough trough the other layers that do contain weights.

Perhaps the most important design decision is the size of the latent space. Smaller latent vectors generally result in worse reconstructions, conversely larger latent vectors often lead to better reconstructions. The choice of the size of the latent space is thus very dependent on the use case of the auto-encoder. For denoising auto-encoders and anomaly detection tasks, it may be sufficient to reduce the size of the input only slightly during the encoding step. In these cases a very small latent vector is undesirable as it is likely to yield worse reconstructions. By contrast, if the latent representation serves as input for another model, picking the correct size is entirely dependent on the task of the other model. Here a more compressed representation may be desirable as it reduces the amount of information extraction that still must be performed by the other model. If the latent representations are used as input for conventional clustering techniques it is desirable to have an amount of latent variables that is within a reasonable range (e.g. higher than 10 but below 100, dependent on the size of the dataset). When auto-encoders serve as an input to another neural model, the optimal latent space can be selected based on the quality of the reconstructions (if we assume the decoder is functioning perfectly). Simply put, if the reconstructions look decent, there must be enough information in the latent representation to be used in the other model, and the latent space was sufficiently large.

If the goal of the auto-encoder is to create an interpretable latent space, the best choice is likely to use a variational auto-encoder.

12 Examples Using the MNIST Dataset

In this section we perform a number of small-scale experiments to show the how the design of the auto-encoder influences its performance. For this purpose we use the MNIST dataset [4]. This dataset consists of 70,000 grayscale images of handwritten digits and is a popular choice for basic experiments among AI researchers.

We split the dataset into a train, validation and test set (80%, 10%, 10% respectively) and trained 9 neural networks until convergence. As a comparison, we also included 3 examples of the commonly used PCA dimension reduction technique. The tested neural architectures consist of a fully connected (linear) architecture without activation functions, a fully connected architecture with activation functions, and a convolutional neural network. For each architecture we train the network with 3 different latent space sizes (2, 4 and 8 latent variables). We configure the PCA method to also reduce the data to 2, 4 and 8 variables.

All images in the dataset consist of 28×28 pixels. Depending on the model architecture we treat the pixel values of the image as either a vector or a matrix. For the fully connected architectures, as well as the commonly used PCA method, we flatten the input 28×28 image, resulting in a vector of 1×784 pixel values. For a convolutional architecture we keep the image in its original matrix form so that convolutions can better capture the spatial relationships between the pixels in the images, in all directions (i.e. horizontal or vertical).

In Fig. 4 we show the reconstructions of a sample for each of the methods and each tested latent space size. The results clearly show that the reconstruction quality increases as more latent variables are used. We also observe the difference in quality between the different architectures. The fully connected models, without linear activation functions, show the worst results, which are even worse than the PCA method. This is expected, as a linear network is likely to only approximate PCA. The non-linear models, both fully connected and convolutional, show the best results, with the convolution network performing slightly better than the fully connected network. Here the strength of convolutional models becomes clear, as the convolutional networks outperform the fully connected networks while having significantly less parameters (approximately 270,000 for the convolutional networks versus 400,000 for the fully connected networks). We thus see that convolutional neural networks can outperform fully connected neural networks despite having less parameters. This difference in the number of parameters generally causes convolutional networks to be more computationally efficient and converge faster. Additionally, this reduction in computational cost may allow us to further increase the depth/size of the network and potentially improve its performance further (Fig. 3).

In order to highlight the fact that auto-encoders do not preserve the relationship between input samples in the latent space, an additional example is provided. We encode a sample image, as well as the rest of the training dataset, to its latent representation, and look for the images that are closest to the sample image in the latent space. We plot the top 5 closest images in Fig. 5, and observe that images 3, 4 and 5 are not similar to our sample image at all (Fig. 4).

We also compare the spread of the values of the latent space of auto-encoders and variational auto-encoders (Fig. 6) to show the differences between both models. To do so we first construct a variational auto-encoder with a latent space of 8 values that uses a similar convolutional architecture as the normal auto-encoder. We than encode all the entries in the training set into their latent representation and create a boxplot for each latent variable. We observe that for the normal auto-encoder the latent variables have mean values that deviate from 0, have larger

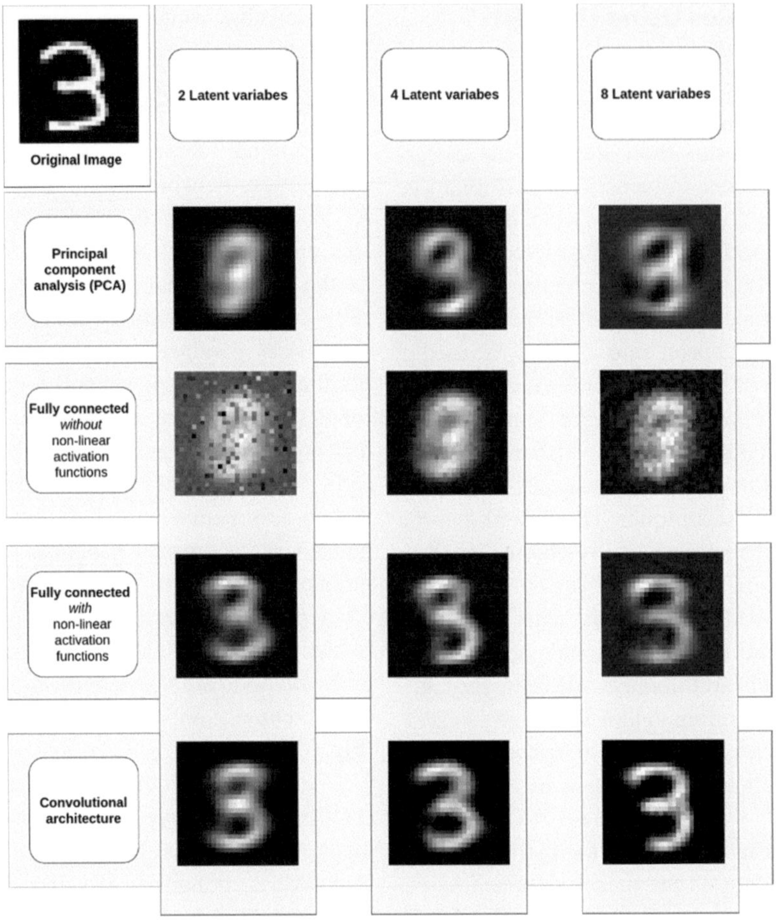

Fig. 3 Reconstructions created using PCA or auto-encoders under different configurations

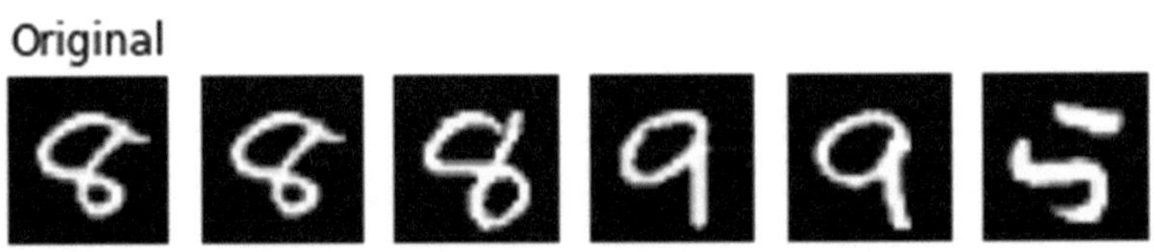

Fig. 4 Examples of digits most similar to the original sample (left) in terms of latent representation

standard deviations, larger confidence intervals and that the mean value of the variables is often not located at the center of the confidence interval. For the variational auto-encoder we observe that each latent variable does indeed appear to be normally distributed, as was enforced during the training of the VAE.

13 Demonstrator Use Case of an VAE for the Electrocardiogram: The FactorECG

Many studies use deep neural networks to interpret electrocardiograms (ECGs) with high predictive performances, some focusing on

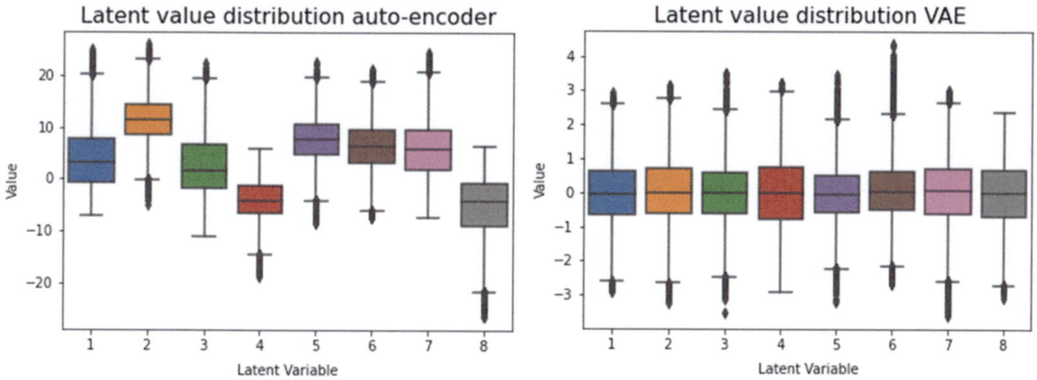

Fig. 5 Boxplots of each latent variable of latent representations of the MNIST dataset created using an auto-encoder (left) and a variational auto-encoder (right)

tasks known to be associated with the ECG (e.g., rhythm disorders) and others identifying completely novel use cases for the ECG (e.g., reduced ejection fraction) [31–34]. Most studies do not employ any technique to provide insight into the workings of the algorithm, however, the explainability of neural networks can be considered a essential step towards the applicability of these techniques in clinical practice [35, 36]. In contrast, various studies do use post-hoc explainability techniques, where the 'decisions' of the 'black box' DNN are visualized after training, usually using heatmaps (e.g.., using Grad-CAM, SHAP or LIME) [37]. In these studies, usually some example ECGs were handpicked, as these heatmap-based techniques only work on single ECGs. Currently employed post-hoc explainability techniques, usually heatmap-based, have limited explainable value as they merely indicate the temporal location of a specific feature in the individual ECG. Moreover, these techniques have been shown to be unreliable, poorly reproducible and suffer from confirmation bias [38, 39].

Variational auto-encoders can be used to overcome this by constructing a DNN that is inherently explainable (i.e. explainable by design, instead of investigating post-hoc). One example is the FactorECG, which is part of a pipeline that consists of three components: (1) a variational auto-encoder that learned to encode the ECG into its underlying 21 continuous factors of variation (the FactorECG), (2) a visualization technique to provide insight into these ECG factors, and (3) a common interpretable statistical method to perform diagnosis or prediction using the ECG factors [19]. Model-level explainability is obtained by varying the ECG factors (i.e. latent traversals), while generating and plotting ECGs, which allows for visualization of detailed changes in morphology, that are associated with physiologically valid underlying anatomical and (patho)physiological processes. Moreover, individual patient-level explanations are also possible, as every individual ECG has its representative set of explainable FactorECG values, of which the associations with the outcome are known. When using the explainable pipeline for interpretation of diagnostic ECG statements, detection of reduced ejection fraction and prediction of one-year mortality, it yielded predictive performances similar to state-of-the-art 'black box' DNNs. Contrary to the state-of-the-art, our pipeline provided inherent explainability on which ECG features were important for prediction or diagnosis. For example, ST elevation was discovered to be an important predictor for reduced ejection fraction, which is an important finding as it could limit the generalizability of the algorithm to the general population. We have also extended the FactorECG methodology and developed a technique called Query based Latent Space Traversals (qLST) which can be used to relate

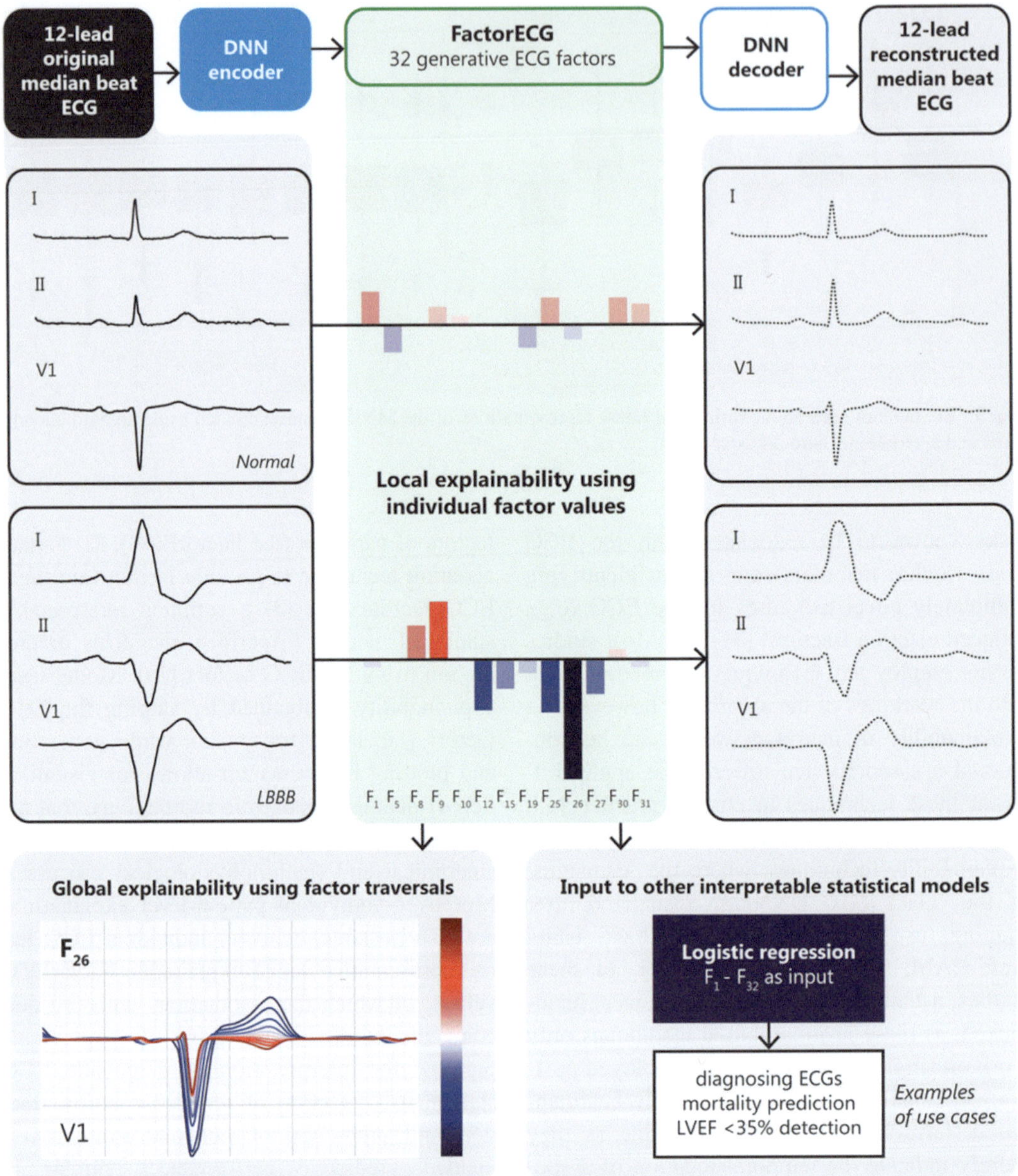

Fig. 6 Illustration of the FactorECG explainable pipeline for ECG interpretation. The VAE consists of three parts, the encoder, the latent space (FactorECG) and the decoder. The model can be made explainable locally (as the individual values of the ECG factors for each ECG are known) and globally (by using factor traversals the influence of individual factors on the ECG morphology can be visualized). Usually, the factors are entered into simple statistical models, such as logistic regression, to perform the task at hand

multiple latent variables to a disease class at once or to explain existing black box classifiers [15].

A longstanding assumption was that the high-dimensional and non-linear 'black box' nature of the currently applied ECG-based DNNs was inevitable to gain the impressive performances shown by these algorithms on conventional and novel use cases. Variational auto-encoders allow for reliable clinical interpretation of these models without performance reduction, however, while also broadening their applicability to detect novel features in many other (rare) diseases, as they provide significant dimensionality reduction. The application of such methods will lead to more confidence in DNN-based ECG analysis, which will facilitate the clinical implementation of DNNs in routine clinical practice.

Glossary

Activation function In neural networks, (non-linear) activation functions are used at the output of neurons to convert the input to an 'active' or 'not active' state. An activation function can be a simple linear or sigmoid function or have more complex arbitrary forms. The Rectified Linear Unit (ReLU) function is currently the most popular choice. In neural networks, (non-linear) activation functions are used at the output of neurons to convert the input to an 'active' or 'not active' state. An activation function can be a simple linear or sigmoid function or have more complex arbitrary forms. The Rectified Linear Unit (ReLU) function is currently the most popular choice.

Back propagation Is a widely used technique in the field of machine learning that is used during the training of a neural network. The technique is used to update the weights of the neural network based on the calculated loss, effectively allowing it to 'learn'.Is a widely used technique in the field of machine learning that is used during the training of a neural network. The technique is used to update the weights of the neural network based on the calculated loss, effectively allowing it to 'learn'.

(mini-) Batch A small set of data samples that is fed through the network at once during training. A too small batch size may lead to instability while a too large batch size may lead to depletion of computer resources.A small set of data samples that is fed through the network at once during training. A too small batch size may lead to instability while a too large batch size may lead to depletion of computer resources.

Convolution Common building block of various neural networks. Convolutional neural networks can be considered the current 'state of the art' of neural networks applied to various data sources. Convolutional layers in a neural network a apply a learned filter to the input data which improves the ability of neural networks to comprehend spatial structures. Convolutions can be applied in 1 dimensional (signal/timeseries data) and 2 dimensional (images) forms.Common building block of various neural networks. Convolutional neural networks can be considered the current 'state of the art' of neural networks applied to various data sources. Convolutional layers in a neural network a apply a learned filter to the input data which improves the ability of neural networks to comprehend spatial structures. Convolutions can be applied in 1 dimensional (signal/timeseries data) and 2 dimensional (images) forms.

Decoder Part of the (variational) auto-encoder that decodes the given latent vector into a reconstruction of the original dataPart of the (variational) auto-encoder that decodes the given latent vector into a reconstruction of the original data

Dimension The dimension of data is the size of the dataset or vector, for a grayscale image this is the height × the width in pixels (e.g. 28 × 28), for an RGB-color image, a third dimension of size 3 is added (e.g. (28 × 28 × 3)The dimension of data is the size of the dataset or vector, for a grayscale image this is the height × the width in pixels (e.g. 28 × 28), for an RGB-color image, a third dimension of size 3 is added (e.g. (28 × 28 × 3)

Encoder Part of the (variational) auto-encoder that encodes the provided data into the latent vectorPart of the (variational) auto-encoder that encodes the provided data into the latent vector

Explainability The ability of a (trained) observer to interpret the inner workings of a model. Neural networks are generally considered to be to complex to comprehend by humans and are treated as an 'unexplainable' black box. The lack of explainability is a major issue in many of the current clinical applications of neural networks.The ability of a (trained) observer to interpret the inner workings of a model. Neural networks are generally considered to be to complex to comprehend by humans and are treated as an 'unexplainable' black box. The lack of explainability is a major issue in many of the current clinical applications of neural networks.

Fullyconnected or linear layer Common building block of neural networks in which every node (or every datapoint) in the input is connected to every node in the output of the layer. Through the weights that are associated with each connection the layer is able perform linear transformations of the input data. Together with non-linear activation functions, fully connected layers make up the most basic forms of neural networks.Common building block of neural networks in which every node (or every datapoint) in the input is connected to every node in the output of the layer. Through the weights that are associated with each connection the layer is able perform linear transformations of the input data. Together with non-linear activation functions, fully connected layers make up the most basic forms of neural networks.

KL Divergence The Kullback-Leiber Divergence is a measure of similarity between two distributions.The Kullback-Leiber Divergence is a measure of similarity between two distributions.**Loss function** The loss function of the network defines the training objective of the neural network. The loss, the output of the loss function, is progressively minimized through backpropagation, allowing the network to learn and be optimized for its training objective.The loss function of the network defines the training objective of the neural network. The loss, the output of the loss function, is progressively minimized through backpropagation, allowing the network to learn and be optimized for its training objective.

MNIST A commonly used dataset consisting of image of handwritten digits. MNIST is often used for small scale experiments because of the simplistic nature of the data.A commonly used dataset consisting of image of handwritten digits. MNIST is often used for small scale experiments because of the simplistic nature of the data.

PCA Principal component analysis. A technique commonly used for dimension reduction. The technique involves the calculation ofPrincipal component analysis. A technique commonly used for dimension reduction. The technique involves the calculation of

Posterior collapse A phenomenon that can occur during the train of variational autoencoder through which the reconstruction accuracy of the network decreases dramatically if the KL-divergence reduces to much.A phenomenon that can occur during the train of variational autoencoder through which the reconstruction accuracy of the network decreases dramatically if the KL-divergence reduces to much.

Vector A vector is a single row or column of numbers.A vector is a single row or column of numbers.

Matrix A set consisting of multiple rows and columns of numbers.A set consisting of multiple rows and columns of numbers.

Convergence A neural network has reached convergence when further training does no longer improve the model.A neural network has reached convergence when further training does no longer improve the model.

MSE loss Mean Squared Error loss, a measure of difference between two data instances such as images or timeseries. The MSE loss is a common loss function that is used to minimize the reconstruction error in auto-encoders.Mean Squared Error loss, a measure of difference between two data instances such as images or timeseries. The MSE loss is a common loss function that is used to minimize the reconstruction error in auto-encoders.

Latent variable A variable that is not directly observed in the data but can be inferred through the usage of a model from other variables that are observed directly. In the case of auto-encoders we refer to the variables in the vector extracted after applying the encoder of the auto-encoder as latent variables.A variable that is not directly observed in the data but can be inferred through the usage of a model from other variables that are observed directly. In the case of auto-encoders we refer to the variables in the vector extracted after applying the encoder of the auto-encoder as latent variables.

Disentanglement The disentanglement of latent variables refers to the process of separating the influence of each latent variable on the reconstructed data.The disentanglement of latent variables refers to the process of separating the influence of each latent variable on the reconstructed data.

References

1. Hinton GE, Zemel RS. Autoencoders, minimum description length and Helmholtz free energy. p. 8.
2. Hinton GE, Salakhutdinov RR. Reducing the dimensionality of data with neural networks. Science. 2006;313(5786):504–7. https://doi.org/10.1126/science.1127647.
3. Using autoencoders for mammogram compression. PubMed. https://pubmed.ncbi.nlm.nih.gov/20703586/. Accessed 31 Jan 2022.
4. Lecun Y, Bottou L, Bengio Y, Haffner P. Gradient-based learning applied to document recognition. Proc IEEE. 1998;86(11):2278–324. https://doi.org/10.1109/5.726791.
5. Baldi P, Hornik K. Neural networks and principal component analysis: learning from examples without local minima. Neural Netw. 1989;2(1):53–8. https://doi.org/10.1016/0893-6080(89)90014-2.
6. Mohd Sagheer SV, George SN. A review on medical image denoising algorithms. Biomed Signal Process Control 2020;61:102036. https://doi.org/10.1016/j.bspc.2020.102036.
7. Gondara L. Medical image denoising using convolutional denoising autoencoders. In: 2016 IEEE 16th international conference on data mining workshops (ICDMW), Barcelona, Spain, Dec 2016, pp 241–46. https://doi.org/10.1109/ICDMW.2016.0041
8. Lu X, Tsao Y, Matsuda S, Hori C. Speech enhancement based on deep denoising auto-encoder. In: Proceedings of interspeech, Jan 2013. p. 436–40.
9. Jifara W, Jiang F, Rho S, Cheng M, Liu S. Medical image denoising using convolutional neural network: a residual learning approach. J Supercomput. 2019;75(2):704–18. https://doi.org/10.1007/s11227-017-2080-0.
10. Nawarathne T et al. Comprehensive study on denoising of medical images utilizing neural network based auto-encoder. Feb 2021. arXiv:2102.01903 [eess]. Accessed 30 Jan 2022. Available http://arxiv.org/abs/2102.01903
11. Shvetsova N, Bakker B, Fedulova I, Schulz H, Dylov DV. Anomaly detection in medical imaging with deep perceptual autoencoders. IEEE Access. 2021;9:118571–83. https://doi.org/10.1109/ACCESS.2021.3107163.
12. Wei Q, Shi B, Lo JY, Carin L, Ren Y, Hou, R. Anomaly detection for medical images based on a one-class classification. In: Medical imaging 2018: computer-aided diagnosis, Houston, United States, Feb 2018. p 57. https://doi.org/10.1117/12.2293408
13. Hinton GE, Krizhevsky A, Wang SD. Transforming auto-encoders. In: Artificial neural networks and machine learning—ICANN 2011, Berlin, Heidelberg, 2011. p. 44–51.
14. Fabius O, van Amersfoort JR. Variational Recurrent auto-encoders. arXiv:1412.6581 [cs, stat], Jun 2015. Accessed 31 Jan 2022. Available http://arxiv.org/abs/1412.6581
15. Vessies MB et al. Interpretable ECG classification via a query-based latent space traversal (qLST). arXiv:2111.07386 [cs, eess], Nov 2021, Accessed 31 Jan 2022. Available http://arxiv.org/abs/2111.07386
16. Kingma DP, Welling M. Auto-encoding variational Bayes. arXiv:1312.6114 [cs, stat], May 2014. Accessed 30 Jan 2022. Available http://arxiv.org/abs/1312.6114
17. Higgins I et al.: β-VAE: learning basic visual concepts with a constrained variational framework. 2017. p. 22.
18. Van Steenkiste T, Deschrijver D, Dhaene T. Generating an explainable ECG beat space with variational auto-encoders. arXiv:1911.04898 [cs, eess,

stat], Nov 2019. Accessed 30 Jan 2022. Available http://arxiv.org/abs/1911.04898

19. van de Leur RR et al. Inherently explainable deep neural network-based interpretation of electrocardiograms using variational auto-encoders. Cardiovasc Med. 2022;preprint. https://doi.org/10.1101/2022.01.04.22268759.
20. Kim J-Y, Cho S. BasisVAE: orthogonal latent space for deep disentangled representation. Sep 2019. Accessed 30 Jan 2022. Available https://openreview.net/forum?id=S1gEFkrtvH
21. Chen RTQ, Li X, Grosse R, Duvenaud D. Isolating sources of disentanglement in variational autoencoders. arXiv:1802.04942 [cs, stat], Apr 2019. Accessed 30 Jan 30 2022. Available http://arxiv.org/abs/1802.04942
22. Asperti A, Trentin M. Balancing reconstruction error and Kullback-Leibler divergence in variational autoencoders. arXiv:2002.07514 [cs], Feb 2020. Accessed 30 Jan 2022. Available http://arxiv.org/abs/2002.07514
23. Lucas J, Tucker G, Grosse R, Norouzi M. Understanding posterior collapse in generative latent variable models. 2019. p. 16.
24. Shao H et al. Control VAE: controllable variational autoencoder. arXiv:2004.05988 [cs, stat], Jun 2020. Accessed 30 Jan 2022. Available: http://arxiv.org/abs/2004.05988
25. Guo X, Gichoya JW, Purkayastha S, Banerjee I. CVAD: a generic medical anomaly detector based on Cascade VAE. arXiv:2110.15811 [cs, eess], Jan 2022. Accessed 30 Jan 2022. Available http://arxiv.org/abs/2110.15811
26. Cakmak AS et al. Using convolutional variational autoencoders to predict post-trauma health outcomes from actigraphy data. arXiv:2011.07406 [cs, eess], Nov 2020. Accessed 25 Jan 2022. Available http://arxiv.org/abs/2011.07406
27. Ministerie van Volksgezondheid WS. Guideline for high-quality diagnostic and prognostic applications of AI in healthcare—Publicatie - Data voor gezondheid. 28 Dec 2021. https://www.datavoorgezondheid.nl/documenten/publicaties/2021/12/17/guideline-for-high-quality-diagnostic-and-prognostic-applications-of-ai-in-healthcare. Accessed 01 Feb 2022.
28. Wang Y, Yao H, Zhao S. Auto-encoder based dimensionality reduction. Neurocomputing. 2016;184:232–42. https://doi.org/10.1016/j.neucom.2015.08.104.
29. He K, Zhang X, Ren S, Sun J. Identity mappings in deep residual networks. In: Computer vision—ECCV, Cham. 2016. p. 630–45. https://doi.org/10.1007/978-3-319-46493-0_38.
30. Chen H, et al. Low-dose CT with a residual encoder-decoder convolutional neural network. IEEE Trans Med Imaging. 2017;36(12):2524–35. https://doi.org/10.1109/TMI.2017.2715284.
31. van de Leur RR, et al. Automatic triage of 12-lead ECGs using deep convolutional neural networks. J Am Heart Assoc. 2020;9(10): e015138. https://doi.org/10.1161/JAHA.119.015138.
32. Attia ZI, et al. Screening for cardiac contractile dysfunction using an artificial intelligence-enabled electrocardiogram. Nat Med. 2019;25(1):70–4. https://doi.org/10.1038/s41591-018-0240-2.
33. van de Leur RR, et al. Discovering and Visualizing disease-specific electrocardiogram features using deep learning: proof-of-concept in phospholamban gene mutation carriers. Circ Arrhythm Electrophysiol. 2021;14(2): e009056. https://doi.org/10.1161/CIRCEP.120.009056.
34. Ribeiro AH, et al. Automatic diagnosis of the 12-lead ECG using a deep neural network. Nat Commun. 2020;11(1):1760. https://doi.org/10.1038/s41467-020-15432-4.
35. Goodman B, Flaxman S. European Union regulations on algorithmic decision-making and a 'right to explanation.' AIMag. 2017;38(3):50–7. https://doi.org/10.1609/aimag.v38i3.2741.
36. Markus AF, Kors JA, Rijnbeek PR. The role of explainability in creating trustworthy artificial intelligence for health care: a comprehensive survey of the terminology, design choices, and evaluation strategies. J Biomed Inform. 2021;113: 103655. https://doi.org/10.1016/j.jbi.2020.103655.
37. Hughes JW, et al. Performance of a convolutional neural network and explainability technique for 12-lead electrocardiogram interpretation. JAMA Cardiol. 2021;6(11):1285–95. https://doi.org/10.1001/jamacardio.2021.2746.
38. Hooker S, Erhan D, Kindermans P-J, Kim B. A benchmark for interpretability methods in deep neural networks. arXiv:1806.10758 [cs, stat], Nov 2019. Accessed 31 Jan 2022. Available http://arxiv.org/abs/1806.10758
39. Adebayo J, Gilmer J, Muelly M, Goodfellow I, Hardt M, Kim B. Sanity checks for saliency maps. arXiv:1810.03292 [cs, stat], Nov 2020, Accessed 31 Jan 2022. Available http://arxiv.org/abs/1810.03292

Artificial Intelligence

John H. Holmes

Abstract

The history of artificial intelligence is a long one, even going back to the ancient Greeks who sought to mimic human intelligence in a machine, the Automaton. However, much of what we consider to be the story of artificial intelligence encompasses only the last 75 years, when the field of research and practice of artificial intelligence was named as such by the giants in the discipline at the time. This chapter reviews this history, focusing on deductive inference, rather than machine learning; it begins with the proposal for a summer institute on artificial intelligence in 1955, through the development of deductive, rule-based approaches to machine-driven inference, including methods for how these approaches were realized on computers. These approaches, realized as knowledge-based systems, found their manifestation a number of domains, including medical decision making, clinical education, population health surveillance, data representation and integration, and clinical trial support. This history provides the reader with an "family tree" of sorts that shows the evolution of artificial intelligence through the past seven decades and its application to medicine and public health.

Keywords

Artificial intelligence · Rule-based systems · Knowledge acquisition · Knowledge representation · Knowledge-based systems · Deductive inference

The quest has been long for ways to mimic the way humans (and other living organisms, but for now we will focus only on humans) act in response to some environmental phenomenon. This quest has manifested in many ways over the course of history, starting with the ancient Greeks' conception of the Automaton, a machine that acted like a human, and its extension into early conceptualizations of robots that persist to this day. It seems natural that in addition to human behavior, one would consider that thought and intention should be a part of these ideas- that an automaton or a robot would be able to *think*, that is, act intelligently, because after all, that is what humans do. However, no one can really argue that "intelligence" programmed into a machine (computer or otherwise) is not artificial,

J. H. Holmes (✉)
Department of Biostatistics, Epidemiology, and Informatics, University of Pennsylvania Perelman School of Medicine, 401 Blockley Hall, 423 Guardian Drive, Philadelphia, PA 19104, USA
e-mail: jhholmes@pennmedicine.upenn.edu

F. W. Asselbergs et al. (eds.), *Clinical Applications of Artificial Intelligence in Real-World Data*,
https://doi.org/10.1007/978-3-031-36678-9_14

in the sense that it is manufactured and in some way imitates human intelligence.

In this chapter, we acknowledge that artificial intelligence is a very broad domain, including rule- and knowledge-based systems as well as numerous species of machine learning. However, we focus on the former, as manifested in the *expert system*. Expert systems are also known as "rule-based systems", or "knowledge-based systems", or "production systems" (in that they systematically produce a conclusion through a reasoning, typically deductive, process.

In 1955, John McCarthy, Marvin Minsky, Nathaniel Rochester, and Claude Shannon wrote a Proposal for the Dartmouth Summer Research Project on Artificial Intelligence [1]. This was a groundbreaking work in that it was the first time the term "artificial intelligence" was coined. Part and parcel of this was "automatic computing", in retrospect a remarkable idea that would set the stage for work on creating computer systems that reason automatically, like an expert would. These systems would later become known as *expert systems*, in that knowledge obtained from a domain expert could be captured in a language (McCarthy's term) that could compute- that is, be processed by a computer but in such a way that the language could support reasoning. A year after McCarthy's proposal, Allen Newell and Herbert Simon developed a system, Logic Theorist, that could mimic human problem solving [2]. Since the Dartmouth Summer Research Project, a number of definitions of expert systems have been offered:

- "A computer system that emulates, or acts in all respects, with the decision-making capabilities of a human expert [in a limited domain]." Attributed to Feigenbaum
- "A computer system that operates by applying an inference mechanism to a body of specialist expertise represented in the form of 'knowledge'."—Goodall [3]
- "A program intended to make reasoned judgements or give assistance in a complex area in which human skills are fallible or scarce."—Lauritzen and Spiegelhalter [4]
- "A program designed to solve problems at a level comparable to that of a human expert in a given domain."—Cooper [5].

Expert systems have a lengthy history back to 1969, starting with the work of Edward Feigenbaum and Bruce Buchanan with the DENDRAL system, developed at Stanford University in the Heuristic Programming Project. This system was designed to identify unknown organic molecules by analyzing their mass spectra and using knowledge from chemistry. Because of this early work, Feigenbaum is considered the father of expert systems. Three years later, De Dombal developed the first expert system with a medical application, the diagnosis of abdominal pain [6], followed by the work of Edward Shortliffe, Feigenbaum, and Buchanan with the development of MYCIN, an expert system for the diagnosis of a bloodborne infection and recommendations for appropriate antibiotics to treat it [7]. MYCIN was the first to deal with uncertainty, and supported over 400 rules derived from experts; it is considered a landmark system in the history of AI. MYCIN was followed in rapid succession by a number of expert systems for specific clinical applications. This history is explored further in each of the following sections of this chapter.

1 The Anatomy and Physiology of the Generic Expert System

An expert system consists of several components, as shown in Fig. 1. It is helpful to think of the system as an expert consultant that is available to a clinician whenever needed. The knowledge base contains facts, some of which will be obtained from an inanimate source, such as published literature that has undergone peer review or is of equal authority, or even more typically, from consultation with human domain experts during a process known as *knowledge elicitation*. This process can involve interviews, direct observation of experts in action, "think aloud protocols", or other means borrowed from the social sciences. The knowledge base also

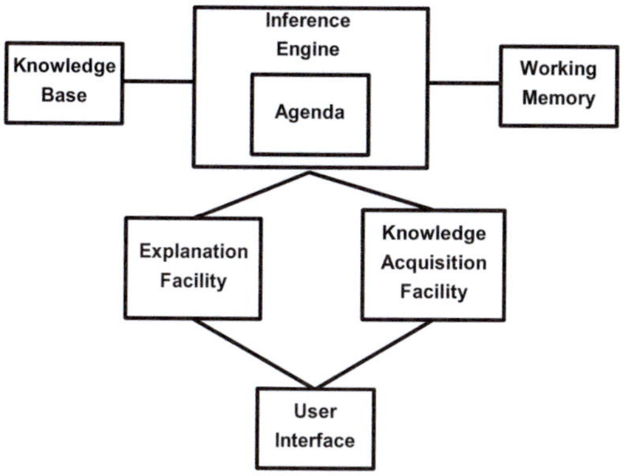

Fig. 1 Schematic of a typical expert system

contains rules, typically expressed in IF–THEN, or antecedent-consequent format. This construction of rules is extremely important for the inference engine which is at the heart of the expert system.

Inference in an expert system is typically deductive, where conclusions follow from premises, and is performed by matching rules and facts with input from the user in the knowledge acquisition facility. Deductive inference follows one of two chaining paradigms. In *forward chaining*, a fact gathered from a user is matched with the antecedent of a rule in in the knowledge base- this causes the rule to be "fired" and the consequent of that rule is then placed in the *agenda*. That consequent now becomes a fact, which itself can be used to match antecedents in the knowledge base and so forth, with additional input from the user, such that a chain is constructed with the ultimate goal of proposing a solution or recommendation back to the user. In clinical systems, just as in clinical reasoning, inference uses *backward chaining*, in that one starts with a hypothesis to be proven or disproven, much like a "rule out" or "rule in" in clinical decision making. In backward chaining, the facts obtained from a user are matched to consequents (as hypotheses), and the inferential chain then works to prove that the antecedents are true (or false). In both cases, there is a working memory that manages the process, which rules are fired, and which facts are included on the agenda. After the system has offered its conclusion, perhaps as a diagnosis, or a recommendation such as a diagnostic procedure to order, an expert system will provide an explanation of its reasoning. MYCIN was the first expert system to include an explanation facility, and has lately been considered a model for new directions in explainable AI.

Creating an expert system is an exercise in knowledge acquisition and the verification and validation of that knowledge. As noted above, the knowledge in an expert system is manifested in rules or facts, either engineered into the knowledge base as a result of the knowledge acquisition process, or obtained from the user in real time, or created through inference in real time by the firing of rules. The process of acquiring knowledge from experts deserves special mention here, and is illustrated in Fig. 2.

Acquiring knowledge from domain experts involves, as noted above, the use of a variety of tools commonly a part of the social scientist's toolkit, such as one would find in ethnography. In addition to the ones mentioned above, these tools also include participant observation, where the person acquiring the knowledge assumes the role of an apprentice to an expert in order to learn her craft. Another tool, more common to the information scientist or librarian is effective searching of the literature, itself considered an "expert". Acquiring knowledge also involves identifying rules and testing them against experts' conceptions of the domain through "what if" scenarios. All of this is conducted by a specially trained knowledge engineer who not

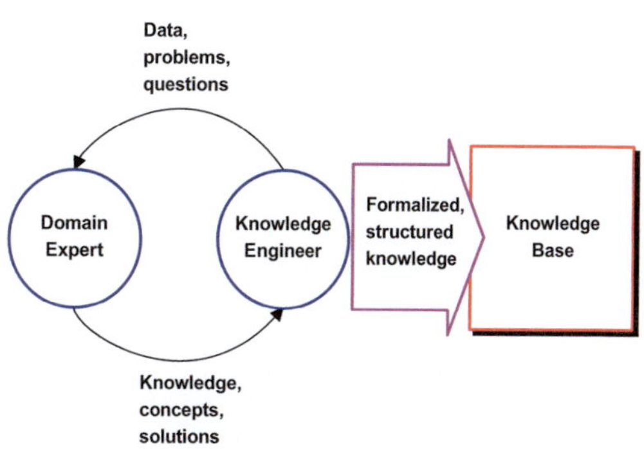

Fig. 2 The knowledge acquisition process

only elicits knowledge from experts but develops computable, formalized representations of that knowledge as a knowledge base. The goal is to create an "expert in a box" that ideally would be undiscernible from a human expert when consulting the system. The evaluation of the expert system, focuses on the verification of the knowledge base (Are the rules in the correct form? Was the system built correctly?) and the validation of the knowledge base as well (Do the rules lead to a correct answer? Was the correct system built?).

It should be evident that knowledge engineering is the Achilles' Heel of any expert system. A breakdown in the specification of rules, or a very large rulebase, can lead to "brittleness", as described by John Holland, where lengthy inferential chains can break, leading to incorrect inferences with catastrophic implications, especially in clinical settings [8]. This is not to say that expert systems do not have a place in clinical applications. As noted below, they are used frequently in medicine, although as a broader type of rule-based system that does not necessarily involve lengthy inferences, is used as frequently in the form of alerts and reminders in electronic health record systems. Broadly speaking, expert systems are a species of *knowledge-based systems*, in that at their heart, expert systems are constructed around a knowledge base. In this chapter, we will use the more inclusive term (abbreviated as "KBS") to refer to any system that uses knowledge to reach a conclusion, offer advice, or make a recommendation. A generic KBS is illustrated in Fig. 3.

The advantages of a KBS are several: Wide distribution of scarce expertise, ease of modification and maintenance, consistency of answers,

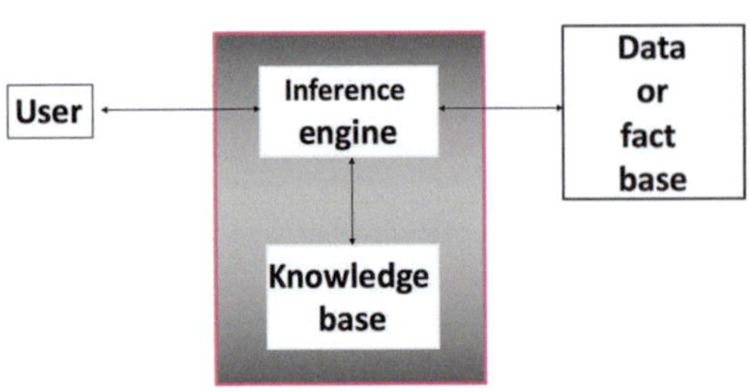

Fig. 3 A generic knowledge-based system

perpetual accessibility, preservation of expertise, solution of problems involving incomplete data, and (usually, but not always) the explanation of solution. However, these advantages come at a cost. First, they are expensive to produce and maintain. In addition, answers might not always be correct for a given clinical problem, and a KBS lacks "common sense". Finally, with few notable exceptions, the KBS cannot learn; this capability is afforded only to knowledge-based systems that incorporate machine learning, which is beyond the scope of this chapter.

This chapter continues with a description of knowledge-based systems as they have been developed for specific clinical or health-related domains: decision support, clinical education, data representation and integration, and clinical trial support. Where appropriate, the history of these systems is discussed as well.

Decision support. In busy or complicated clinical settings, it is often difficult to make consistently accurate and appropriate decisions about diagnosis, treatment, and ongoing management of patients. For this reason, clinical decision making has been and continues to be a target of AI research, application development, and implementation, and the earliest knowledge-based systems focused on diagnosis. The earliest system was INTERNIST-1, which was developed in 1974 by Jack Myers in the 1970s at the University of Pittsburgh for the purposes of training medical students in clinical diagnosis [9]. INTERNIST-1 supported a very broad knowledge base, but it did not find its way into clinical use. Perhaps the best-known early system is MYCIN, developed by Edward Shortliffe, working with Bruce Buchanan at Stanford University. MYCIN was a backward-chaining expert system that focused on decision support for treatment of bacterial infections by capturing information about the bacteria to perform classification, and then recommending an appropriate antibiotic to treat the infection [7].

In the 1980s, an extension and modification to INTERNIST-1, called CADUCEUS, an expert system was created for treating bacterial infections. It was developed at the University of Pittsburgh by Harry Pople with an extensive knowledge base elicited from Jack Myers [10].

Rather than being limited to blood-borne infections, as was MYCIN, CADUCEUS focused on a much broader domain, and supported diagnosis support in as many as 1000 diseases. INTERNIST-1 was also the foundation for another system, the Quick Medical Reference (QMR), developed in the 1980s by Randall Miller, also for use in medical education [11]. Another early system was PUFF, an expert system designed (and put into clinical practice) to analyze pulmonary function tests [12].

Since these early efforts, decision support has been a focus of knowledge-based systems, with many applications in a broad spectrum of clinical applications. Perhaps the broadest use of KBS is in the electronic health record, which supports alerts and reminders to clinicians in real time as they provide care. Even though many such systems are not framed in the architecture of the typical expert system, which relies on chaining to arrive at conclusions (and hence, decisions or recommendations), they are still knowledge-based systems in that they rely on rules, derived from evidence from experts and other sources; they have long captured the attention of clinicians and informaticians, and the work of Safran [13] and Shellum [14] are two early examples. Alert and reminder systems are typically developed using Medical Logic Modules specified in the Arden Syntax [15, 16], which lends a high degree of expressivity to rigorous and specific rule specification [15, 17]. One example of an alert system in pediatrics is CHICA, which was developed to screen patients in while waiting to be seen by the physician so she can optimize her time with the patient [18]. Many other applications have been developed for specific care domains, such as pharmacy, drug prescribing, and adverse event monitoring [19–23], psychiatry [19], infectious disease [20], antibiotic therapy [21–23], anesthesiology [24], intensive care [25, 26], dermatology and obstetrics [27]. In addition, KBS alerts are finding application in remote monitoring and self-reporting of psychiatric symptoms [28], and management of heart failure [29], and diabetes [30]. In addition to the wide application domain of KBS, they have been accepted by physicians as usable and useful in decision support. For example, internal medicine residents judged a decision support system based on DXplain to offer additional or alternative diagnoses in response to heir inputs to the system, and they generally welcomed the possibility of having the system available in practice [31].

Clinical education. As noted above, knowledge-based systems occupied pride of place in the early history of artificial intelligence. Jack Myers' work on INTERNIST-1, CADUCEUS, and QMR truly laid groundwork for the numerous educational and training systems [32]. For example, QMR was incorporated onto a clinical workstation for training students; this system was augmented with material from Scientific American Medicine and anatomic and other images on videodisc [33]. Wolfram's appraisal of INTERNIST-1 and QMR was instrumental in publicizing the value of the latter in undergraduate medical education, even to the extent that it could serve as an "electronic textbook of medicine" [34]. Over the past several decades, there have been numerous calls for incorporating KBS diagnostic decision support systems training in medical education [35], radiology [36], hepatology [37, 38], respiratory failure [39], psychiatry [40], clinical case teaching [41], neonate stabilization prior to transport [42, 43], physical therapy [44], evaluating urinary incontinence [45], and diabetic patient education [46]. Especially with the growth of non-traditional pedagogical methods, such as distance learning and increasing use of multimedia, there is every reason to believe that KBS will continue to play an important role in clinical training.

2 Population Health Surveillance

Public health practitioners and researchers have long been interested in novel ways to conduct disease and risk surveillance. Traditional methods such as manual or even computerized methods of surveillance, which rely on time-consuming data collection, analysis, and dissemination, often fail in providing rapidly actionable information that could identify and forestall emerging infectious or other diseases. As a result, AI, and especially KBS, has attracted the attention of the public health and informatics communities, most recently with the COVID-19 pandemic. One notable example of an expert system in this domain is an expert system that provides clinical guidelines for COVID-19 diagnosis and management, particularly in low-resource settings [47]. Two other expert systems developed for use during the pandemic offer promise for future applications, One used fuzzy logic for early assessment of hypoxemia in COVID-19 [48], and another provides early detection of disease outbreaks with a system that uses a continuously updating knowledge base [49].

However, the COVID-19 pandemic is just one example of a domain where KBS has been applied to population health surveillance. For example, Staudt, et al. developed and evaluated an expert system-based intervention to reduce alcohol use [50]. Another example is a system that performed surveillance using the EHR during the 2002 Winter Olympics; the authors proposed this system as a path toward biosurveillance and improved communication between public health agencies [51]. More broadly, and particularly applicable to the increasing development of health information networks, is a proposal for incorporating expert systems into comprehensive health surveillance networks [52] Finally, a very useful review of AI in global health proposes a conceptual framework for the development of strategies for global AI development and employment [53].

Data representation and integration. Ontologies provide robust frameworks for the integration of data from multiple sources and of different types, not only in terms of their ability to represent concepts but enforce the relationships between those concepts through the use of embedded axioms, or rules. As such an ontology can be used as the structural framework for a KBS. One example is the Unified Medical Language System, which supports domain ontologies with rules that facilitate the creation of knowledge bases in the UMLS that can be used in developing decision support systems [54]. In addition, ontologies themselves can be used as a knowledge base, such as has been accomplished by Ahmed Benyahia, et al. [55], where the ontology-based KBS supported a telemonitoring system that incorporates auscultation sounds in the decisions made by the system. Another remote monitoring application using an ontology as a knowledge base focuses on chronic obstructive pulmonary disease and chronic kidney disease [56]. Other applications include diagnosis [57], knowledge acquisition [58, 59], clinical guideline authoring and retrieval [60–63], evaluation of disability [64], and ultrasound diagnosis in obstetrics [65].

Clinical trial support. Knowledge-based systems have been used in the design and administration of clinical trials. For example, the selection of a clinical trial that is appropriate for a patient can be difficult unless guided by rules that can assist with that process [66–68]. Two early examples of systems that assist with the design of trial protocols is OPAL, which is intended to identify errors in protocol authoring [69] and the Design-A-Trial system which generates a protocol based on an automated interview with the investigator [70]. Several investigators have created such systems to help clinicians identify trials by mapping patient features to the selection criteria for breast cancer clinical trials [71], renal cell carcinoma [72], heart failure [73], and serial graded exercise electrocardiographs [74]. Another example of this application uses natural language processing in the evaluation of patient features to identify cohorts of candidate subjects for clinical trials [75]. The KBS can also be a useful tool in designing a clinical trial where disease progression models need to be taken into account. Such models constitute a knowledge base that could be incorporated in an expert system that would assist a clinical trial designer [76], especially important in complex diseases that manifest a complicated progression [77]. One such example is provided in [78], in which there is the opportunity for community participation of experts in maintaining and enriching the knowledge base.

Another application of KBS is the measurement of response in a multicenter clinical trial can be complex, especially where images are used in this process: there can be considerable variation due to random measurement error, for example. In one study, a KBS was used to guide brain tumor response to radiation therapy and improve on the assessment of that response through MRI; although this study involved a small sample of subjects, the results suggested some promise [79]. Another study using a KBS to monitor progression of disease; in this case, visual analysis of scans for bone metastasis in prostate cancer showed more promise [80]. In addition to response to treatment, trialists are concerned about evaluating side effects, adverse events, and toxicity. A useful review looked at reviewed several KBS that have been used to predict carcinogenic toxicity in clinical trials [81]. Even though individually these systems have demonstrated suboptimal predictive performance, the accepted recommendation is to use them collectively as a composite model using other knowledge sources, including expert advice in real time.

3 Summary

This chapter has offered a view of AI that focuses on knowledge-based approach, especially expert systems. Such systems are at the top of the "family tree" of AI, whether framed chronologically or in terms of scientific inquiry or advancement. In short, it could be argued that KBS are "where it all began", but one must also remember that this domain is not static. Rather than the mere specification and storage of rules, a KBS includes an inference engine of some type- one that reasons with the knowledge in the system and that added to the system by a user in time. The earliest attempts at AI all took into account this requirement that systems must reason- like humans reason- in response to the demands of a current situation, be it a clinical encounter, or student training, or a pandemic. This requirement continues to dominate the field to this day and is manifested in the many machine learning approaches that have been developed over the past 10 years. However, it is good to consider the contributions that efforts manifested in the knowledge-based system branch of the AI family tree- as early as some of these were, continue to influence the development of AI methods and applications.

References

1. McCarthy J, Minsky ML, Rochester N, Shannon CE. A proposal for the dartmouth summer research project on artificial intelligence. AI Mag. 2006;27(4):12–4.
2. Gugerty L. Newell and Simon's logic theorist: historical background and impact on cognitive modeling. In: Proceedings of the human factors and ergonomics society annual meeting; 2006. p. 880–84.
3. Goodall A. Guide to expert systems. Oxford: Learned Information; 1985.
4. Lauritsen SM, Kristensen M, Olsen MV, et al. Explainable artificial intelligence model to predict acute critical illness from electronic health records. Nat Commun. 2020;11(1):3852.
5. Cooper G. Current research directions in the development of expert systems based on belief networks. Appl Stoch Models Data Anal. 1989;5:39–52.
6. de Dombal FT, Leaper DJ, Staniland JR, McCann AP, Horrocks JC. Computer-aided diagnosis of acute abdominal pain. Br Med J. 1972;2(5804):9–13.
7. Buchanan BG, Shortliffe EH. Rule based expert systems: The Mycin experiments of the Stanford heuristic programming project. Reading MA: Addison Wesley; 1984.
8. Holland JH. Escaping brittleness: the possibilities of general-purpose learning algorithms applied to parallel rule-based systems. In: Machine learning: an artificial intelligence approach San Francisco. San Francisco: Morgan-Kaufman; 1986.
9. Miller RA, Pople HEJ, Myers JD. Internist-1, an experimental computer-based diagnostic consultant for general internal medicine. N Engl J Med. 1982;307(8):468–76.
10. Banks G. Artificial intelligence in medical diagnosis: the INTERNIST/CADUCEUS approach. Crit Rev Med Inform. 1986;1(1):23–54.
11. Miller RA, Masarie FEJ. Use of the Quick Medical Reference (QMR) program as a tool for medical education. Methods Inf Med. 1989;28(4):340–5.
12. Aikins JS, Kunz JC, Shortliffe EH, Fallat RJ. PUFF: an expert system for interpretation of pulmonary function data. Comput Biomed Res. 1983;16(3):199–208.
13. Safran C, Rind DM, Davis RB, et al. A clinical trial of a knowledge-based medical record. Medinfo MEDINFO. 1995;8(Pt 2):1076–80.
14. Shellum JL, Freimuth RR, Peters SG, et al. Knowledge as a service at the point of care. In: AMIA annual symposium proceedings; 2016. p. 1139–48.
15. Hripcsak G. Writing Arden syntax medical logic modules. Comput Biol Med. 1994;24(5):331–63.

16. Poikonen J. Arden syntax: the emerging standard language for representing medical knowledge in computer systems. Am J Health-Syst Pharm AJHP Off J Am Soc Health-Syst Pharm. 1997;54(3):281–4.
17. Johnson KB, Feldman MJ. Medical informatics and paediatrics. Decision-support systems. Arch Pediatr Adolesc Med. 1995;149(12):1371–80.
18. Anand V, Biondich PG, Liu G, Rosenman M, Downs SM. Child health improvement through computer automation: the CHICA system. Stud Health Technol Inform. 2004;107(Pt 1):187–91.
19. Bronzino JD, Morelli RA, Goethe JW. OVERSEER: a prototype expert system for monitoring drug treatment in the psychiatric clinic. IEEE Trans Biomed Eng. 1989;36(5):533–40.
20. Chizzali-Bonfadin C, Adlassnig KP, Koller W. MONI: an intelligent database and monitoring system for surveillance of nosocomial infections. Medinfo MEDINFO. 1995;8(Pt 2):1684.
21. Pestotnik SL, Evans RS, Burke JP, Gardner RM, Classen DC. Therapeutic antibiotic monitoring: surveillance using a computerized expert system. Am J Med. 1990;88(1):43–8.
22. Evans RS, Classen DC, Pestotnik SL, Clemmer TP, Weaver LK, Burke JP. A decision support tool for antibiotic therapy. Proc Symp Comput Appl Med Care 1995;651–55.
23. Pittet D, Safran E, Harbarth S, et al. Automatic alerts for methicillin-resistant Staphylococcus aureus surveillance and control: role of a hospital information system. Infect Control Hosp Epidemiol. 1996;17(8):496–502.
24. Gorges M, Winton P, Koval V, et al. An evaluation of an expert system for detecting critical events during anesthesia in a human patient simulator: a prospective randomized controlled study. Anesth Analg. 2013;117(2):380–91.
25. Herasevich V, Kor DJ, Subramanian A, Pickering BW. Connecting the dots: rule-based decision support systems in the modern EMR era. J Clin Monit Comput. 2013;27(4):443–8.
26. Lau F. A clinical decision support system prototype for cardiovascular intensive care. Int J Clin Monit Comput. 1994;11(3):157–69.
27. Seitinger A, Rappelsberger A, Leitich H, Binder M, Adlassnig K-P. Executable medical guidelines with Arden Syntax-Applications in dermatology and obstetrics. Artif Intell Med. 2018;92:71–81.
28. Goulding EH, Dopke CA, Michaels T, et al. A smartphone-based self-management intervention for individuals with bipolar disorder (LiveWell): protocol development for an expert system to provide adaptive user feedback. JMIR Form Res. 2021;5(12): e32932.
29. Seto E, Leonard KJ, Cafazzo JA, Barnsley J, Masino C, Ross HJ. Developing healthcare rule-based expert systems: case study of a heart failure telemonitoring system. Int J Med Inf. 2012;81(8):556–65.
30. Katalenich B, Shi L, Liu S, et al. Evaluation of a remote monitoring system for diabetes control. Clin Ther. 2015;37(6):1216–25.
31. Bauer MA, Berleant D. Usability survey of biomedical question answering systems. Hum Genomics. 2012;6(101202210):17.
32. Siegel JDPTA. Computerized diagnosis: implications for clinical education. Med Educ. 1988;22(1):47–54.
33. Skinner C, Bormanis J. A multipurpose teaching workstation using expert systems, CD ROM and interactive laserdisc. Proc Annu Symp Comput Appl Med Care 1992;831–32.
34. Wolfram DA. An appraisal of INTERNIST-I. Artif Intell Med. 1995;7(2):93–116.
35. King AJ, Cooper GF, Hochheiser H, Clermont G, Visweswaran S. Development and preliminary evaluation of a prototype of a learning electronic medical record system. In: AMIA annual symposium proceedings, vol. 2015, issue 101209213; 2015. p. 1967–75.
36. Canade A, Palladino F, Pitzalis G, Campioni P, Marano P. Web-based radiology: a future to be created. Rays. 2003;28(1):109–17.
37. Molino G, Ripa Di Meana V, Torchio M, Console L, Torasso P. Educational applications of a knowledge-based expert system for medical decision making in hepatology. Ital J Gastroenterol 1990;22(2):97–104.
38. Console L, Molino G, Ripa di Meana V, Torasso P. LIED-liver: Information, education and diagnosis. Methods Inf Med 1992;31(4):284–97.
39. Cutrer WB, Castro D, Roy KM, Turner TL. Use of an expert concept map as an advance organizer to improve understanding of respiratory failure. Med Teach. 2011;33(12):1018–26.
40. do Amaral MB, Satomura Y, Honda M, Sato T. A psychiatric diagnostic system integrating probabilistic and categorical reasoning. Methods Inf Med 1995;34(3):232–43.
41. Fontaine D, Le Beux P, Riou C, Jacquelinet C. An intelligent computer-assisted instruction system for clinical case teaching. Methods Inf Med. 1994;33(4):433–45.
42. Heermann LK, Thompson CB. Prototype expert system to assist with the stabilization of neonates prior to transport. In: Proceedings of the AMIA annual fall symposium, vol. 9617342. American Medical Informatics Association; 1997. p. 213–7.
43. LeFiore JL, Anderson M. Effectiveness of 2 methods to teach and evaluate new content to neonatal transport personnel using high-fidelity simulation. J Perinat Neonatal Nurs. 2008;22(4):319–28.
44. Junkes-Cunha M, Cardozo G, Boos CF, de Azevedo F. Implementation of expert systems to support the functional evaluation of stand-to-sit activity. Biomed Eng Online. 2014;13(101147518):98.
45. Koutsojannis C, Lithari C, Hatzilgeroudis I. Managing urinary incontinence through hand-held

real-time decision support aid. Comput Methods Programs Biomed. 2012;107(1):84–9.
46. Levy M, Ferrand P, Chirat V. SESAM-DIABETE, an expert system for insulin-requiring diabetic patient education. Comput Biomed Res Int J. 1989;22(5):442–53.
47. Banjar HR, Alkhatabi H, Alganmi N, Almouhana GI. Prototype development of an expert system of computerized clinical guidelines for COVID-19 diagnosis and management in Saudi Arabia. Int J Environ Res Public Health. 2020;17(21).
48. Comesana-Campos A, Casal-Guisande M, Cerqueiro-Pequeno J, Bouza-Rodriguez JB. A methodology based on expert systems for the early detection and prevention of hypoxemic clinical cases. Int J Environ Res Public Health 2020;17(22).
49. Feng R, Hu Q, Jiang Y. Unknown disease outbreaks detection: a pilot study on feature-based knowledge representation and reasoning model. Front Public Health. 2021;9(101616579): 683855.
50. Staudt A, Freyer-Adam J, Meyer C, Bischof G, John U, Baumann S. The Moderating effect of educational background on the efficacy of a computer-based brief intervention addressing the full spectrum of alcohol use: randomized controlled trial. JMIR Public Health Surveill. 2022;8(6): e33345.
51. Gundlapalli AV, Olson J, Smith SP, Baza M, et al. Hospital electronic medical record-based public health surveillance system deployed during the 2002 Winter Olympic Games. Am J Infect Control. 2007;35(3):163–71.
52. Tamang S, Kopec D, McCoffie T, Levy K. Developing health surveillance networks: an adaptive approach. Stud Health Technol Inform 2006;121(ck1, 9214582):74–85.
53. Hadley TD, Pettit RW, Malik T, Khoei AA, Salihu HM. Artificial intelligence in global health—A framework and strategy for adoption and sustainability. Int J MCH AIDS. 2020;9(1):121–7.
54. Achour SL, Dojat M, Rieux C, Bierling P, Lepage E. A UMLS-based knowledge acquisition tool for rule-based clinical decision support system development. J Am Med Inform Assoc. 2001;8(4):351–60.
55. Ahmed Benyahia A, Hajjam A, Andres E, Hajjam M, Hilaire V. Including other system in E-Care telemonitoring platform. Stud Health Technol Inform 190(ck1, 9214582):115–17.
56. Bellos C, Papadopoulos A, Rosso R, Fotiadis DI. Clinical validation of the CHRONIOUS wearable system in patients with chronic disease. In: Annual international conference of the IEEE Engineering in Medicine and Biology Society. IEEE Engineering in Medicine and Biology Society. 2013. p. 7084–87.
57. Bertaud Gounot V, DOnfack V, Lasbleiz J, Bourde A, Duvauferrier R. Creating an ontology driven rules base for an expert system for medical diagnosis. Stud Health Technol Inform. 169(ck1, 9214582):714–18.
58. Cheah YN, Abidi SS. Health expert's tacit knowledge acquisition and representation using specialised healthcare scenarios. Stud Health Technol Inform. 2000;77(ck1, 9214582):837–41.
59. Cheah YN, Abidi SS. Healthcare knowledge acquisition: An ontology-based approach using the extensible markup language (XML). Stud Health Technol Inform. 2000;77(ck1, 9214582):827–31.
60. De Clercq E, Moreels S, Bossuyt N, Vanthomme K, Goderis G, Van Casteren V. Routinely-collected general practice data from the electronic patient record and general practitioner active electronic questioning method: a comparative study. Stud Health Technol Inform. 2013;192(ck1, 9214582):510–14.
61. Iglesias N, Juarez JM, Campos M. Comprehensive analysis of rule formalisms to represent clinical guidelines: Selection criteria and case study on antibiotic clinical guidelines. Artif Intell Med. 2020;103(bup, 8915031):101741.
62. Moskovitch RSY. A multiple-ontology customizable search interface for retrieval of clinical guidelines. Stud Health Technol Inform. 2004;101(ck1, 9214582):127–31.
63. Shalom E, Shahar Y, Taieb-Maimon M, Martins SB, Vaszar LT, et al. Ability of expert physicians to structure clinical guidelines: Reality versus perception. J Eval Clin Pract. 2009;15(6):1043–53.
64. Gaspari M, Roveda G, Scandellari C, Stecchi S. An expert system for the evaluation of EDSS in multiple sclerosis. Artif Intell Med. 2002;25(2):187–210.
65. Maurice P, Dhombres F, Blondiaux E, et al. Towards ontology-based decision support systems for complex ultrasound diagnosis in obstetrics and gynecology. J Gynecol Obstet Hum Reprod. 2017;46(5):423–9.
66. Dassen WR, Mulleneers R, Frank HL. The value of an expert system in performing clinical drug trials. Comput Biol Med. 1991;21(4):193–8.
67. Fink E, Kokku PK, Nikiforou S, Hall LO, Goldgof DB, Krischer JP. Selection of patients for clinical trials: an interactive web-based system. Artif Intell Med. 2004;31(3):241–54.
68. Papaconstantinou C, Theocharous G, Mahadevan S. An expert system for assigning patients into clinical trials based on Bayesian networks. J Med Syst. 1998;22(3):189–202.
69. Musen MA, Rohn JA, Fagan LM, Shortliffe EH. Knowledge engineering for a clinical trial advice system: uncovering errors in protocol specification. Bull Cancer (Paris). 1987;74(3):291–6.
70. Wyatt JC, Altman DG, Healthfield HA, Pantin CF. Development of Design-a-Trial, a knowledge-based critiquing system for authors of clinical trial protocols. Comput Methods Programs Biomed. 1994;43(3–4):283–91.
71. Ash N, Ogunyemi O, Zeng Q, Ohno-Machado L. Finding appropriate clinical trials: Evaluating encoded eligibility criteria with incomplete data. In: Proceedings. AMIA symposium; 2001. p. 27–31.
72. Gore ME, Bellmunt J, Eisen T, Escudier B, et al. Evaluation of treatment options for patients with advanced renal cell carcinoma: assessment

of appropriateness, using the validated semi-quantitative RAND Corporation/University of California, Los Angeles methodology. Eur J Cancer. 2012;48(7):1038–47.
73. Jonnalagadda SR, Adupa AK, Garg RP, Corona-Cox J, Shah SJ. Text mining of the electronic health record: an information extraction approach for automated identification and subphenotyping of HFpEF patients for clinical trials. J Cardiovasc Transl Res. 2017;10(3):313–21.
74. Long JM, Slagle JR, Leon AS, et al. An example of expert systems applied to clinical trials: analysis of serial graded exercise ECG test data. Control Clin Trials. 1987;8(2):136–45.
75. Chen L, Gu Y, Ji X, et al. Clinical trial cohort selection based on multi-level rule-based natural language processing system. J Am Med Inform Assoc. 2019;26(11):1218–26.
76. Malogolowkin MH, Horowitz RS, Ortega JA, et al. Tracing expert thinking in clinical trial design. Comput Biomed Res Int J. 1989;22(2):190–208.
77. Haag U. Knowledge representation for computer-aided planning of controlled clinical trials: The PATriCIa project. Methods Inf Med. 36(3):172–78.
78. Barrett JS, Nicholas T, Azer K, Corrigan BW. Role of disease progression models in drug development. Pharm Res. 2022;39(8):1803–15.
79. Clarke LP, Velthuizen RP, Clark M, Gavira J, et al. MRI measurement of brain tumor response: comparison of visual metric and automatic segmentation. Magn Reson Imaging. 1998;16(3):271–9.
80. Haupt F, Berfing G, Namazian A, et al. Expert system for bone scan interpretation improves progression assessment in bone metastatic prostate cancer. Adv Ther. 2017;34(4):986–94.
81. Dearden JC. In silico prediction of drug toxicity. J Comput Aided Mol Des. 2003;17(2–4):119–27.

Machine Learning in Practice—Clinical Decision Support, Risk Prediction, Diagnosis

Amy Nelson and Parashkev Nachev

Abstract

Making clinical decisions about individual patients relies on intelligence drawn from statistical models fitted to populations. The approach embodied in evidence-based medicine, the current gold standard, is founded on the application of simple, comparatively rigid models to coarse, low-dimensional data. Reflecting a blend of prior beliefs about biological form and historical limits to tractable model complexity, this approach is far from what the nature of clinical problems demands and what contemporary machine learning could conceivably deliver. Here we examine the fundamentals of diagnostic, prognostic, and prescriptive models in medicine—whether simple or complex—and provide a rationale for and an approach to introducing machine learning to real-world practice across medicine. We focus on conceptual and ethical aspects we identify as the primary obstacles to innovation in this rapidly emerging field.

Keywords

Machine learning in healthcare · Evidence-based medicine · High-dimensional modelling · Machine phenotyping · machine prescription · Medical ethics · Equity modelling

1 Introduction

Few technologies have promised as transformative an impact as machine learning, or threatened to deliver it as quickly. There is a pervasive sense that our powers are here developing faster than our understanding of what we should—and should not—do with them, and that they will soon be great enough for public consensus on their application to be an urgent necessity. Arriving at such a consensus is obstructed by widespread conceptual unclarities about what machine learning is, what it does, and why it must be brought into the world. In the realm of practical medical applications, the problem is amplified by commensurate conceptual unclarities about what medicine is, what it does, and why it needs to change. The air of mystique clinging to the field encourages others to multiply the questions rather than to answer them, to expand the problems rather than to contract their solutions, to magnify the hypothetical risks of the new rather than to expose the certain failures

A. Nelson · P. Nachev (✉)
UCL Queen Square Institute of Neurology, UCL, London, UK
e-mail: p.nachev@ucl.ac.uk

F. W. Asselbergs et al. (eds.), *Clinical Applications of Artificial Intelligence in Real-World Data*,
https://doi.org/10.1007/978-3-031-36678-9_15

of the old. The result is a great deal of talk, but very little in which decisions about action could be securely grounded. Rather than survey specific applications of machine learning to the cardinal tasks of risk prediction, diagnosis, treatment selection, and prognosis—a field evolving so quickly a textbook falls out of date before it is written—here we examine the fundamental nature of these tasks, the rationale for applying machine learning to them, and the opportunities and risks new modelling technologies introduce in practice, with special attention to ethical considerations.

2 The Nature of Machine Learning

Machine learning is not sharply demarcated from conventional analytic methods [6, 14]. We should review the characteristics that are unique to it or specifically amplified, for the others require no clarification. Though naturally mathematical in form, it is helpful to describe machine learning in broader terms, not merely to make it accessible to non-specialists but also more brightly to illuminate the underlying generalities.

A learning machine embodies a set of *rules* for transforming *data,* for a given *purpose*, to satisfy some *criterion,* yielding a *representation* or a *model* of the data. It departs from conventional mathematical models primarily in its *complexity*: the number of parameters and the size of the space from which they are drawn. Other features follow consequentially:

- *Data-dependence*: The more complex a model, the more likely its parameter space will breach the bounds of intuitive surveyability. What information cannot be specified a priori must be drawn from the data itself.
- *Solution*: The probability of finding an analytic solution rapidly diminishes with increasing model complexity, leaving approximate numerical, typically iterative, approaches as the only option.
- *Evaluation*: The ability of a model to generalise to unseen instances of the data on which it has been trained becomes harder to determine the more complex it is, and the less intuitive its structure. This makes performance on unseen data the key evaluative metric.
- *Stability*: The conjunction of heavily data-dependent specification and approximate solving results in greater propensity to change with the introduction of new data or a new algorithmic approach.

A machine capable of effecting a transformation is an *agent*, and its ability naturally intelligible as a *power* [12]. Further differentiation depends on the autonomy of acquisition and application. The power of a conventional machine can only be *first-order*, for it is externally prescribed; that of a learning machine is *second-order*, for it is autonomously acquired. Most machines exhibit only *one-way* powers—they *cannot* choose *not* to act—but an especially complex learning machine may have *partial two-way* power if its application is itself conditionally gated. Such a power is only partially two-way because the conditional gating will generally be context-specific. It is easy to see how these features bring machine learning systems closer to biological agents, where two-way, second-order powers are more commonly encountered. But the two remain distinct, and the distinction is critical to our applications, as we shall see.

To determine the appropriate role of machine learning in the clinical domain, we should consider the kind of learning these tasks demand. Any input–output data transformation can be distinguished by the nature of the inputs, the nature of the outputs, and the criterion the transformation attempts to satisfy.

2.1 Inputs and Outputs

The natural descriptive complexity of human beings—across health and disease—means the appropriate model—at least in theory—will usually be a multivariate one, indeed constrained in its dimensions more by the available data and compute rather than intrinsic dimensionality [18]. Where the inputs are many, they may correspond to different features of the problem—static models—or the same feature replicated over time—dynamic models—forming time series. The inputs may have a superordinate structure, as in multi-instance learning, or each may denote an individual instance to be handled independently. The outputs are often few—one in binary classification, for example—in reflection of the relative poverty of the space of possible clinical actions. Where the outputs are many, they may correspond to multiple features of the solution—multi-label models—or the same feature replicated in order—sequence models. An output may be any kind of number or set of categories, as the target output space demands. Outputs may exhibit a structure more complex than a linear sequence: a hierarchy for example. The characteristics of neither side of the transformation limits the other: a model may instantiate any combination of inputs and outputs. Clinical scenarios arise across the full space of possibility here.

Note medicine's preoccupation with simple, typically univariate, "biomarkers" as inputs to decision-support models reflects not biological reality but the exigencies of deriving and validating variables in the clinical realm and a prior belief in the essential simplicity of biological phenomena [16]. As machine learning relaxes the constraints arising from the former, and the value of greater model flexibility becomes apparent, belief in the latter is likely to erode. Equally artificial is preservation at the modelling stage of differences in the input modalities: there is no biological reason for segregating (say) imaging and biochemical inputs, indeed there may be useful interactions only a cross-modal model could conceivably capture [1, 4]. Again, practice is here coloured by historical limitations on model flexibility.

2.2 Criteria

The simplest transformational criterion—faithful recovery of the original input from the output—though at first sight trivial is, as we shall see, definitional of architectures destined to dominate the field [13]. More common is the fidelity of the predicted association between sets of variables falling into binary or multinomial classes (classification), or across a real number line (regression), or the establishment of new associations (reinforcement learning). In supervised models, the criterion seeks to impose an order defined by a subset of the features of the data, such as a particular variable, usually in line with a specific purpose, in unsupervised and semi-supervised models, the externally imposed order is absent or weaker respectively. The transformation itself may simply seek to find a more compact representation of the data distribution; if so, the degree of compactness will also be a part of the criterion [5]. Such "generative" models may seek to impose properties on the representation other than compactness, as downstream tasks demand. More commonly, the transformation will seek to magnify a region of interest in the space of data features so that a decision boundary may be robustly drawn. The transformation achieved by such "discriminative" models is kin with standard statistical classification and regression.

3 Reasoning with Medical Data

The choice of transformation is guided by the intended application. In general, the aim is to establish a *connection* between one set of facts and another for a given purpose. The categories here broadly correspond with their logical counterparts: *deduction, induction, inference, and synthesis.* Common use, especially of the term inference, is loose, but there are important distinctions here it pays to preserve [12, 23].

3.1 Deduction

Within a closed, completely specified system of relations, the connection between one fact and another is logically prescribed. All conclusion is here deduction. Where the system is complex—chess, for example—the space of possible solutions may be so large that the principles of modelling may resemble those applied to open, incompletely specified systems. Where the objective is to compete with another player—a human being, for example—the model may be helpfully informed by empirical aspects outside the system itself. But the problems here are fundamentally deductive, and rarely applicable to the biological systems of concern to us.

3.2 Induction

Most relations of interest in the clinical realm arise within open, incompletely specified systems. Here the mode of connection is inductive: from a set of observed associations, we derive a regularity that might be used to *describe* the association more compactly than reciting the data, and to *predict* unseen observations, from the past or in the future. Since induction may always be altered by new observations, it is naturally qualified probabilistically, indexed by our confidence. Most models in machine learning are used inductively, indeed they are pieces of induction themselves. We shall see that induction is central to prognostic or risk prediction models in medicine.

3.3 Inference

Though inference is often used where prediction is meant, there is an important distinction stricter use of the term helps to preserve. To infer something is not merely to predict it, but to ***adopt a position*** *that is asserted to* ***explain*** *it* [23]. Both elements are essential. The element of adopting a position is why we may succeed or fail to predict something but not succeed or fail to infer it, and we may hesitantly or confidently predict something but not hesitantly or confidently infer it. Inference implies a decisive commitment, even if the grounds for it may be probabilistic. The element of explanation is why prediction is paraphrased as what *will happen* or *has happened*, while inference is paraphrased as what *must happen* or *must have happened.* To put it in more mathematical terms, to predict something is to derive an expectation from a model, to infer something is to assert that a given model is the correct one, or at least has no superior. Prediction hopes its model is good, inference insists it is the best. This formulation places inference at the heart of diagnostic and prescriptive models, though not prognosis or risk prediction.

It should be noted that causation is typically something inferred, though causal relations may be posited within a purely inductive framework. Inferences to causality are no different from other kinds, and merely imply adopting a specific position about a set of modelled relations. To call a model causal is usually to imply it is used for inference, but inference generally need not be to causes.

Inference is commonly claimed in conventional statistical analyses, and rarely in machine learning. But in the former it typically rests on (even if good statisticians reject the notion [11]) an unjustified a priori assumption that the space of possible models is small, and that one therefore only needs to reject a few models to leave a single one standing. Machine learning explores a wider space, and so its grounds for inference are actually stronger. We develop this point in the next section.

3.4 Synthesis

A generative model may be used to synthesise data that resembles the input data but is identical with no instance of it. Unconditional synthetics may be used in place of data limited by procedural circumstances such as privacy constraints; conditional synthesis provides a potentially powerful method of dealing with data missingness or imbalance. But since possession of good generative models typically implies the knowledge we need imputation or rebalancing to acquire, we are rarely in a position to make use of them. Representations drawn from generative models, rather than their synthetic outputs, can augment inductive or inferential tasks, either explicitly through structured data-driven phenotyping, or implicitly by augmentation of the models themselves, as we shall see.

4 The Nature of Clinical Tasks

A system does not need to be very complex to cease to be intuitively surveyable. Indeed, it is simple for us to create synthetic examples, such as the game of Go, where the limits of intuition are easily reached. The complexity of the natural world is bound to vary, but there are no grounds to suppose that much of it, let alone most of it, should be easy to navigate. The only option open to a disinterested, dispassionate observer is to demand an exploration of the full space of possibilities for any system under study. Where this space is intuitively navigable, there is no need for anything other than conventional analytic methods; where it is not, we need alternative methods that do not merely test hypothetical models but also survey the space of hypothetical possibility. Only then can we have confidence in our chosen model.

Note that our concern is not just with the dimensions of the search space, but also with the complexity of the solution. The problem might be less that we are looking for a needle in a haystack than that we are looking for a collection of *many* needles, intricately arranged. Simple, serially mechanistic causal models certainly explain some systems, but the general paradigm of causation does not limit the size of what must be properly seen as a *causal field* of many contributory factors [15]. So the model itself might be too complex to be intelligible, even if it could be intuitively formulated.

Where intuition cannot penetrate the space of possible models or the model itself, it needs to be replaced by a mathematical process. Conversely, intuition may be discarded without harm even where its guidance is adequate, for a well-crafted model should converge on a simple solution if it is what the data command. Its explanatory characterisation of a simple causal field should be as good as that of a simple model, but it may also apprehend a complex causal field opaque to human understanding. Machine learning, then, is not a niche, exotic method for modelling the world: in making fewer assumptions and rendering greater complexity accessible it is *theoretically* superior to all others. That it might be easier to misuse in practice than simpler methods cannot change this theoretical truth. Contrary to frequently expressed opinion, machine learning is no more a transient fashion than differential calculus or linear algebra: it is here to stay because the critical difficulties it overcomes have no other plausible solution.

While superiority in many uses is generally conceded, machine learning is often argued to be weaker in inference than conventional analytic approaches. This view is mistaken. As we have seen, questions of inference arise *only* once questions of prediction are satisfactorily answered. A poorly predictive model is even poorer grounds for inference, for if individual cases are weakly predicted it is even less likely the model is the correct one. Conventional analysis often tries to wriggle out of this by arguing that the residual uncertainty is utterly unpredictable, i.e. that it is “noise”. But one cannot conclude this without having plausibly explored the space of all possible models, and the assertion is instantly undermined by finding a single model with greater generalisable predictive power. So the argument rests on not applying the technique—machine learning—it seeks to reject out of hand. This is neither valid nor intellectually honest.

To understand why medicine needs machine learning, we need to remind ourselves of what practicing medicine entails. The marginal case of public health aside, the object of medicine is the *individual* patient. The primary task of the clinician is to *predict* the natural history of the patient’s disorder and to *prescribe* the best treatment for it, if a treatment is indeed available and needed. Since patients usually present with disorders that are new to them, the only available predictive or prescriptive intelligence is from *other* patients. For most of its history, medicine has drawn such intelligence informally, more or less tacitly embodied in the practice of the clinician. Its natural form is the recognition of similarities and differences, along such dimensions as the clinician can observe clinically or measure with investigations, defining *clusters* of patients with multiple kindred constitutional and pathological features.

The desire to formalise this process, to render it perspicuous enough to be replicated and standardised, has shifted contemporary medicine to a different model [9, 21]. Rather than relying on many clinical or investigational features, contemporary "evidence-based medicine" seeks to discard all but a few critical "biomarkers" of disease, defined not by local similarity but by the global average of a large, relatively undifferentiated group. It is exemplified by conventional epidemiological studies, where an individual's propensity to develop a disease, characterised by a small number of demographic and clinical features, is assumed to deviate randomly from some average value the study seeks to determine for the group as a whole. It is exemplified further by the standard paradigm for interventional studies—the randomised controlled trial—where the response to an intervention is determined by comparing large treated and untreated groups again reductively characterised, and shown to be unbiased only with respect to the few recorded features.

Such formalisation can never be fully perspicuous or replicable until the clinician is removed from it altogether, and the management of the patient is stated wholly in terms of features of the patient alone. Statements of this kind are subject to two severe constraints. First, for the statement to be practically useful it needs to be compact, and to invoke features that are objectively defined. It is generally no good to give a list of (say) 500 criterial features of a disorder, or to include ones whose detection presupposes skill that itself cannot be stated without reference to a clinician. Second, for the statement to be testable within conventional analytic techniques it needs to be aggressively parsimonious, for beyond a few dozen putative explanatory variables such techniques tend to fail, even with large datasets. Evidence-based medicine thus passes the biological world through an artificial filter, yielding a caricature shaped more by incidental practical limitations than by the subject matter itself.

So distorted a picture would be resisted were it inimical to the natural temperament of science. But relatively simple, serially-organised chains of causation are encountered often enough outside biology for the prototype relation to be reasonably assumed within it. Some aspects of biology *are* indeed mechanistically simple, encouraging us to think the rest should be construable on the same model. Nonetheless, the belief biology is more like horology than meteorology is clearly not justifiable a priori: it needs to be determined empirically, case-by-case [18]. Such determination can only be done with the aid of analytic methods that render great complexity adequately surveyable. Let us now consider why such methods are likely to be needed more widely than is currently held.

5 Model Requirements

Had evidence-based medicine been the success it was promised to be, hospitals would have fully transitioned to the production line model managers have sought to impose, and clinicians would be spending more time developing care algorithms than seeing patients. In reality, little of medicine has been rendered impersonally rule-governed, *nomothetic*, not because the profession is resistant to change but because the management of the individual patient, outside niche disciplines, is not specifiable in this way. The actions of a contemporary physician are often *justified* by pointing to diagnostic features, or reasoning from supposed mechanistic relations, but such justification rarely provides a *recipe* a non-expert could follow with comparable effect.

Moreover, the fundamental nature of biological systems makes a simplicity of organisation unlikely beyond marginal cases, for four interrelated reasons:

First, the information content of the human genome—no more than 3×10^9 bits [20]:

roughly the capacity of an old-fashioned compact disk—is not only shuffled by the reproductive process at each generation, but also far too small in proportion to the complexity of the body to yield the comprehensive "manual" a uniform mechanistic description presupposes. External factors certain to vary widely across individuals will therefore determine a great deal of biology.

Second, that both feedback and interdependence between multiple contributory elements are near universal across biological mechanisms means there will always be *multiple* comparably good "configurations" for any pathway: this is an inescapable feature of any multi-parameter interactive optimisation problem [19]. There are no evolutionary drivers for mechanistic homogeneity across individuals, so biological solutions that are unique, or found only in a small minority, need not be uncommon. In short, biology is indifferent to "overfitting" across the species.

Third, there is evolutionary pressure to keep the genetic code compact because the propagation of fitness information is inversely related to the number of coding elements [14]. The genetic contribution to the final biological form must thus be encoded in the *interactions* between many genes rather than each gene in isolation, or a few in linear combination. Even where the causal field appears relatively restricted, the form of the representation is likely to require complex modelling.

Fourth, there is biological pressure to keep physiological causality compact too because the difficulty of optimising a system scales with the complexity of its specification. The causal contribution of each physiological feature will tend to be dependent on many others, requiring modelling of their high-dimensional interactions.

In sum, not only is the presumption of simplicity unjustified, the fundamental constitution of the biological makes great complexity overwhelmingly probable. Much of biology may not be knowable in the way a simple mechanistic system is knowable, and what is knowable is likely to require high-dimensional modelling to predict and comprehend. We should now consider what this implies for predictive and inferential models in medicine as applied to risk prediction, diagnosis, treatment selection, and prognosis.

6 The Optimal Model

It follows from the preceding that however they might be created, useful models in medicine will commonly exhibit the following features.

First, models with adequate individuating power will tend to be high-dimensional, locating each individual on many axes of variation. Note it is not merely the number of input variables that needs to be large, but the minimum size of the representation within the most compact parts of the model.

Second, an individual will be better informed by the nearest neighbourhood of patients, rather than a simple population mean, where the neighbourhood is not known a priori, but is defined in the modelling process itself, and may well lie amongst a very rich field of different modelled modes.

Third, it is perfectly possible for the instantiation of some biological function in any one individual to have no helpfully informative neighbours whatsoever. Even the best possible model will mistakenly view such instances as noise. When addressed to the individual, both inferences and deterministic predictions will thus always be insecure. The task of medicine is rarely to identify definitively the one true model, but rather incrementally to optimise the fidelity of the models it uses, updating them with each and every biological instance. Unsurprisingly, this reflects how clinical expertise is personally developed.

Fourth, models in medicine will nearly always be probabilistic, not merely in their predictions but in the handling of the causal relations that underlie them. Not only will one typically estimate a distribution—rather than an expected value—for any prediction, the factors invoked in explaining it will also be probabilistically defined. The classification of patients into either outcome or causal categories will generally be blurred, at least at the boundaries.

Fifth, a model complex enough to absorb the intricacies of the underlying biology might not be easily intelligible. Biology is under no pressure to be easily intelligible: indeed, the opposite is true, for evolution is naturally more concerned with maintaining opacity to adversaries than with enabling perspicuity to clinicians.

Sixth, though its placebo effects may be greater, inference will generally be less secure than prediction here, for the dimensionality of the space of possible models makes it difficult to be confident of excluding all alternatives. Predictive models will therefore dominate the field, and risk predictive and prognostic models will advance faster than diagnostic or prescriptive tasks.

7 Clinical Applications

The present focus of machine learning in medicine is determined less by clinical need than by the dominant direction of technical innovation. Machine vision leads the way technically; machine radiology is its most obvious translation clinically. But the application of machine learning ought to be dictated by the clinical problems most likely to benefit from it, and the size of the potential impact of solving them better than current methods allow. A focus so realigned would be guided by the following considerations.

First, though the space of biological problems is near-universally high-dimensional, the picture yielded by the investigational instrument we use in a given clinical setting need not be. This is obvious where the result is a single variable, but may be obscure where the variables are many, and the signal is intrinsically low-dimensional either because of correlations between them, or because most of the variation is incidental to the clinical picture. The classification of mammograms, for example, though satisfying for the machine visionary does not segregate closely with the tumour genetics and other cellular factors on which patient survival ultimately depends [3]. For machine learning to be most useful we need the dimensionality of the underlying biology to be accessible through the investigational method *and* to be maximally material to the clinical outcome of interest.

Second, the marginal benefit of introducing machine learning to a clinical field depends on the *difference* between the complexity of the problem and the simplicity of the best current solution. In areas of medicine so complex that decision-making is left to *tacit* clinical experience—gait assessment in movement disorders, for example—the machine is compelled to compete with a real neural network—the clinician's brain—that will always be hard to match. Far greater margins are available where clinical practice is formalised into (usually highly reductive) algorithms of one kind or another: in short, where medicine is already in a sense *mechanised* even if the algorithms are not embodied digitally.

Third, the advantage of machine learning also depends on the *accessibility* to a human expert of the biological relationships being modelled. A radiologist has direct, easy, immediate access to images, but not to the multi-modal covariance of multiple investigations, or conjunctions of imaging and complex clinical phenotypes. The less human-surveyable the data, the greater the machine's advantage, for human experts are here compelled to reduce each modality, and only link them thereafter.

These considerations leave radiology—at least when treated in isolation from deeper clinical management—some way behind the areas of greatest potential benefit. Here we give three general examples that ought to receive greater attention than they so far have.

7.1 Disease Stratification and Prognosis

The statistical framework of evidence-based medicine has compelled a reductive specification of the observed factors—clinical or investigational—in which the risk of disease or its progression are generally grounded. But if such models are too simple to be adequately individuating, the kind of "personalised" medicine universally agreed to be desirable will need high-dimensional models integrating information across a wide multiplicity of factors. Where the relations between the material factors are complex, a model's predictions may not be intelligible in the linear, threshold-defined manner of the "risk-factors" so commonly referred to in conventional medicine. Instead, the clinician will simply have to refer to the model itself, and the causal field of factors it surveys in forming its predictions. That it is the model, and not a limited set of factors, on which our confidence rests does not alter the fundamental measure of fidelity: the accuracy of predictions made on unseen, out-of-sample data.

7.2 Interventional Inference and Prescription

The context of intervention adds to the foregoing case only a few more factors—how, if at all, the patient is treated. And here the usual reductive models should be analogously expanded to include all potential determinants of the clinical outcome. Equally, a complex model rather than a set of factors will now guide an individual's prescription, for the demands of individuation in stratification and prognosis must extend to treatment too. Inference to the question of whether or not an intervention works *in general*, also requires high-dimensional modelling, for it is only once individual variability is adequately captured that the specific effect of the treatment can be reliably isolated [1, 24].

7.3 Clinical Pathways

A blend of ideology, logistics, and reproducibility compels hospitals to follow a production line model of operation, where patient care is delivered along a set of stereotyped sequential steps. Such pathways tend to be simple—a small set of decision variables guiding a narrow plurality of management options—and are reinforced by equally reductive sets of "key performance indicators". Since patients, unlike cars on a production line, are not identical in their design, the alternative of multi-dimensional "clinical fieldways", guiding patient not along a linear path but across a multiplicity of planes of management, is likely to improve on the status quo. This evolution naturally proceeds from our revised notions of risk, prognosis and treatment.

8 Ethical Aspects

Machine learning is widely held to pose unique ethical problems that impede its application to medicine, indeed may render some forms of it wholly unsuited to the domain [2, 17]. The objections are commonly taken to be self-evident, and their conceptual foundations are rarely examined in depth. This is a large topic, in need of dedicated treatment: here we may only draw attention to a set of important misconceptions relevant to our specific focus. We shall see that far from a threat to medical ethics, machine learning is an important part of its defence.

We should begin by noting that ethics is generally concerned with ends more than means. Since machine learning changes the intellectual instruments of medicine rather than its objectives, its ethical implications form a comparatively minor part of medical ethics. Five comparatively neglected aspects nonetheless require consideration.

First, the value of a *change* in any clinical practice cannot be determined without a comparison between the old and the new. Concerns about the *possible* infelicities of machine learning need to be moderated by the *manifest* infelicities of medicine as it is practised now. We have shown contemporary medical management to be very far from any reasonable conception of the ideal, whereas the direction of travel machine learning promotes is unequivocally towards it. From a moral perspective, at this foundational level, the critical question is less whether or not we should introduce machine learning in medicine but why we have not done it already.

Second, machine learning, in the well-founded applications discussed above, does not seek to replace tacit human expertise, but the crude, simple algorithms currently used to codify it. The competition here is not between man and machine, but between two different kinds of model differing in flexibility and expressivity. The models of conventional evidence-based medicine are no less mechanical for being expressible on paper: they still prescribe a relation in a form that leaves the clinician out of the equation [10, 21]. The critical question, then, is whether or not a complex model may be *systematically* worse than a simple one. *Given the right modelling architecture*, a complex model need not perform worse than a simple one trained on the same data, and where it fails it should fail with the same grace. If the model is capable of absorbing complex patterns of variation across the population, it may systematically perform better for some subpopulations over others. Imagined as tailoring, a simple model will cut everyone a universally ill-fitting, generic suit, whereas a complex model will cut a close-fitting suit for those it knows sufficiently well. But for no-one should the suit be any worse than the generic, and the variation in fit overall, across the entire population, both systematically and randomly, will naturally be smaller. From an ethical perspective, escalating model complexity has no major inevitable negative consequences, indeed the opposite.

Third, far from a novelty, the act of replacing human decision-making by algorithms is widespread in medicine, *indeed it is what evidence-based medicine demands.* That machine learning algorithms are generally embodied in machines—rather than intuitive flow diagrams—changes no aspect of their status conceptually. Those in opposition to the mechanisation of medicine have already irretrievably lost the war, so waging a battle against machine learning is a pointless exercise. Moreover, the strongest criticism against conventional evidence-based medicine—that it is absurdly reductive—is precisely what machine learning seeks to address. Machine learning *humanises* what is *already* mechanical: it does not supplant human expertise but improves what has already been ceded. And human experts will always retain control over whether or not an algorithm is applied, exactly as they do now. So this aspect presents no new ethical problems either.

Fourth, the widespread objection that complex models are "black boxes" is misguided. The transformation effected by a deterministic model, however complex, is openly and unambiguously specified by its parameters, as is that effected by a stochastic model except that the output there is probabilistic within some known interval. Yes, the behaviour of a complex model may not be easily predictable under all possible circumstances, but that is either a property of the problem, not the model, or is addressable by the right kind of model-building and evaluation. What the objectors here are insisting on is not really intelligibility but a particular, very narrow, notion of it. As we have said, nothing in biology compels it to be intelligible to anyone, so imposing an arbitrarily low barrier is wholly unjustified. In any event, if a well-designed machine learning model converges on a complex solution, then it is because the necessary explanation *is* complex and the desire for easy intelligibility cannot be satisfied whatever the method. We should, of course, recommend the use of the most parsimonious model to hand, but to place any kind of ceiling is fundamentally wrong. The priority here is generalizable fidelity, for the patient's concern is obtaining the right treatment not knowing how it is done.

Those who nonetheless object to the use of inscrutable models need reminding that clinicians are often inscrutable themselves. When a clinician acts, the relation between the state-of-affairs and the action is rarely causal, for someone else in possession of the same facts and the same putative rules of application may act differently. Were it not so, all of medicine would by now have been reduced to simple algorithms executable by agents whose only function—and expertise—is in providing the inputs. Rather, clinical action is normally justified by giving *reasons*, in a way that is akin to pointing to a complex model's latent variables. But whereas we can explicitly specify the parameters of a model, we cannot peer inside the head of a clinician: we can only take his or her word for it. We need not doubt the clinician's sincerity, of course, but a reason does not necessarily yield an adequate explanation of what took place, nor need it render the action replicable on another occasion, for much of the knowledge may be tacit. So those who demand absolute transparency by implication condemn clinicians themselves.

Fifth, we should step back to reflect on the circumstances in which we naturally demand explanations for phenomena. Imagine an event we do not understand but know cannot recur. It is pointless to ask for an explanation, for it both has no use and cannot be tested anyway. We do not, for example, ask for an explanation of the *specific* circumstances leading to rain last Thursday, not because it will never rain again but because the weather is so complex the circumstances of *that* particular day are unlikely ever to be repeated and cannot be recreated. The notion of explanation comes into play only once an event may recur, for it is only then that *generalizability* across time and kindred events matters.

Now imagine we have generalisability *without* explanation: a wholly opaque "oracle" that tells us the future and how it can be altered to any end. Adding explanation has no material value here, for generalisability is what explanation is supposed to buy us in the first place, and if we have it already there is no need to write the cheque. Yes, it might satisfy our curiosity, soothe our vanity, ease our mistrust, but none of these things can be a clinician's primary concern. From an ethical perspective, then, the nature of the generalizable intelligence brought onto clinical problems does not matter: all we care about is its fidelity.

9 Quantifying Model Equity

Indeed, careful reflection on one crucial aspect of medical ethics—*epistemic equity:* the equitable distribution of the knowledge used to guide clinical care—shows that complex modelling is essential to quantifying disparities in care.

Recall that the primary focus of medicine is—and always has been—the *individual* patient. Its task is to achieve the best possible individual outcome, through the most appropriate individual intervention. Equity of care then translates to pursuing with equal vigour and fidelity the optimal possible outcome for everyone. Equity implies neither equality of *treatment*—stroke complicated by pneumonia requires different treatment from stroke alone—nor equality of *outcome*—stroke complicated by massive haemorrhage will inevitably carry a worse prognosis. Indeed, since each patient is unique—in health and disease—clinical management ought to be specifically tailored to each individual, with the widely pursued—if rarely achieved—aim of delivering personalised care.

How do we quantify equity? For each individual, we must measure the difference between the *achieved outcome* and the *individual optimal possible outcome*, what might be termed the **individualised outcome loss (IOL)**. Medicine is equitable when each patient's achieved outcome is equally close to his or her individual optima, i.e. the IOL is the same across the population; it is inequitable when there is variation, i.e. the IOL differs across the population. Systematic variation related to variables of ethical concern—e.g. age and sex—then identifies ethically important inequity.

How do we measure the IOL? The achieved outcome is directly measurable, but the individual possible must be assumed or inferred. Evidence-based medicine defines the current gold standard for doing this [21]. The ideal possible outcome is here determined by the *population average*, defined by few features and drawn from large, presumptively homogeneous, cohorts. It is widely argued that the objectivity, reproducibility, the formal rigour of the approach provides the most unbiased guide. This view is mistaken. At the limit of infinite data, simple, low-dimensional models can only minimize the bias in our estimates of the *parameters of the underlying distribution*, reductively described, *not* the inaccuracy of our estimates of the individual optimal [8]. Each individual estimate will be biased in direct proportion to the individual's distance from the group average, and that bias will be *entrenched* rather than reduced with further data.

Moreover, systematic biases affecting subpopulations characterised by complex conjunctions of demographic and clinical characteristics can never be detected, for the underlying models are too simple to expose them. In sum, evidence-based medicine—as currently practised and advocated—*guarantees* inequity, even at the limit of infinite data, and ensures that where systematic it remains invisible to external observers (Fig. 1).

Is there an alternative? As we have seen, machine learning models render tractable the multiplicity of clinical and physiological variables in which a patient's individuality is naturally grounded. The reference for the optimal possible outcome can then be defined not by the global mean of the population, crudely parameterised, but by the local centroid of the *neighbourhood* (Fig. 2). This naturally reduces the IOL because the distance to the local centroid will generally be shorter. Moreover, it makes care *more* equitable, because variations in the distance to a well-defined local centroid will generally be smaller than variations to a point fixed for the entire distribution. But the improvement can be uneven: where, for whatever reason, the neighbourhood is inadequately characterised, the reference will move either to a distant neighbourhood or the global mean, yielding substantially worse performance than for those in other neighbourhoods, even if likely no worse than using the mean.

The introduction of machine learning can thus not only improve care, but also render it more equitable. Enhanced equitability is a catalyst for the adoption of machine learning in healthcare, not the inhibitor many believe it to be. But we need a principled framework for *detecting*, and *quantifying* the impact of any model—complex or simple—on the equitability of care, so that the ethical fidelity of machine learning models can be evaluated and optimised. Such a framework must expose the relation between the performance of a model used to guide care and a patient's location on an axis of ethical concern, such as membership of a specific cluster of demographic features: what we might call *ethical model calibration* by analogy with conventional model calibration. Lack of

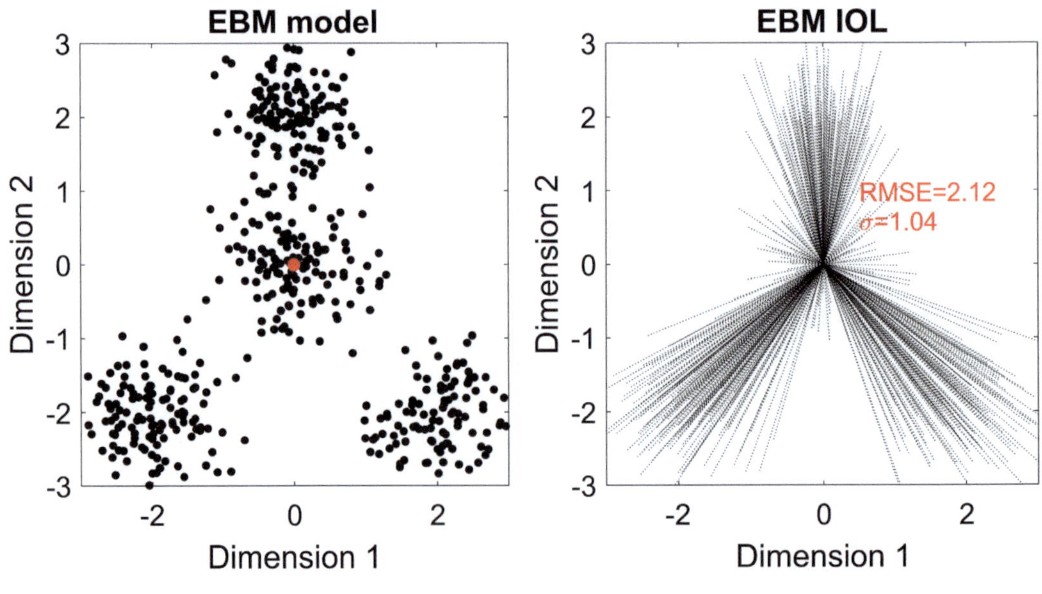

Fig. 1 Simulation illustrating the individualised outcome loss in a population described along two dimensions (black points) when the average of the population (red point) is taken as the reference for the optimal possible outcome within the standard evidence-based medicine (EBM) framework. The loss is proportional to a patient's distance from the population average (right plot), which may systematically disadvantage those falling within distinct clusters of the population. The loss, quantified by the root mean squared error (RMSE) also varies substantially (as captured by standard deviation, σ)

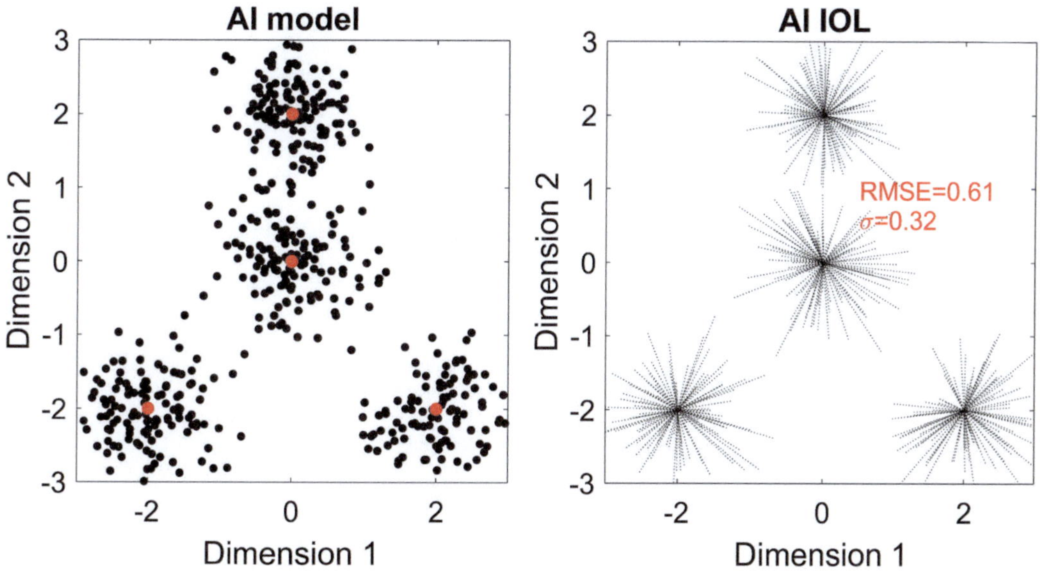

Fig. 2 Simulation illustrating the individualised outcome loss when the local centroids (red) are taken as references for the optimal possible outcome. The loss is proportional to a patient's distance from the centroid, which will typically be less than to the average. Note loss variation is much diminished and less systematic, but depends on well-characterised neighbourhoods

equitability in guiding care is then revealed by comparatively worse performance for patients lying on one part of the dimension of ethical interest compared with another, identifying the region where adjustment to the model is required, and enabling comparisons between the ethical fidelity of rival models.

Note the descriptive landscape within which a subpopulation is located need be neither simple nor confined to features of recognized ethical concern, such as demographics. A subpopulation defined by the complex interaction of multiple, previously unknown, features such as polygenic risk profiles, has no weaker claim to equity than any other. Indeed, in the presence of disordinal interactions, inequity with respect to any single feature may be obscured. A sincere attempt at ethical calibration inevitably requires a segmentation of the population at the finest granularity the available data can sustain, supported by "intersectional" interactions between multiple features. We have proposed such *representational ethical model calibration* as the definitive solution to quantifying epistemic equity in any model used in healthcare, whether simple or complex [8].

Note that detecting inequity is only the first step to eliminating it, and the optimal form of any remedial action is both unsettled and likely to vary case-by-case. In no circumstances, however, may the solution involve *less* detailed knowledge of the population than the baseline, for improving the outcomes for any given subpopulation could not plausibly be achieved by greater ignorance of it. Remediation here will typically take the form of seeking more data on the underserved group, and ensuring the model has sufficient flexibility to capture its distinctive features: in short, more, not less, machine learning. Of course, remediation may also involve architectural adjustments to the model that rebalance its attention more equitably or otherwise modify its operation [7, 22]. Such redistributive modification may involve a compromise between equity and the performance of specific groups or the population as a whole that itself requires ethical examination and justification. But here we enter the familiar realm of equitable allocation in the context of limited resources, for which the conceptual equipment is well established.

We should also note that ethical model calibration, at least statically, cannot distinguish the limits to IOL imposed by knowledge from those imposed by biology. Further investigation that brings better data and/or more felicitous models is needed, and even then, any judgement will always be open to revision.

10 Conclusion

Reflection on the fundamental nature of medicine, and the demands on the diagnostic, prognostic, and prescriptive models it implies, shows that machine learning provides the only plausible path to achieving optimal outcomes for individual patients. The notion of "personalised care" is pleonastic: medical care has always been about the individual, and if it has drawn intelligence from crudely parameterised populations, it is only because it has lacked the empirical, conceptual, and technical equipment to do better. Now that the pre-requisites for deploying complex modelling in medicine—large scale data, flexible yet robust algorithms, and powerful compute—are in place across many clinical domains, it is incumbent on us to deliver its potentially transformative benefits. Success here is increasingly impeded less by technology, evolving at break-neck speed, than by misconceptions about the correct approach to extracting intelligence from clinical data and applying it to the cardinal tasks of medicine. Adopting what we argue is the correct perspective will be crucial to disseminating machine learning across medicine. The necessary adjustment is more radical than much of the current discourse—preoccupied with technical and narrowly conceived ethical considerations—suggests, and requires reconsideration not just of modelling but of the practice of medicine itself.

References

1. Acosta JN, Falcone GJ, Rajpurkar P, Topol EJ. Multimodal biomedical AI. Nat Med. 2022;28(9):1773–84.
2. Amann J, Blasimme A, Vayena E, Frey D, Madai VI, The Precise4Q Consortium. Explainability for artificial intelligence in healthcare: a multidisciplinary perspective. BMC Med Inf Decis Mak. 2020;20(1):310. https://doi.org/10.1186/s12911-020-01332-6
3. Autier P, Boniol M. Mammography screening: a major issue in medicine. Eur J Cancer. 2018;90:34–62. https://doi.org/10.1016/j.ejca.2017.11.002.
4. Baltrušaitis T, Ahuja C, Morency L-P. Multimodal machine learning: a survey and taxonomy. IEEE Trans Pattern Anal Mach Intell. 2018;41(2):423–43.
5. Bengio Y, Courville A, Vincent P. Representation learning: a review and new perspectives. IEEE Trans Pattern Anal Mach Intell. 2013;35(8):1798–828.
6. Bishop, C. Pattern recognition and machine learning. Springer; 2006. http://www.amazon.ca/exec/obidos/redirect?tag=citeulike09-20&path=ASIN/0387310738
7. Buolamwini J, Gebru T. Gender shades: intersectional accuracy disparities in commercial gender classification. In: Proceedings of the 1st conference on fairness, accountability and transparency; 2018. p. 77–91. https://proceedings.mlr.press/v81/buolamwini18a.html
8. Carruthers R, Straw I, Ruffle JK, Herron D, Nelson A, Bzdok D, Fernandez-Reyes D, Rees G, Nachev P. Representational ethical model calibration. NPJ Digit Med. 2022;5(1):1–9.
9. Cochrane AL. Effectiveness and efficiency: Random reflections on health services. 1972
10. Greenhalgh T, Howick J, Maskrey N. Evidence based medicine: a movement in crisis? BMJ. 2014;348.
11. Greenland S, Senn SJ, Rothman KJ, Carlin JB, Poole C, Goodman SN, Altman DG. Statistical tests, P values, confidence intervals, and power: a guide to misinterpretations. Eur J Epidemiol. 2016;31(4):337–50. https://doi.org/10.1007/s10654-016-0149-3.
12. Hacker PMS. Human nature: the categorial framework. Wiley; 2007.
13. Hinton GE, Salakhutdinov RR. Reducing the dimensionality of data with neural networks. Science. 2006;313(5786):504–7.
14. MacKay D. Information theory, inference, and learning algorithms. Cambridge University Press; 2003.
15. Mackie JL. The cement of the universe. Oxford: Clarendon Press; 1974.
16. Mayeux R. Biomarkers: potential uses and limitations. NeuroRx. 2004;1(2):182–8.
17. Mittelstadt B. Principles alone cannot guarantee ethical AI. Nat Mach Intell. 2019;1(11), Article 11. https://doi.org/10.1038/s42256-019-0114-4
18. Nachev P, Rees G, Frackowiak R. Lost in translation. F1000Research. 2019;7:620. https://doi.org/10.12688/f1000research.15020.2
19. Noble D. Dance to the tune of life: biological relativity. Cambridge University Press; 2016.
20. Rands CM, Meader S, Ponting CP, Lunter G. 8.2% of the human genome is constrained: variation in rates

of turnover across functional element classes in the human lineage. PLoS Genet. 2014;10(7):e1004525. https://doi.org/10.1371/journal.pgen.1004525
21. Sackett DL, Rosenberg WMC. On the need for evidence-based medicine. J Public Health. 1995;17(3):330–4. https://doi.org/10.1093/oxfordjournals.pubmed.a043127.
22. Sagawa S, Koh PW, Hashimoto TB, Liang P. Distributionally robust neural networks for group shifts: on the importance of regularization for worst-case generalization. 2020. https://doi.org/10.48550/arXiv.1911.08731
23. White AR. Inference. Philos Q. 1971;21(85):289–302.
24. Xu T, Rolf Jäger H, Husain M, Rees G, Nachev P. High-dimensional therapeutic inference in the focally damaged human brain. Brain. 2018;141(1):48–54. https://doi.org/10.1093/brain/awx288.

Machine Learning in Practice—Evaluation of Clinical Value, Guidelines

Luis Eduardo Juarez-Orozco, Bram Ruijsink, Ming Wai Yeung, Jan Walter Benjamins and Pim van der Harst

Abstract

Machine learning research in health care literature has grown at an unprecedented pace. This development has generated a clear disparity between the number of first publications involving machine learning implementations and that of orienting guidelines and recommendation statements to promote quality and report standardization. In turn, this hinders the much-needed evaluation of the clinical value of machine learning studies and applications. This appraisal should constitute a continuous process that allows performance evaluation, facilitates repeatability, leads optimization and boost clinical value while minimizing research waste. The present chapter outlines the need for machine learning frameworks in healthcare research to guide efforts in reporting and evaluating clinical value these novel implementations, and it discusses the emerging recommendations and guidelines in the area.

Keywords

Machine learning · Artificial intelligence · Clinical applications · Evaluation · Guidelines · Standards

1 Introduction

The exponential growth in machine learning-based research in medical sciences has created a novel picture in the traditional horizon of proof-implementation-evaluation-regulation efforts. Given its relative novelty and trendy buzz words, the *corpus* of first-line publications (proof-of-concept and first performance) in this area has expanded beyond what can be effectively covered and filtered by the average human observer in search for the latest developments in any given area of expertise. Moreover, free distribution services and an open-access archives housing non-peer reviewed reports further expand the body of potentially valuable information available to the interested parties.

L. E. Juarez-Orozco · B. Ruijsink · M. W. Yeung · P. van der Harst (✉)
Department of Cardiology, Heart and Lungs Division, University Medical Center Utrecht, Utrecht, The Netherlands
e-mail: P.vanderHarst@umcutrecht.nl

L. E. Juarez-Orozco
Turku PET Centre, University of Turku, 20520 Turku, Kiinamyllynkatu 4-8, Finland

B. Ruijsink
Imaging Sciences and Biomedical Engineering, King's College London, St Thomas' Hospital, London WC2R 2LS, United Kingdom

M. W. Yeung · J. W. Benjamins · P. van der Harst
Department of Cardiology, University of Groningen, University Medical Center Groningen, Groningen, The Netherlands

F. W. Asselbergs et al. (eds.), *Clinical Applications of Artificial Intelligence in Real-World Data*,
https://doi.org/10.1007/978-3-031-36678-9_16

Such disparity between the number of publications involving ML analytics in clinical research and the number of guidelines generated to ensure quality, standardize their report and harmonize their interpretation is presently unique. In the last few years, a substantial amount of grants and initiatives have been promoted to boost the development of solid, stable, interpretable and user-friendly implementations of ML in medicine, yet unifying frameworks are still missing. The need for a ML framework in healthcare research is best understood in the present disconnection between the data science and the clinical medicine realms, and it presently represents a crucial gap in the further development of ML-based health care. Consequently, roadmaps for the development of novel ML systems dedicated to tasks well-defined by clinicians as well as mechanisms to evaluate their effect in the "real-world" and on accepted hard endpoints are strongly needed. Consequently, international standards and guidelines to inform, orient and evaluate the use and incorporation of ML in clinical research are beginning to emerge.

In the present chapter, we outline the need for ML frameworks to orient and guide efforts in reporting and evaluating the clinical value and relevance of ML-based implementation studies in healthcare. Thereon, we discuss the emerging standards to this effect and underline the necessity for international guidelines that bridge the knowledge gaps in this relatively novel multi-expertise area of development.

2 The Need for Frameworks in Ml-Based Clinical Research

The recent interest in ML-oriented research has created a unique horizon of information available to researchers with massive amounts of first publications and only a very few "accepted" clinical implementations. ML-based tools have been increasingly proposed to aid in clinical decision making through the generation of diagnostic and prognostic estimates. Yet, the largest proportion of these advances are merely theorical and the clinical implementation bottleneck has strengthened the notion that robust structured are needed to inform, guide and also evaluate the incorporation of ML analytics in clinical research.

Several are the contributors to the landscape of ML clinical research such as a wide variety of ML algorithms, the initial lack of standards for conducting or reporting ML studies, and even absence of standard conceptualizations or terms in ML studies, all of which have deepened the clear disconnection between the two constitutional areas involved in it, namely: ML researchers/developers and clinicians. This reflects consequently in the detachment from other health researchers, health services, research organisms, regulatory bodies and patients.

Furthermore, the unparalleled growth in ML research publications in medical science traces to a series of core circumstances. For example, there is an increasing offer of ML courses, open code and free resources, big datasets and application libraries for the experimentation with and use of ML algorithms. Second, there are no strict patents for untrained models and therefore isolated experimentation with optimized versions of a model can easily take place and become reported as proof-of-concept. Third, the initial lack of ML expertise of reviewers posed an accessible threshold for original ML publications with the natural interest in a novel area of development. Finally, new journals and journal derivations have emerged with specific focus on ML research and its applications. Figure 1 depicts contrasts the proportions in the publication profile of machine learning clinical research against that of another known area of relatively recent methodological developments, i.e. genetics.

Furthermore, the pace of ML-based developments poses specific challenges related to organized data storage and ownership, preprocessing, quality evaluation, patenting and commercialization of algorithms (for example, as medical devices). Virtually all ML-based studies and model training have been performed in current retrospective data, and the size of the utilized datasets varies widely from a few hundreds to millions of datapoints, which greatly influences the quality, replicability and therefore generalizability of reported clinical applications.

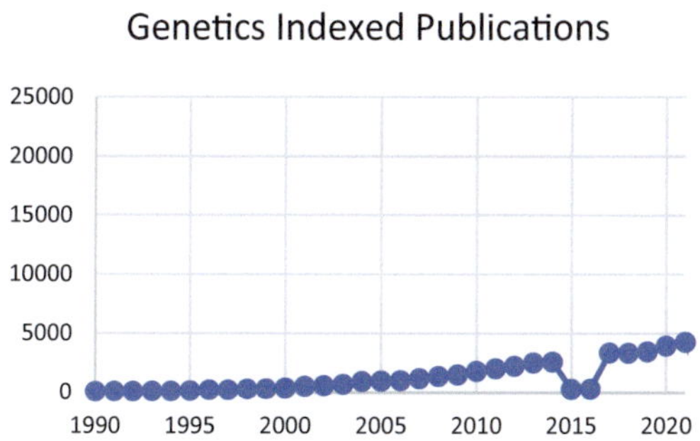

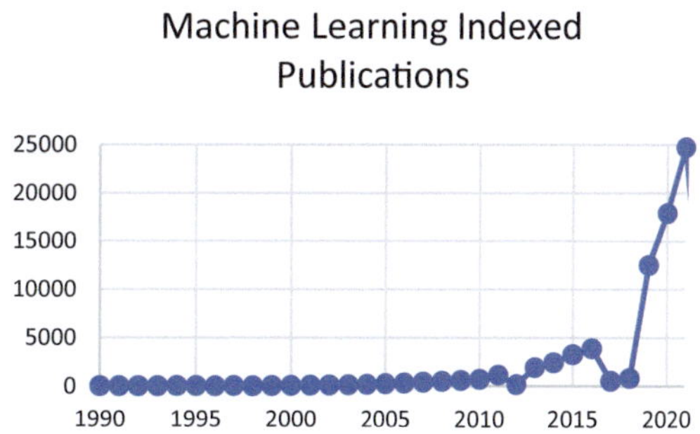

Fig. 1 Comparative scatter graphs on the number of Medline indexed clinical publications with the term *genetics* vs *machine learning* since 1990. Notice the exponential increase in machine learning publications

Hence, when considering the exponential growth in ML first studies with limited translation to clinical settings, the disconnection between developers and clinicians, the variety in quality and reporting techniques and the increasing need for reliable and high-quality clinical implementations, the need for ML *frameworks* in clinical research aimed at maximizing the value of such analytics and reducing the waste in oriented research is paramount [1, 2].

Figure 2 proposes a framework for ML systems development and highlights the areas where the current necessity for evaluation, recommendations and guidelines emerge.

Once initial development and reporting of ML applications has taken place, a continuous process of evaluation is warranted, especially with highly adaptive systems such as those based in ML where training can be updated and performance improved. This monitoring task should couple with specific recommendations and guidelines in the form of checklists or standards. This in order to orient the path to implementation in real clinical settings and minimize the loss of valuable ML research due lack of clarity on the ulterior objective and applicability potential. The ML framework once again can link relevant efforts to the next step in the process and reduce the disconnection between the predominantly data science-dependent initial developments (originating from lack of awareness of the clinical context) and the predominantly clinically oriented vision of the later stages in the framework (restricted by a lack of understanding of ML analytics and their potential).

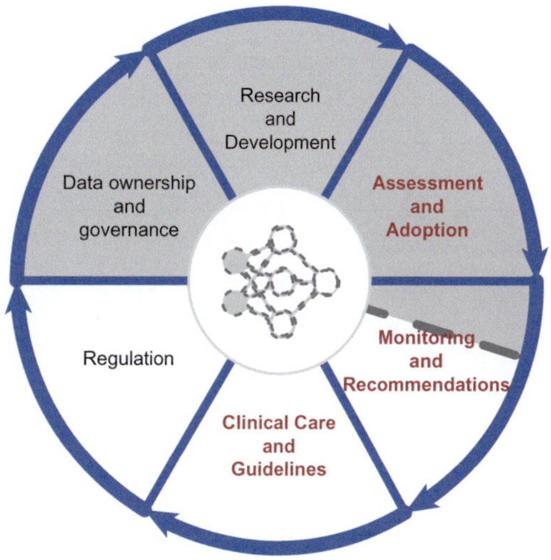

Fig. 2 The cycle of ML-based applications development from inception and data to clinical care and regulation. Note that assessment and monitoring represent crucial concepts for guideline generation in the mid and later stages of the continuous cycle presented

3 Evaluation and Monitoring in Clinical Ml Research

The known horizon of applicability of ML analytics has been suggested in several fronts concerning medical sciences [3, 4]. And overall, evaluation remains a ubiquitous process at every

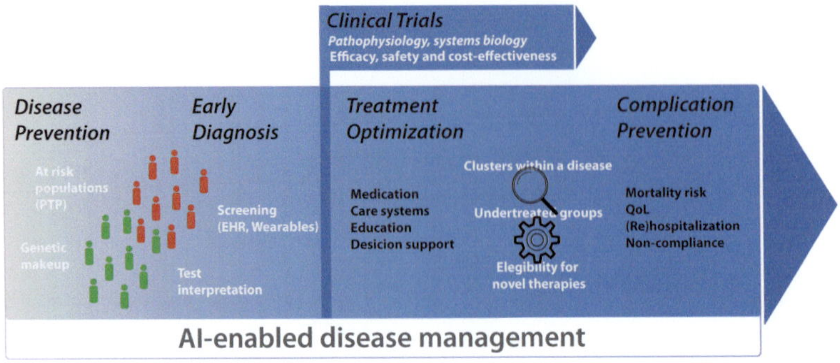

Fig. 3 Horizon of ML applicability. Every section conveys an area where ML performance and added value must be continuously evaluated. Within time, the areas that draw the largest benefits from ML and those where classic analytical approaches suffice will become apparent

level of clinical implementation ranging from early disease detection to improvements in hard clinical endpoints. Ultimately, this will allow the identification of the areas in which unequivocal benefit can be obtained through the implementation of ML analytics. Figure 3 shows the horizon of applicability and some of the tentative tasks where ML is expected to deliver relevant gains in clinical research.

The evaluation of ML applications after initial development (and publication) should constitute a continuous process that allows performance characterization, facilitates repeatability, orients optimization and maximizes clinical value while minimizing research waste at every point of the applicability horizon. In this sense, it would be ideal for involved professionals to display both clinical and data science knowledge, a conjunction still sparsely found in this developing area.

The biggest challenges with regards to ML research evaluation are currently found in two aspects, one is reporting and the other is the lack of clear paths to clinical translation. In the former, adequate reporting promotes verification ease and reproducibility. It facilitates the avoidance of redundant efforts, while also maximizing the proportion of proofs-of-concept that may progress to full-blown clinical tools or accessible blueprints. And notably, there is some evidence suggesting that the utilization of reporting standards can increase confidence in published findings and improve the adequacy of decisions made around evaluated interventions [5]. Novel reporting standards and checklists will be discussed in a later section. For the latter, emerging recommendations and toolkits to orient the creation of ML systems intended to ultimately be used as medical devices (software as medical device [SaMD]) can simultaneously facilitate evaluation of stablished standards. Once more, an ML framework is fundamental to identify design and delivery issues to be considered for evaluation and recommendation purposes in the route of studies that aim to advance clinical applications [6].

Once the robustness and validity trained ML models have been demonstrated. Their effects on the "real-world" can be explored in several ways. One of these, are retrospective analyses of the clinical consequences of the implementation of the model. An example of this can be found in the estimation of the number of advanced imaging studies that may be spared through optimized selection of patients for further diagnostic testing in coronary artery disease. For example, Overmars et al. [7] demonstrated a rate of nearly 50% of normal CT, CMR and SPECT findings in a cohort of roughly 7000 patients with CT and 3000 with CMR/SPECT, which represents a well-balanced big dataset for the identification of positive and negative cases with coronary artery disease. Of note, they achieved only a discrete performance able to identify < 20% of negative cases with a high probability (>90%). Another study by Benjamins et al. [8] placed the scope on the identification of patients that demonstrate myocardial ischemia through PET imaging and those who ultimately underwent early revascularization through ML analysis of clinical and CT data. The subtext proposes that utilization of advanced imaging can be optimized by means of ML in order to spare unnecessary scans that pose a radiation and economic burden. In an earlier report by Juarez-Orozco et al. [9] this concept was also explored through the identification of patients with regional and global ischemia on PET from the ML analysis of simple and accessible clinical variables.

Real-world evaluation therefore has renewed importance in the development and evaluation of ML applications because presently the theoretical demonstrations of performance and clinical value have been formulated from retrospective datasets due to their accessibility and size. A crucial interest therefore exists in organizing the prospective evaluation of retrospectively generated ML models and eventually of prospectively generated ML applications.

Varying examples of such enthusiasm have been the analysis by Khera et al. [10], which retrospectively evaluated electronic health records from more that 750,000 patients from a clinical data registry (Chest Pain–MI Registry of the National Cardiovascular Data Registry in the United States from the American College of Cardiology) through ML to discriminate in-hospital mortality after an acute myocardial infarction. The modeled data included patient demographics, medical history, comorbidities, home medications, electrocardiogram findings, and initial medical presentation and laboratory values. Notably, ML modelling was compared to the current standard model for myocardial infarction mortality built within the registry involving 9 variables integrated through logistic regression. And interestingly, ML models did not substantively improve discrimination of the outcome, although they offered a marginal advantage in analyzing patient at highest risk. Their results suggest that traditional analytics may be sufficient to evaluate such data deeming ML likely unnecessary, while proposing that data from current electronic health records may be rather insufficient in depth or quality in order to extract the most benefit from complex analytics. Another example is the study by D'Ascenzo et al. [11], which evaluated ML in the prediction of all-cause death, recurrent acute myocardial infarction, and major bleeding after an acute coronary syndrome from a pooled dataset (composed by the BleeMACS and the RENAMI registries) aggregating more than 19,000 patients. This study showed acceptable performance of four ML models and also utilized an external validation sample, which translates in a quality criterium. However, it offered no direct comparison to simpler analytics or other accepted risk models based on traditional statistics. A third case is found in the registry of fast myocardial perfusion imaging with next generation single photon emission computed tomography SPECT (REFINE-SPECT) [12]. This registry is a multicenter contribution into a comprehensive clinical-imaging database including 290 individual imaging variables merged with clinical variables from patients undergoing SPECT myocardial perfusion imaging due to suspected or known coronary artery disease. And remarkably, it also includes a prognostic cohort followed for the occurrence of major adverse cardiac events and has stated the aid in the development of new artificial intelligence tools as one its main objectives. These initiatives demonstrate the range of approaches to retrospective data and underline the need for continuous evaluation of reporting and quality to underpin advancements to clinical implementation.

In-silico experiments (simulation studies) represent an alternative for evaluation of proposed ML applications. And although not predominant, reports have been dedicated to dissect and therefore balance out the working assumption that ML-based implementations outperform traditional statistical approaches in every analytical setting. It has become increasingly clear that this may not be the case and that research, evaluation and emerging recommendations in this realm must contrast and specify the areas where the largest benefit of ML implementation is expected. Whether we are able to characterize and control the tradeoff between complexity and interpretability will determine the place that ML will occupy in years to come either as a specialization within medical research or as another adaptable tool in our analytical arsenal.

More broadly, an exemplary structure in the process of *clinical evaluation* of a (ML) software as medical device (SaMDs, see ahead) is considered by the FDA and the International Medical Device Regulators Forum (IMDRF). This process evaluates whether there is a valid clinical association, whether a (ML) model adequately processes input into adequate output, and whether the model achieves the intended purpose in the intended target population and clinical context [13].

Overall, we still fundamentally lack studies that demonstrate how the prospective use of ML applications can substantially improve patient care, while high-quality reporting and the creation of development pathways in ML frameworks offer the best possibilities to organize and deploy adequate evaluation and monitoring of ML applications. Emerging recommendations and guidelines for the conduction and reporting of ML clinical research will be discussed ahead.

4 The Issue of Interpretabiliy

Interpretability or explainability in ML analytics remains a main area of criticism. The notion that every complex abstraction made by ML models should be not only accessible but comprehensible to the user is partially justified given that responsibility remains deposited in the clinician. A lack of explainability in systems involved in clinical decisions places a threat to core ethical values (autonomy, beneficence, nonmaleficence and justice) in biomedicine, which in turn may produce negative consequences in public health [14]. Notably, interpretability may not represent a solely technological obstacle; it also it invokes legal, ethical, and societal queries in need of thorough exploration.

In other areas of medical research, structured reporting and regulations are available underpinning the reliability of techniques such as laboratory analytics or genetic studies. Such structures do not yet exist in ML. The need for interpretability in ML varies with the type of ML used. Deep learning models, which learn complex associations through 1000s of connections, are inherently hard to interpret. Less complex ML models (for example decision trees or SVMs) are more easily understood.

Several approaches exist to establish (some degree of) interpretability of ML models. Interpretation steps can be integrated into the model itself, or added as a post-hoc analysis, and can provide understanding on a global level, or at the level of individual predictions or even individual features. A traditional method for model interpretation is the use of partial dependence plots (PDP) [15]. PDPs plots the impact of a single features' value on prediction outcomes. However, as the feature-size of models increased significantly over the last years, interpretation of PDPs become more challenging. Therefore, feature importance ranking (FIR) has become increasingly useful. FIR establishes the importance of each feature in the ML model on the global model prediction error and ranks them accordingly. This ranking allows to identify the most relevant features in predictions. Another approach to weight feature importance is the use of Shapley Values (SHAP) [16]. SHAP originates from game theory, and measures the contribution of each 'player' (feature) to the game (i.e. improves or deteriorates the predictions). A plot of all the values together subsequently visualizes the additive contribution of each feature to the prediction. A different approach to interpretability is the use of global surrogates for a ML model [17]. After training the ML model, a second interpretable model (i.e. linear model or decision tree) is trained on the dataset and outcome predictions (the surrogate model). By design this surrogate model provides an interpretation of the most relevant characteristics of the decisions made by the ML algorithm. Local surrogate (LIME) [18], is a variant to surrogate models. Instead of explaining the full model, LIME aims to explain the relative important of different features for the individual predicted outcome. In image classification tasks, classification activation maps (CAMs) [19] can be used. CAMs provide 'attention maps' that highlight the most important areas that affected model predictions. Uncertainty estimations can also be used to provide some intuition about model decisions [20, 21]. While not directly introducing interpretability, epistemic and aleatoric uncertainty measures can help to value the quality of predictions and identify potential weaknesses in model design. Moreover, uncertainty labels can be used to provide effective iterative sample selection in continuous learning algorithms [22].

Many more solutions are and have been developed to provide some degree of interpretability for ML models. However, the increasing complexity of developed models seems to make interpretation evermore challenging. Some researchers therefore argue to shift the use of ML away from 'black box' models, and instead focus on developing interpretable models [23]. In particular in medicine, such an approach could significantly reduce the significant challenges for large scale ML implementation.

5 Reporting Statements, Checklists and Position Papers in MI Research

Once understood the need and relevance of establishing ML frameworks that facilitate the creation, evaluation and monitoring of ML applications, a number of documents have emerged that exemplify the efforts to harmonize and safeguard the quality of new reports.

Some have the form of extensions of previously established quality statements and some represent de novo documents. Here we discuss some of the core characteristics of these statements and checklists. Table 1 enlists statements and checklists gathered in the Enhancing the QUAlity and Transparency Of health Research (EQUATOR) network and dedicated to address the incorporation of ML-oriented research. This network represents a well-established global initiative with the aim of improving the quality of research and its derived publications (https://www.equator-network.org).

5.1 CONSORT-AI

The consolidated standard of reporting trials (CONSORT) represents a guideline for reporting randomized trials. Its current version dates from to 2010 and aims to ensure transparency in the evaluation of novel through randomizes study setups. Its ML extension was triggered by the unmet need to prospectively evaluate ML applications to demonstrate their real-world impact. Consequently, the CONSORT-AI focuses on the reporting of clinical trials evaluating interventions with a ML-based component.

Table 1 Statements considered by the EQUATOR network for different types of research reporting and their extensions for the integration of ML analytics

Area of application	Statement	AI/ML extension
Randomized trial	CONSORT	CONSORT AI
Study protocols	SPIRIT	SPIRIT AI
Diagnostic/prognostic studies	STARD TRIPOD	STARD-AI* TRIPOD-AI* and PROBAST-AI*
Observational studies	STROBE	PRIME CHECKLIST (CV imaging)
Systematic reviews and meta-analysis	PRISMA	–
ML modelling	–	MI-CLAIM
Biomedical image analysis challenges	–	BIAS
Decision support systems driven by artificial intelligence	–	DECIDE-AI*

The asterisk marks those statements that are under development and for which a protocol for their creation has been published

The original CONSORT considers 25 reporting items and the CONSORT-AI has selectively generated extensions in 14 items according to the needs triggered by ML implementation in clinical trials. In general, CONSORT-AI extensions are found for the following sections:

1. Title and abstract. Indicate that the intervention involves machine learning and specify the type of model.
2. Background and objectives. Explain the intended use of the ML intervention in the context of the clinical pathway (purpose and users).
3. Participants. Describe inclusion/exclusion criteria for input data.
4. Interventions. Describe the version of the ML application, how input data was acquired, how missing and low-quality data was handled, whether human-ML interaction took place and level of expertise required, specify the output of the ML intervention and explain how the outputs contributed to decision-making (clinical effect).
5. Harms. Describe any analysis of performance errors and how errors were identified.
6. Funding. State if the ML application can be accessed and its restrictions.

Notably, the CONSORT-AI was developed simultaneously with the SPIRIT-AI extension (see ahead) and as other standard of the sort it attempts to assist a myriad of users such as researchers, clinicians and editors to more easily understand and appraise the quality of a clinical trial involving ML. CONSORT-AI was simultaneously published in three high-impact journals in 2020 [24–26].

5.2 SPIRIT-AI

The statement for standard protocol items: recommendations for interventional trials (SPIRIT) was published in 2013 with the objective to improve the completeness of clinical trial protocol reporting through recommendations for the minimum set of items expected. The novel SPIRIT-AI extension represents a guideline to reporting clinical trial protocols (as opposed to their results, which are addressed by the CONSORT-AI) that evaluate ML-based interventions [27].

The SPIRIT-AI extends 15 items (from the 33 originally contemplated in SPIRIT) that should be reported in addition the SPIRIT components. These items follow a similar profile as the one described for the CONSORT-AI.

5.3 STARD-AI

The Standards for Reporting of Diagnostic Accuracy Studies (STARD) statement is a widely accepted set of reporting standards developed to improve completeness and transparency in studies reporting diagnostic accuracy. Its most recent iteration was published in 2015 and a protocol for its artificial intelligence extension is now available [28].

The STARD-artificial intelligence (STARD-AI) steering group has expressed there are unique issues arising from ML-based diagnostic analytics such as an unclear methodological and therefore diagnostic interpretation (e.g. isolated performance, performance comparison against other models or humans, characteristics of validation datasets), a lack of a standardized nomenclature (e.g. model vs. algorithm, vs. machine learning), and heterogeneity of performance parameters (e.g. AUC, F1 scores, predictive values). Most importantly, they have recognized that such issues should be surmounted at the validation stage (i.e. echelon 2 and 3 of the proposed ML framework) to allow for adequate downstream evaluation of real-world benefits.

5.4 TRIPOD-ML and PROBAST-AI

The Transparent Reporting of a multivariable prediction model of Individual Prognosis Or Diagnosis (TRIPOD) statement and the Prediction model Risk Of Bias ASsessment Tool (PROBAST) were designed to improve the reporting and critical appraisal of prediction models for diagnostic and prognostic purposes. Their respective extensions to cover prediction model studies that applied machine learning analytics are being prepared through a Delphi procedure [29]. They will be published in two complementary papers one dealing with the statement and another dealing with the explanation and elaboration details. Furthermore, they will feature an online tool to maximize accessibility and ease of deployment.

5.5 DECIDE-AI

The Developmental and Exploratory Clinical Investigation of DEcision Support systems driven by Artificial Intelligence (DECIDE-AI) project [30] will develop a new reporting guideline for early-stage evaluation of ML-based clinical decision support systems. The expected benefits include promotion of consistency, comprehensiveness and reproducibility in novel ML systems with clinical support applicability potential with emphasis in the experience of the human users.

The focus of the DECIDE-AI project can be found on initial small-scale algorithm performance, its safety profile, its human-oriented evaluation, and the preparation for large-scale clinical trials.

5.6 PRIME-Checklist

The proposed requirements for cardiovascular imaging-related machine learning evaluation (PRIME) checklist [31] is an interesting initiative also considered in the EQUATOR network with implementation focus on cardiovascular imaging studies employing ML analytics given the success demonstrated in image processing solutions.

It organizes the relevant reporting components in seven sections (Study plan design, data standardization, ML model selection, model assessment, model evaluation, model replicability and reporting limitations) and aims to reduce errors and biases in ML-based image analysis algorithms.

Notably, it recognizes that increasing model complexity increases the risk for inconsistencies in the interpretation and reporting of ML-based (imaging) studies. Moreover, the authors consider that the growing use of ML platforms increases the need to reduce such risk.

5.7 BIAS

The transparent reporting of biomedical image analysis challenges (BIAS) initiative emerged from the increase in these organized challenges which have delivered interesting proofs-of-concept in ML research. Moreover, these challenges provide an ambient of benchmarking algorithms on large common data sets with the noticeable problem that their reporting seems to hamper interpretation and reproducibility of the presented results.

The BIAS recommendations try to address the divergence between the impact of these novel challenges and their effective quality control regardless of the implementation field, image modality or task [32].

5.8 MI-Claim

The minimum information about clinical artificial intelligence modeling (MI-CLAIM) checklist [33] represents a suggested set of minimal requirements in reporting ML application generation, triggered by emerging interpretability problems and pitfalls in generalizability of ML research based on suboptimal documentation.

The MI-CLAIM process consists of reporting 6 sections. These and their subcomponents are namely:

1. Study design including clinical setting, performance metrics, population composition and current reference performance.
2. Data parcellation for model training and testing.
3. Optimization and final model selection.

4. Performance evaluation.
5. Model examination.
6. Reproducible pipeline.

Hence, the MI-CLAIM advances the notion of documentation standardization that can aid clinical and data science researchers in contact with emerging ML tools.

All the aforementioned initiatives show high concordance on their conceptual structure and their differences hinge on specific application necessities. Overall, reporting statements, reporting and quality checklists and recent position papers echo fundamentals aspects in the evaluation and promotion of high-quality ML applications. Moreover, they provide structures that can inform development pathways for novel ML solutions with minimization of errors and research waste. These fundamentals recurrently link to the need for clear documentation through explicit reporting of ML components and their objectives, exhaustive description of their data origins, broad characterization of their performance with consideration of the theoretical and clinical settings, and referral to the code to maximize ease of replicability and generalization.

Of note, all evaluation and quality initiatives link with the base model of scientific research quality and hierarchy in which the realm of ML should be currently inserted to facilitate their development and refinement over time. Also, this will allow the characterization of gaps in knowledge and tendencies in corresponding literature over time. Figure 4 proposes a schematic model of this integration.

As such, the number of ongoing or recently published initiatives to strengthen the incorporation of ML analytics through high-quality, extensive and clarity-oriented reporting statements is increasing. One issue that cannot be ignored is that these statements and recommendations should be prompted to the community of ML researchers both in the data science and clinical spectrum. Otherwise, there is a risk that these aids however comprehensive and useful may be only considered in isolation and that

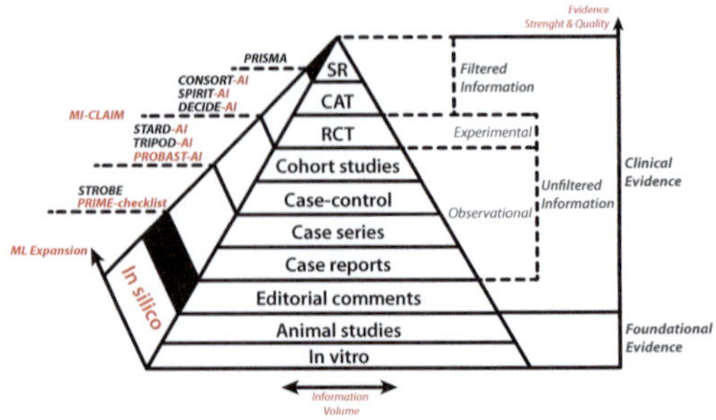

Fig. 4 Modified pyramid of scientific research hierarchy. The expansion of the base model depicts the type of studies for which machine learning-oriented recommendations and standards have been generated or are still missing

their sheer number will continue to increase. This would dilute their practical effect and deliver a similar situation as the one currently witnessed with first publications in ML research.

6 Guidelines

The use of diagnostic and prediction tools in the real-world clinical setting may appear distant, yet this view emerges from the traditional behavior of the development of analytical tools seen in the past (see sections above). Emerging recommendations for reporting ML clinical research should promote the convergence of the clinical and computer science communities in order to bridge the disconnection between developers and clinicians. There is a clear lack of international guidelines for the utilization and implementation of ML in clinical research, nevertheless the need for them is evident and we elaborate on the expected structures and describe how this could be envisioned for the near future.

One starting point could be the consideration of ML as a specialization area mean to deal with any sort of input in different and adaptive ways. This would require the theoretical basis and applicable resources proper of an independent knowledge area. In this case, a unique society with international reach for the study and implementation of ML in medical sciences would be the preference with divisions according to the types of models of types of input to be analyzed. Alternatively, ML research and implementation could be considered as an area of added value in every already existing knowledge or specialization areas. This would have the advantage of initiation ease and the disadvantage of effort fragmentation due to lack of cross talk between specializations. In this latter case, there could be extensions to existing reporting guidelines and recommendations in clinical and health sciences to integrate ML-based methods.

Notably, there seems to be efforts in both directions with the generation of statements and recommendations by established networks and journals (see above), and the expansion of ML-dedicated symposiums and congresses such as the European Society of Cardiology Digital Summit which took place for the first time in 2019.

An international task force may be helpful considering authors of proof-of-concept ML clinical studies in several areas of medical specialty underlining imaging, pathology, cardiology, genetics, public health and others. The intention could be to distill the concepts and standards grounding good practices in ML clinical research with help from the aforementioned position statements from varying medical societies (e.g. EANM/EACVI) based on the utilization of criteria informed by expert opinion and empirical data.

Thereon, it will be necessary to identify reports aiming to standardize the evaluation and quality of ML-based clinical studies such as the PRIME-checklist. Importantly, cross-applicability to any specialty areas in medical sciences should be central.

Furthermore, a structural approach with ML dedicated committees in every area of sub-specialization subject to election and replacement should be considered much in the same way that society board leadership functions currently. An example of this can be found in the new journal European Heart Journal: Digital Health, Nature: Machine Intelligence.

7 Regulatory Aspects

Regulation of ML in health-care is still in its infancy [34]. ML software is currently regulated through the medical device regulations in both the European Union (EU) and United States (US). However, the unique characteristics of ML algorithms, mean that these regulations do not suffice. For example, the existing regulatory frameworks for medical devices necessitate re-authorisation for all changes in ML algorithms. Continuous learning, in which ML algorithms learn from new data and keeps improving performance over time, therefore requires a rewrite of the regulatory rule books.

Although no concrete laws are yet in place to regulate ML, the EU and US have taken provisional steps in developing regulatory frameworks for (medical) AI in 2021. The European Commission (EC) has published the Artificial Intelligence Act [35]. This act creates the first legal framework on A and aims to "*guarantee the safety and fundamental rights of people and businesses, while strengthening AI uptake, investment and innovation across the EU.*" It encompasses all areas of AI, including healthcare AI, which it regards as a 'high risk' application. The FDA published its Artificial Intelligence/Machine Learning (AI-ML)-Based Software as a Medical Device (SaMD) Action Plan [13]. The FDA's action plan aims to create a framework to "*enable to provide a reasonable assurance of safety and effectiveness while embracing the iterative improvement power of artificial intelligence and machine learning-based software as a medical device.*"

The EU AI Act provides comprehensive, sector-specific and cross-sector regulations for implementation of AI algorithms. Instead, the US AI Action Plan sustains from comprehensive regulation of ML, but delegates responsibility of regulation to specific federal agencies, while providing general principles including a mandate to avoid overregulation. Some of the main areas of focus of these regulatory frameworks are data quality and algorithmic bias, risk assessment and mitigation systems, continuous learning and transparency.

7.1 Data Quality and Algorithmic Bias

Biases exist widely in healthcare data, both in historical datasets, as well as current healthcare usage [36]. ML systems may perpetuate biases presented in the data, which could lead to wrong outcomes or systematic underperformance in certain population groups [37].

Both the US and European regulators acknowledge the importance of mitigating bias in medical ML. The EU AI Act requires that data used for ML must be subject to appropriate data-governance and must meet high standards of quality. For example, data must be relevant, representative, free of errors and complete, also with regard to all patient groups to which the ML is applied. Moreover, specific geographical, behavioural (socio-economic) or functional characteristics need to be reflected in the data. As the EU encompasses multiple states with different ethnic representations, this might mean require retraining of algorithms using EU, or even country/region-specific, datasets. The FDA's AI Action Plan is less detailed, but states that ML systems must be well suited for a racially and ethnically diverse intended patient population, without specifying exact regulations on how to ascertain such appropriateness.

7.2 Continuous Learning and Post-market Risk Assessment

One of the unique features of ML resides in the continuous or adaptive learning that can be exploited post-authorisation to improve future performance. Current regulations have not been designed for adaptive systems. The EU and US 2021 AI regulation frameworks for the first time introduce the possibility of continuous learning in ML software.

The FDA proposes submission of a predetermined 'change control plan' for ML software. This plan must include 'what' aspects might undergo change through learning, 'how' the algorithm will change through learning and 'how' safety and effectiveness are ensured. The adaptivity of ML software can encompass changes in performance, as well as changes in indications of use, for example extending to a new patient population. Larger changes that involve significant deviations from original use or increase the power of the AI, for example transforming it from a low-risk application (support-algorithms) to a high-risk application (diagnostic algorithms) necessitate re-authorisation [38].

The EU regulations are again more specific and stipulating detailed prerequisites for continuous learning, that need to be submitted to the regulator prior to approval. These include the goals of continuous training, the technology used and the design of a systematic post-market monitoring system to monitor changes in the algorithm. This monitoring system is an active process that obligates manufacturers to collect, document and analyse data to monitor performance of its ML software throughout its lifetime. Furthermore, the AI act states that ML tools will need to maintain appropriate levels of accuracy and robustness with respect to the state-of-art of that time. These regulations means that manufacturers will carry greater and on-going responsibility for their tools to enable trust and mitigate potential risks early.

7.3 Transparency

Transparency regarding ML is important to enable users to evaluate the appropriate use-case of the software in their clinics and mitigate risks. The EU AI Act provides a regulatory framework to assure transparency. It states that detailed documentation needs to be provided regarding the instructions of use and characteristics of the AI software, including capabilities and limitations of performance, as well as a detailed description of the training, validation and test data, cybersecurity issues and the expected lifetime of ML.

The FDA's AI Action Plan, states similar regulatory requirements albeit being less specific; it affirms that users should be able to understand the benefits, risks and limitations of ML software through reporting of issues of usability, trust and accountability.

Both regulatory bodies express the desire to provide a public registry of approvals of AI systems to ensure transparency, trust and facilitate regulatory oversight. The FDA already holds a public registry with statements for each approved medical device [35]. An EU-wide database for AI software is intended to be established in the coming years.

The initial steps laid out in the EU's AI Act and FDA's AI Action give a roadmap for future regulations on ML. The two regulations share a set of core values and principles regarding implementation of AI in healthcare. The next years will see efforts to translate the current plans into laws for regulation and authorisation of fast-evolving capacities of ML in the medical field.

8 Conclusions

Machine learning as the base of novel artificial intelligence research in healthcare has grown dramatically but there is still limited translation to clinical settings. The current disparity between the number of initial publications and orienting guidelines hinders clinical evaluation in the real-world. Therefore, machine learning *frameworks* in clinical research are needed to maximize analytical value and reduce research waste. Emerging recommendations statements mostly constitute extensions from existing standards (form the EQUATOR Network) and regulatory initiatives aim to establish clear paths to clinical translation.

References

1. Mateen BA, Liley J, Denniston AK, Holmes CC, Vollmer SJ. Improving the quality of machine learning in health applications and clinical research. Nat Mach Intell. 2020;2(10):554–6. https://doi.org/10.1038/s42256-020-00239-1.
2. Vollmer S, Mateen BA, Bohner G, et al. Machine learning and AI research for patient benefit: 20 critical questions on transparency, replicability. Ethics Effective. December 2018. https://doi.org/10.48550/arxiv.1812.10404.
3. Deo RC. Machine learning in medicine. Circulation. 2015;132(20):1920–30. https://doi.org/10.1161/CIRCULATIONAHA.115.001593.
4. Benjamins JW, Hendriks T, Knuuti J, Juarez-Orozco LE, van der Harst P. A primer in artificial intelligence in cardiovascular medicine. Netherlands Hear J. 2019;27(9):392–402. https://doi.org/10.1007/S12471-019-1286-6/FIGURES/5.
5. Glasziou P, Altman DG, Bossuyt P, et al. Reducing waste from incomplete or unusable reports of biomedical research. Lancet. 2014;383(9913):267–76. https://doi.org/10.1016/S0140-6736(13)62228-X.
6. Vollmer S, Mateen BA, Bohner G, et al. Machine learning and artificial intelligence research for patient benefit: 20 critical questions on transparency, replicability, ethics, and effectiveness. *BMJ*. March 2020;l6927. https://doi.org/10.1136/bmj.l6927
7. Overmars LM, van Es B, Groepenhoff F, et al. Preventing unnecessary imaging in patients suspect of coronary artery disease through machine learning of electronic health records. Eur Hear J Digit Heal. 2022;3(1):11–9. https://doi.org/10.1093/ehjdh/ztab103.
8. Benjamins JW, Yeung MW, Maaniitty T, et al. Improving patient identification for advanced cardiac imaging through machine learning-integration of clinical and coronary CT angiography data. Int J Cardiol. 2021;335:130–6. https://doi.org/10.1016/j.ijcard.2021.04.009.
9. Juarez-Orozco LE, Knol RJJ, Sanchez-Catasus CA, Martinez-Manzanera O, van der Zant FM, Knuuti J. Machine learning in the integration of simple variables for identifying patients with myocardial ischemia. J Nucl Cardiol. 2020;27(1):147–55. https://doi.org/10.1007/s12350-018-1304-x.
10. Khera R, Haimovich J, Hurley NC, et al. Use of machine learning models to predict death after acute myocardial infarction. JAMA Cardiol. 2021;6(6):633. https://doi.org/10.1001/jamacardio.2021.0122.
11. D'Ascenzo F, De Filippo O, Gallone G, et al. Machine learning-based prediction of adverse events following an acute coronary syndrome (PRAISE): a modelling study of pooled datasets. Lancet. 2021;397(10270):199–207. https://doi.org/10.1016/S0140-6736(20)32519-8.
12. Slomka PJ, Betancur J, Liang JX, et al. Rationale and design of the REgistry of Fast myocardial perfusion Imaging with NExt generation SPECT (REFINE SPECT). J Nucl Cardiol. 2020;27(3):1010–21. https://doi.org/10.1007/s12350-018-1326-4.

13. U.S. Food and Drug Administration. Software as a Medical Device (SAMD): clinical Evaluation guidance for industry and food and drug administration staff. FDA Guide; 2017. p. 1–32. https://www.fda.gov/media/100714/download
14. Amann J, Blasimme A, Vayena E, Frey D, Madai VI. Explainability for artificial intelligence in healthcare: a multidisciplinary perspective. BMC Med Inform Decis Mak. 2020;20(1):310. https://doi.org/10.1186/s12911-020-01332-6.
15. Friedman JH. Greedy function approximation: a gradient boosting machine. Ann Stat. 2001;29(5). https://doi.org/10.1214/aos/1013203451
16. Shapley LS. Notes on the N-person game—II: the value of an N-person game. RAND Corporation; 1951. https://doi.org/10.7249/RM0670
17. Lakkaraju H, Kamar E, Caruana R, Leskovec J. Interpretable & explorable approximations of black box models. July 2017. http://arxiv.org/abs/1707.01154
18. Ribeiro MT, Singh S, Guestrin C. Why should i trust you? In: Proceedings of the 22nd ACM SIGKDD international conference on knowledge discovery and data mining. New York, NY, USA: ACM; 2016. p. 1135–44. https://doi.org/10.1145/2939672.2939778
19. Zhou B, Khosla A, Lapedriza À, Oliva A, Torralba A. Learning deep features for discriminative localization. IEEE Conf Comput Vis Pattern Recognit. 2016;2016:2921–9.
20. Vranken JF, van de Leur RR, Gupta DK, et al. Uncertainty estimation for deep learning-based automated analysis of 12-lead electrocardiograms. Eur Hear J Digit Heal. 2021;2(3):401–15. https://doi.org/10.1093/ehjdh/ztab045.
21. Puyol-Antón E, Ruijsink B, Baumgartner CF, et al. Automated quantification of myocardial tissue characteristics from native T1 mapping using neural networks with uncertainty-based quality-control. J Cardiovasc Magn Reson. 2020;22(1):60. https://doi.org/10.1186/s12968-020-00650-y.
22. Ruijsink B, Puyol-Antón E, Li Y, et al. Quality-aware semi-supervised learning for CMR segmentation. 2021. p. 97–107. https://doi.org/10.1007/978-3-030-68107-4_10
23. Rudin C. Stop explaining black box machine learning models for high stakes decisions and use interpretable models instead. Nat Mach Intell. 2019;1(5):206–15. https://doi.org/10.1038/s42256-019-0048-x.
24. Liu X, Rivera SC, Moher D, Calvert MJ, Denniston AK, SPIRIT-AI and CONSORT-AI Working Group. Reporting guidelines for clinical trial reports for interventions involving artificial intelligence: the CONSORT-AI extension. BMJ. 2020;370:m3164. https://doi.org/10.1136/bmj.m3164
25. Liu X, Cruz Rivera S, Moher D, Calvert MJ, Denniston AK, SPIRIT-AI and CONSORT-AI Working Group. Reporting guidelines for clinical trial reports for interventions involving artificial intelligence: the CONSORT-AI extension. Nat Med. 2020;26(9):1364–74. https://doi.org/10.1038/s41591-020-1034-x
26. Liu X, Cruz Rivera S, Moher D, Calvert MJ, Denniston AK, SPIRIT-AI and CONSORT-AI Working Group. Reporting guidelines for clinical trial reports for interventions involving artificial intelligence: the CONSORT-AI extension. Lancet Digit Heal. 2020;2(10):e537–e48. https://doi.org/10.1016/S2589-7500(20)30218-1
27. Cruz Rivera S, Liu X, Chan A-W, et al. Guidelines for clinical trial protocols for interventions involving artificial intelligence: the SPIRIT-AI extension. Nat Med. 2020;26(9):1351–63. https://doi.org/10.1038/s41591-020-1037-7.
28. Sounderajah V, Ashrafian H, Golub RM, et al. Developing a reporting guideline for artificial intelligence-centred diagnostic test accuracy studies: the STARD-AI protocol. BMJ Open. 2021;11(6): e047709. https://doi.org/10.1136/bmjopen-2020-047709.
29. Collins GS, Dhiman P, Andaur Navarro CL, et al. Protocol for development of a reporting guideline (TRIPOD-AI) and risk of bias tool (PROBAST-AI) for diagnostic and prognostic prediction model studies based on artificial intelligence. BMJ Open. 2021;11(7): e048008. https://doi.org/10.1136/bmjopen-2020-048008.
30. DECIDE-AI: new reporting guidelines to bridge the development-to-implementation gap in clinical artificial intelligence. Nat Med. 2021;27(2):186–87. https://doi.org/10.1038/s41591-021-01229-5
31. Sengupta PP, Shrestha S, Berthon B, et al. Proposed requirements for cardiovascular imaging-related machine learning evaluation (PRIME): a vhecklist. JACC Cardiovasc Imaging. 2020;13(9):2017–35. https://doi.org/10.1016/j.jcmg.2020.07.015.
32. Maier-Hein L, Reinke A, Kozubek M, et al. BIAS: transparent reporting of biomedical image analysis challenges. Med Image Anal. 2020;66: 101796. https://doi.org/10.1016/j.media.2020.101796.
33. Norgeot B, Quer G, Beaulieu-Jones BK, et al. Minimum information about clinical artificial intelligence modeling: the MI-CLAIM checklist. Nat Med. 2020;26(9):1320–4. https://doi.org/10.1038/s41591-020-1041-y.
34. Muehlematter UJ, Daniore P, Vokinger KN. Approval of artificial intelligence and machine learning-based medical devices in the USA and Europe (2015–20): a comparative analysis. Lancet Digit Heal. 2021;3(3):e195–203. https://doi.org/10.1016/S2589-7500(20)30292-2.
35. European Commission. Proposal for a Regulation of the European Parliament and of the Council laying down harmonised rules on artificial intelligence (artificial intelligence act) and amending certain union legislative acts. https://eur-lex.europa.eu/legal-content/EN/TXT/?uri=CELEX:52021PC0206. Published 21 Apr 2021. Accessed 23 May 2022.
36. Lavizzo-Mourey RJ, Besser RE, Williams DR. Understanding and mitigating health

inequities—Past, current, and future directions. N Engl J Med. 2021;384(18):1681–4. https://doi.org/10.1056/NEJMP2008628.

37. Puyol-Antón E, Ruijsink B, Harana JM, et al. Fairness in cardiac magnetic resonance imaging: assessing sex and racial bias in deep learning-based segmentation. Front Cardiovasc Med. 2022;9:859310. https://doi.org/10.3389/FCVM.2022.859310.

38. U.S. Food and Drug Administration. Proposed regulatory framework for modifications to artificial intelligence/machine learning (AI/ML)-based software as a medical device (SaMD)-discussion paper and request for feedback. 2019. https://www.fda.gov/downloads/medicaldevices/deviceregulationandguidance/guidancedocuments/ucm514737.pdf. Accessed 23 May 2022.

Challenges of Machine Learning and AI (What Is Next?), Responsible and Ethical AI

Polyxeni Gkontra, Gianluca Quaglio, Anna Tselioudis Garmendia and Karim Lekadir

Abstract

Research in medical artificial intelligence (AI) is experiencing an explosive growth. This growth highlights the potential of AI to significantly improve healthcare across a wide spectrum of applications such as risk stratification, diagnosis, therapeutics, and resource management among others. However, despite the great promises of medical AI and recent technological advancements, a gap persists in translating and deploying AI solutions within clinical settings. This gap is attributed to the risks and challenges that these promising technologies entail. To bring AI one step closer to the real-word clinical practice, we identify and outline the principal clinical, ethical and socio-ethical risks associated with AI in healthcare, unravelling their potential sources. These risks include potential errors leading to patient harm, risk of bias causing exacerbated health disparities, lack of transparency and trust, as well as susceptibilities to hacking and data privacy breaches. Furthermore, we discuss approaches towards minimizing risks and developing tools that can be safely deployed and routinely used in the clinic. Moreover, we introduce a set of concrete recommendations aimed at mitigating risks and maximizing the advantages presented by medical AI. These recommendations include fostering multi-stakeholder engagement throughout the AI production lifecycle, increased transparency and traceability, exhaustive clinical validation of AI tools, and comprehensive AI training and education for both medical practitioners and the general public. The adoption of such policies stands to significantly influence the trajectory and deployment of AI within clinical practice.

Keywords

Artificial Intelligence (AI) · Healthcare · Medical AI risk analysis · Trustworthy medical AI · Medical AI risk minimization

P. Gkontra (✉) · K. Lekadir
Departament de Matemàtiques i Informàtica, Universitat de Barcelona, Artificial Intelligence in Medicine Lab (BCN-AIM), Barcelona, Spain
e-mail: polyxeni.gkontra@ub.edu

G. Quaglio
Panel for the Future of Science and Technology (STOA), European Parliament, Brussels, Belgium

A. T. Garmendia
Faculty of Medicine, School of Public Health, Imperial College, London, UK

F. W. Asselbergs et al. (eds.), *Clinical Applications of Artificial Intelligence in Real-World Data*,
https://doi.org/10.1007/978-3-031-36678-9_17

1 Trustworthy and Responsible AI

Medical artificial intelligence (AI) holds both great promises and risks. In this chapter, we focus on the latter in an effort to unravel the factors that can hinder the performance and use of medical AI tools leading to serious complications, including patient harm and violations of patients' rights. First, we describe the main risks and challenges associated with medical AI, unraveling their potential sources, and offering mitigations strategies. Subsequently, we shift our focus to approaches towards minimizing risks and developing tools that can be safely deployed and routinely used in the real-word clinical practice. Finally, we provide concrete recommendations towards achieving trustworthy medical AI and bringing medical AI one step closer to the clinic.

1.1 Risks in Medical AI

Despite the great promise of AI in revolutionizing healthcare, by improving its quality and delivery, the adoption of AI in the clinic has been slow. This is mainly related to the severe technical and socio-ethical risks that medical AI has been associated with [15, 24, 35, 74, 84]. These risks hamper AI adoption in the clinic as they might cause harm to patients and citizens, in addition to eroding the clinicians' and the general public's trust in AI. Therefore, to ensure and accelerate AI use in the clinic, risk assessment, classification and management of AI tools must be an integral part of the AI development, evaluation and deployment processes.

In this chapter, we focus on the main risks and challenges associated with medical AI. These can be roughly divided into seven categories (Fig. 1):

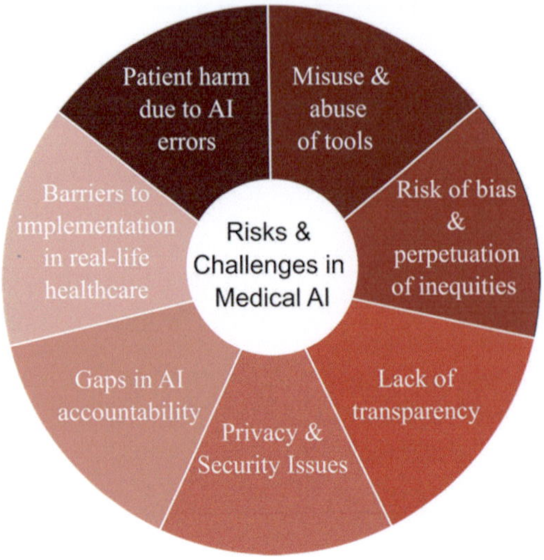

Fig. 1 Main risks and challenges in medical AI

1. Patient safety issues due to AI errors
2. Misuse and abuse of medical AI tools
3. Risk of bias in medical AI and perpetuation of inequities
4. Lack of transparency
5. Privacy and security issues
6. Gaps in AI accountability
7. Barriers to implementation in real-world healthcare.

1.1.1 Patient Safety Issues Due to AI Errors

AI is expected to improve patient safety by reducing human errors and enabling prediction, prevention, and detection of health adverse events [10]. Nonetheless, at the same time, novel risks for patient harm can emerge due to medical AI failures. These include: (1) patients with life-threatening conditions not being diagnosed leading to failure to begin treatment on-time (false negatives), (2) patients being incorrectly classified to the diseased population leading to unnecessary treatments or procedures (false positives), and (3) incorrect scheduling and prioritisation of interventions, particularly in the emergency departments and surgery.

The main causes for AI failures are:

- noise and artefacts in AI's clinical inputs, measurements, and labels
- the distribution shift problem, i.e., shifts in the distribution between training and real-world data

- the Frame Problem, i.e., inability to identify and handle unexpected changes in clinical contexts and environments.

More precisely, noisy data can greatly affect the performance of AI models. Both scanning errors, typically depending on the experience of the operator, the cooperation of the patient, and the clinical environment (e.g. emergency room) [93], as well as low quality data labels used during training can lead to inaccuracies in the AI results [52]. Particularly in the case of deep learning models, noisy labels have been reported as the main challenges for the subsequent AI adoption in the clinic [16, 60].

The second category of common AI error sources includes the distribution shift problem [112]. This term refers to incorrect results being produced by the AI system due to shifts between the distribution of the AI training and validation data, and that of the real-world data produced in the clinic. This is a well-known AI issue demonstrated in different medical domains. For instance, in the cardiology domain, a recent study revealed scanner-related bias and accuracy drop in performance of AI models in the task of segmenting cardiac structures from cardiac magnetic resonance images (CMR) when provided with CMR from unseen scanners [14]. In the area of ophthalmology, the promising AI system of DeepMind for automated diagnosis of retinal diseases from optical coherence tomography [28] presented a highly increased diagnosis error rate, from 5.5 to 46%, when applied in data from a different device than the one used for training. Apart from scanner-related biases, a multi-center study in the United States has also reported potential hospital-specific biases [131]. The authors built a highly accurate pneumonia diagnosis AI system based on data from two hospitals. The system performed poorly when applied to data from a third hospital.

Moreover, the Frame Problem [76] is one of the major challenges for patient safety. The term was coined by McCarthy and Hayes in 1969 and refers to the difficulty in identifying and describing intuitively obvious non-effects. In the clinic, this can be translated in failure of the AI system to recognize and handle unexpected changes in the environment. For example, mis-classifying a patient as having lung cancer (false positive) because the patient, who is wearing a ring, places his hand on his/her chest during X-ray and the system is trained to recognize circular objects as lesions [129].

If we are to fully harness the potential of medical AI, these failures related to patient safety must be addressed. To this end, there are three main approaches to follow. First, standardized processes for rigorous model evaluation are required to ensure robustness and reliability in novel environments, but also to evaluate data and labels quality. Such processes should involve comprehensive multi-center studies to identify potential instabilities and increase robustness of medical AI models by ensuring their capability to deal with both noisy data and shifts, while maintaining their accuracy even if the data is heterogeneous across populations, hospitals or machines. Moreover, the use of large datasets with trustworthy labels along with strategies for handling noisy labels are imperative. Second, healthcare providers should remain part of the data processing workflow and final decision making. In the near-term, medical AI should be designed and deployed as "augmented intelligence" systems, i.e. supportive solutions and not fully autonomous agents [75]. Third, mechanisms to detect and convey anomalies must be embedded in the tools, along with mechanisms for continuous learning and calibration. Nonetheless, the latter will require human feedback, and therefore, the cooperation of the healthcare providers who will evaluate and document the system's performance including reporting contextual changes and potential errors. The balance between preserving cost and accuracy benefits, and minimizing patient harm is to be studied.

1.1.2 Misuse and Abuse of Medical AI Tools

One main risk factor for misuse of AI tools is the lack of a true understanding of the medical AI technologies on the part of the end-user, i.e. the healthcare providers and citizens. This is mainly related to the limited involvement of those important groups in the medical AI development as current solutions. A recent study [114] evaluating twenty-four medical AI tools found that clinicians are usually consulted only at inconsistent points and, more often, at the later stages of the design (82%, 19/24 tools).

This fact coupled with the general lack of AI literacy in the society [38], but even within the medical community, result in increased chances for misuse and human errors. Recent studies in Australia and New Zealand [102], the United Kingdom [108] and the European Union [102] show that health care professionals receive limited, if any, training regarding AI and utilization of technology-based tools as part of their compulsory curriculum.

Another rising problem is the proliferation of easily accessible web or mobile medical applications whose efficiency and quality regarding potential bias can be questioned. For example, in the domain of skin cancer detection, a plethora of such apps already exists (e.g. Skinvision, MelApp, skinScan and SpotMole to name a few). Nonetheless, a recent study [34] demonstrated efficiency and potential bias issues in the six mobile applications that were evaluated. Despite being a promising solution for remote diagnosis and disease monitoring, the widespread use of online apps may pose a public health risk in the same manner that the online pharmacies have been associated to over-prescription [72]. Lastly, most users ignore the disclaimers of such tools on not being certified medical devices.

To reduce the risk for harmful misuse of medical AI tools, four main mitigation strategies can be followed. First, medical AI technologies should be designed and developed in continuous interaction with the end-user to better integrate end-users' needs and feedback and, thus, maximize their understanding of the technology being developed and its limitations. Second, a compulsory AI curriculum for healthcare providers should be offered by faculties to ensure adequate understanding of the AI techniques and results. Moreover, easily accessible programmes that enhance AI literacy of the society at large have the potential to increase the public awareness and knowledge regarding medical AI and its risks. Finally, there is an urgent need for strict regulatory mechanisms offered by governmental authorities for mobile and online applications to reduce potential misuse and abuse of such technologies by partially or misinformed end-users.

1.1.3 Risk of Bias in Medical AI and Perpetuation of Inequities

In the context of healthcare, Panch et al. defined for the first time the algorithm bias as "the instances when the application of an algorithm compounds existing inequities in socioeconomic status, race, ethnic background, religion, gender, disability or sexual orientation to amplify them and adversely impact inequities in health systems" [89]. To date, several studies have reported algorithmic bias in healthcare,against Black patients in the referral process for additional or specialist care [87], against young females, black and patients/households with low income [104], and against women who are being consistently over-diagnosed for diseases such as depression and under-diagnosed for others, such as cancer [130–71], to name a few.

The sources of bias are several. Bias most commonly occurs due to AI models being trained with biased and unbalanced data. This leads to a significant accuracy drop when the system is applied to unrepresented or underrepresented groups in the training set. One popular example are AI technologies for skin cancer detection. A study evaluated six mobile applications and found that all of them were trained on datasets comprising images from lighter-skin patients, failing to generalize to darker-skin patients [2]. Other examples include the 2002 National Lung Screening Trial for early diagnosis of lung cancer which was trained with data from 53,000 smokers. Only 4% of data were from black individuals [29]. Without mitigation strategies, similar situations that could lead to amplification of healthcare inequalities can occur with AI tools adopted in the fight against Coronavirus Disease 2019 (COVID-19) [66]. Apart from gender and racial biases, data-related bias also stems from the lack of geographical variation in the datasets used for training. In the USA, a recent review [53] revealed that 71% of data used to train deep learning algorithms were based on data only from three states, while in the remaining studies 34 out 50 states were not considered. Such bias might also originate in disparities in access to quality equipment and digital technologies.

Another important source of bias is the human bias. For example, in the evaluation of pain, it has been demonstrated by different studies that reports of pain by black [50] and female patients [101] are not receiving adequate attention. Moreover, women are systematically being diagnosed with most diseases later than males [121]. This issue also results in bias in data labels. This is a particularly important issue as AI models can propagate disparities present in the current health data registries, such as misdiagnosis of specific subgroups [96].

In a nutshell, bias in medical AI has severe implications for healthcare. Therefore, mitigation strategies are necessary at all stages of the AI system development [118]. Startegies include the use of balanced, representative datasets in terms of key attributes such as sex/gender, age, socioeconomics, ethnicity, and geographic location. Moreover, the datasets should also include well-curated labels free of bias in annotation themselves. Beyond the generation of fair datasets, computational approaches such as generation of synthetic datasets to cover under-represented groups or to deal with bias during model design such as adversarial [132] or continuous learning [119] should be explored. Explainable and highly interpretable models are also of paramount importance to detect and tackle bias. But most importantly, AI developers should work closely with clinical experts and healthcare professionals, but also with social scientists, biomedical ethicists, public health experts, as well as patients and citizens from diverse backgrounds, experiences and needs to promote diversity in the field of medical AI. Lastly, the development of a standardized evaluation system, consisting of a set of key performance indicators that jointly evaluate the quality of the training set, accuracy and risk for bias proposed by a recent study [23], can aid ensure the fairness of medical AI.

1.1.4 Lack of Transparency

Transparency is an essential requirement for the adoption of medical AI in clinical practice. It refers to the ability to comprehend how an AI tool works, reaches a decision, and adequately communicate these processes. Medical AI systems even with high accuracy, such as the Google algorithm for breast cancer screening [78], can be potentially harmful if the end-users cannot fully understand how they make decisions [43]. Without transparency, reproducibility and independent evaluation of the systems is hampered. Moreover, identification of sources of errors and subsequent definition of responsibilities are difficult to take place.

AI transparency is closely linked to two concepts: traceability and explainability. The former refers to documenting the entire AI development process in a transparent manner, including tracking how the AI model performs in real-world scenarios after deployment [83]. The latter refers to the ability to transparently explain how the AI system reached a decision rather than viewing it as "black-box". In this direction, Explainable Artificial Intelligence (XAI) has recently emerged as a new field focused on bringing transparency on AI systems by developing novel approaches for explaining and interpreting their decisions [69].

Overall, lack of transparency can hinder the trust in AI predictions and decisions, and therefore, delay their incorporation in the real-world. To tackle these limitations, different avenues exist. First, an "AI passport" that includes all model's key information should be requested for AI medical technologies. Traceability tools to detect and report potential errors and model drift are also essential. Furthermore, to increase explainability, the end-users must be involved in the design and development process to ensure that explanations are clear, helpful and address their needs. Finally, it is essential that regulatory entities require traceability and explainability mechanisms for the tools to provide certification. Nonetheless, explainable AI should at no point mean more flexibility regarding the requirement for rigorous internal and external validation of the models as novel risks might arise [37].

1.1.5 Privacy and Security Issues

A key concern regarding medical AI is privacy and security issues. More precisely, there exist two types of risks in this category; (1) risks regarding the use, sharing, and re-use or re-purposing of patient data without informed consent or knowledge, and (2) risks related to (cyber-) attacks and hacking or fooling of the tools.

A popular example within the first category is the sharing of 1.6 million patients' data from the United Kingdom without their consent from the Royal Free NHS Foundation Trust to the Google-owned AI company DeepMind for the development of an app for diagnosis of acute kidney disease [35]. In this case, there was a clear security bleach as patients had not provided consent, but it is becoming an increasingly alarming issue that patients might provide consent, but not fully understand how their data might be shared or re-used [77]. Furthermore, beyond data re-use, there exists the threat of data repurposing for medical or non-medical purposes, known as "function creep" [59]. Hocking et al. detailed the way patient data are re-purposed within the healthcare domain for the European pharmaceutical industry [49], while data from the COVID-19 contact tracing application of the government of Singapore was used also for criminal investigations [124].

AI systems are also vulnerable to (cyber-) attacks and hacking, while they can be easily fooled [23]. Researchers have demonstrated that they could remotely control AI-powered insulin pumps, which could potentially even lead to the administration of lethal overdoses [56]. Another example in this category is the Düsseldorf University Hospital cyber-attack that rendered the hospital's computer system unusable and resulted in the death of a patient [54]. To further understand the vulnerability of medical AI, we should also consider the issue of potential adversarial attacks, including "one-pixel" attacks, to AI systems based on medical imaging. The term refers to modifying the input provided to the AI model even slightly, for example by just rotating the image [32] or just changing a pixel [107], to intentionally make the system produce a false result. Given that many AI technologies offer binary classification, paired with the current lack of full explainability of deep learning models, these attacks represent significant hazards for the patients.

Due to the serious consequences that privacy and security issues could have, it is essential to adopt mitigation strategies. First, awareness and literacy regarding data privacy, informed consent and cybersecurity are essential. Regulations to address accountability and protect citizens and their rights are also needed. To further avoid exposure of sensitive patient data accidentally or intentionally, we should shift our focus from models that work in a centralized manner, to federated privacy-preserving AI solutions which do not require the data to ever leave the hospital. Lastly, mechanisms to identify attempts to intentionally fool AI systems should continue to be developed [127] and improve.

1.1.6 Gaps in AI Accountability

Modern medical AI systems are challenging the way we understand and define accountability in the healthcare sector. First, given that AI systems cannot be held morally accountable or liable [95] and the elevated number of actors in the development, implementation and use of the solutions, ranging from AI developers to healthcare professionals [109], it is unclear who is to be held accountable or liable for medical AI failures and errors.

Second, the difficulty in identifying the error source and whether it was due to the data used, an algorithmic error, or due to misuse and lack of understanding of the tool's results renders allocation of responsibility even more unclear. In this context, AI accountability is closely related to explainability and transparency, as in cases of errors, it is possible that the one to be held accountable will be the healthcare professional who used a tool but cannot explain his/her decision or error [73]. This is particularly true in the case of assistive tools as it might be considered as consulting a colleague [44].

Third, the lack of a unified ethical and legal standard for AI manufacturers and industries creates further gaps in AI accountability. Currently, while healthcare professionals are usually under strict regulatory responsibilities that can even result in losing their license in cases of errors, AI developers and technologists generally work under ethical codes [122]. The latter have been criticized frequently for being ambiguous and challenging to implement into real-life cases [95].

The current lack of accountability needs to be addressed by novel frameworks and mechanisms that ensure responsibility, prevent such acts from being repeated, and manage reclamations, compensations and sanctions [124]. More precisely, procedures should be put in place to define the roles of clinical users and AI developers when AI-assisted medical decisions result in patient harm. Additionally, regulatory entities specially focused on medical AI must be created. These entities are expected to create and implement regulatory frameworks to guarantee that agents are held accountable in cases of errors.

1.1.7 Barriers to Implementation in Real-World Healthcare

Despite significant advances in the development of medical AI technologies, their actual implementation, integration, and use remain limited with clinicians being characterized as the professionals that traditionally delay in the adoption of novel technologies [94]. The barriers in the realization of medical AI in the clinic are several [30, 86, 106]. First, one of the main obstacles is the high data heterogeneity across clinical sites and electronic health systems. More precisely, health data from different sites have varying quality [62], while a significant part, e.g. referral letters, informs, is unstructured. This leads to rich data remaining ¨locked¨ at individual institutions and becoming unexploitable by AI algorithms.

Second, healthcare professionals are skeptical regarding the way AI medical systems might transform the clinician-patient relationship. On one hand, AI technologies are expected to improve the clinician-patient interaction and make it more patient-centered as they have the potential to help the clinician better engage and include the patient in the decision-making process by allowing them, for example, navigate and discuss through their AI-proposed treatment options [5]. On the other hand, there is the risk that trust towards the clinician might be questioned and shifted towards the AI tools. Furthermore, there exist ethical issues regarding the communication of AI-derived risk scores for high-burden diseases such as cancer or dementia [18, 30].

Third, the lack of integration of the novel AI systems with the tools that healthcare professionals are already familiar with and use in their everyday work makes the adoption of such novel technologies more challenging. Inevitably, the introduction of medical AI tools into everyday practice will result in changes affecting both the healthcare professionals and the patients. Currently, there are concerns regarding the systematic interoperability of AI technologies across clinical sites and health systems, and doubts on whether they can be easily integrated within existing workflows [79] without significant changes to existing clinical practices, care models and training programmes.

For the successful implementation of the medical AI in routine clinical practice to become true, the aforementioned barriers must be overcome. Towards this end, common data protocols must be established as well as mechanisms to handle heterogenous data, including unstructured data, and enhance data interoperability across clinical sites and different electronic health systems. An example in that direction is coming from Europe and is the creation of the so-called European Health Data Space (European Health Data Space 2021). Moreover, clinical guidelines and care models should be adapted to take into account the evolving AI-medicated relationship between patients and clinicians, including personal and ethical issues raising from the communication of AI results. Last, novel AI technologies should be compatible with current tools used at clinical level, such as genetic sequencing, electronic patient records and e-health consultations (Arora 2020).

1.2 Approaches Towards Trustworthy and Responsible AI

To ensure the design, development and deployment of trustworthy and responsible AI solutions in the clinic, we need efficient risk assessment and risk minimization approaches. In this context, hereby, we report self-assessment guidelines to evaluate the trustworthiness of the medical AI systems. Moreover, we detail the requirements for achieving a thorough evaluation of the medical AI; a key requirement for identifying different types of potential risks. We also outline current regulatory frameworks, that could be used to characterise and classify the AI risks based on the severity, probability and harm that they might induce.

1.2.1 Guidelines for Developing Trustworthy Medical AI

To help medical AI to evolve from the experimental and development phase to the deployment phase, guidelines to assess potential risks (and ensure that medical AI tools are robust, safe, ethical and lawful), are imperative. Despite remarkable efforts in the development of guidelines for self-assessing AI, such as TRIPOD-AI [19], CLAIM [82], MINIMAR [47], CONSORT-AI [70], and recommendations on AI algorithm evaluation [61, 91, 92, 97], advancements in guidelines for deploying medical AI technology in real-life clinical practice have been slower.

In Europe, a first self-assessment guide, known as Assessment List for Trustworthy AI (ALTAI), was proposed as recently as 2020 by Europe's High-Level Expert Group on Artificial Intelligence (European Commission 2020). ALTAI assesses seven crucial aspects to evaluate whether an AI system can be considered trustworthy: (1) human agency and oversight, (2) technical robustness and safety, (3) privacy and data governance, (4) transparency, (5) diversity, non-discrimination and fairness, (6) societal and environmental well-being, and (7) accountability. Despite the importance of the ALTAI guideline, it was derived for general AI and does not cover specific risks and challenges relevant to the healthcare domain. In healthcare, the first self-assessment list was provided by Scott et al. [103] in an effort to help physicians determine the readiness of algorithms for use and identify cases where further testing and evaluation are needed. Nonetheless, the assessment list is not that detailed as ALTAI.

More recently, the FUTURE-AI consortium, comprising of a multidisciplinary international group of more than 80 experts from 30 countries around the globe, published a detailed guideline for designing, developing, validating and deploying trustworthy medical AI based on six principles (Fig. 2): (1) **F**airness, (2) **U**niversality, (3) **T**raceability, (4) **U**sability, (5) **R**obustness, and (6) **E**xplainability [63, 64] (Fig. 2):

- Fairness: The principle states that tools must maintain accuracy across sub-populations. To this end, it is recommended to integrate approaches for identifying and correcting for systemic and hidden bias from the early stages of the medical AI lifecycle.

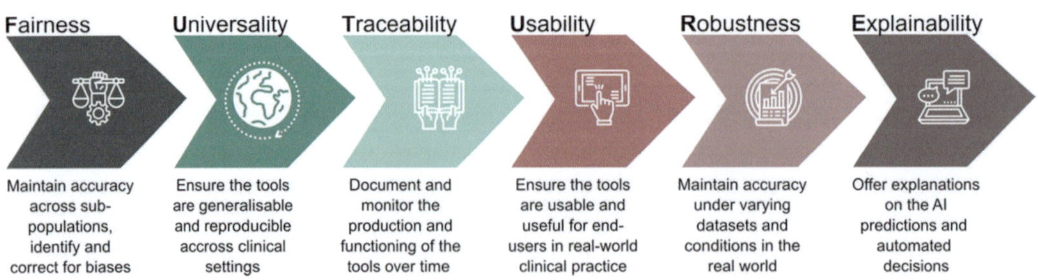

Fig. 2 Guiding principles for trustworthy AI according to the FUTURE-AI guideline for medical AI

- Universality: The principle states that medical AI tools must be universally applicable, interoperable, generalizable and reproducible outside the controlled environment where they were initially developed and tested. This principle translates to tools that can be used across multiple clinical sites and countries.
- Traceability: The principle refers to the requirement of integrating mechanisms for documenting and monitoring the production and functioning of the tools in order to identify and act against potential model and data drifts.
- Usability: The principle refers to tools being user-friendly, effective and useful to real-world clinical practice. Towards this, a human-centered approach putting in the center the end-user and multi-stakeholder engagement throughout the AI production lifecycle should be followed for the development of the tools.
- Robustness: The principle refers to the requirement that the performance of medical AI systems is not be affected by variations in equipment, contexts, operators and/or annotations.
- Explainability: The principle states that the AI systems should provide useful explanations for the model's automated predictions and decisions that will help the end-user understand, inspect and validate of the proposed output.

To assess the AI-based tools in terms of these six principles, the FUTURE-AI guideline consists of 28 recommendations and a self-assessment list in the form of questions that address all currently known risks and challenges in AI in healthcare. FUTURE-AI is dynamic and intended to be constantly updated according to the future developments and needs of the rapidly evolving medical AI field.

1.2.2 Evaluation of Medical AI Technologies

Another important aspect towards bringing medical AI in the clinic is the evaluation process. Currently, evaluation has mainly focused on model performance in terms of accuracy and robustness. Nonetheless, there exist other important aspects to be evaluated related to the specific risks and ethical considerations associated with medical AI, i.e. clinical safety and effectiveness, fairness and non-discrimination, transparency and traceability, as well as privacy and security. In this context, an increasing amount of research is focusing on achieving a multifaceted and objective evaluation of medical AI technologies [61, 91, 92, 97]. The findings of these studies can be roughly summarized into five groups of recommendations that can ensure an improved and thorough assessment of medical AI tools (Fig. 3):

1. *Standardized and universal definition of clinical tasks*

The first step towards building a medical AI tool is the definition of the clinical task that the system is expected to perform. A common definition of the clinical tasks to be performed by the AI tools, such as disease diagnosis, classification or prognosis, can enhance the objective and comparative evaluation of medical AI

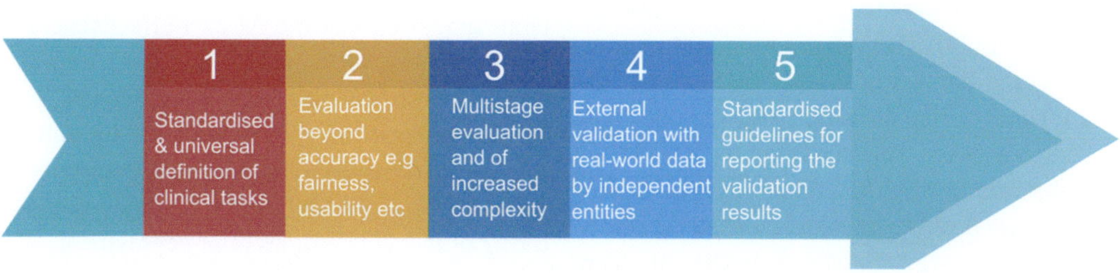

Fig. 3 Approaches for improving the evaluation of medical AI

algorithms and enable their re-usability. To this end, the involvement of non-conflicted entities responsible for defining and updating the definitions of the tasks in light of new information from relevant stakeholders could be particularly helpful. On the contrary, discrepancies in the definition of the tasks to be performed by the medical AI, as it has occurred for COVID-19 diagnosis and classification of its severity [61], makes objective comparison of different algorithms for the same task infeasible. To address this challenge, medical societies, such as the European Society of Cardiology, the European Society of Radiology, or the European Society for Medical Oncology, could propose standardized definitions of diverse clinical tasks in their respective fields of expertise.

2. *Performance evaluation beyond accuracy*

Metrics to evaluate the performance of the models beyond their accuracy are essential to avoid unexpected failures of highly performing models in terms of accuracy. For example, to tackle this limitation, Larson et al. [61] proposed an extended list of aspects for radiology AI models that should be evaluated, including the algorithm's response to unexpected input. The list included questions related to whether the model is reliable, applicable, deterministic, non-distractible, self-aware of limitations, fail-safe, auditable, able to be monitored, and whether it offers an intuitive user interface with transparent logic and a transparent degree of confidence.

Despite the importance of the work of Larson et al., the list fails to assess the technologies in terms of risks related to algorithmic bias and inequality. A work in this direction is that of Barocas et al. [9]. The authors proposed metrics to assess the fairness of algorithms such as statistical parity, group fairness, equalised odds and predictive equality. Seyyed-Kalantari et al. [104] used the true positive rate disparity, i.e. difference in true positive rates, to evaluate state-of-the-art chest X-ray classifiers based on deep learning with respect to patient sex, age, race, and socioeconomic status.

Another important aspect in medical AI evaluation is the perceived usability by the end-user. Elements of interest in the evaluation of medical AI usability are (1) easiness of use without prior training, (2) user's perceived level of mental effort, and (3) offered improvement in clinical efficiency by reducing the required time for information gathering and decision-making. Other usability aspects to be evaluated are the perceived quality of patient-clinician communication, and the explainability and interpretability level of the AI results, among others. To evaluate these elements, questionnaires, such as the System Usability Scale (SUS), could be employed [67]. The SUS, first conceived in the '80s and introduced formally as such in 1996 [13], is a widely used and constantly evolving standardized questionnaire. Example questions of the SUS include how complex the system seemed to the user, and how often he/she would like to use it, among others. In the healthcare domain, researchers evaluated a decision support system powered by AI for depression using such a usability questionnaire [113].

Apart from reliability, robustness, fairness and usability, the medical AI technology should be evaluated in terms of its clinical utility [91]. Furthermore, the cost-effectiveness of medical AI must be evaluated case-by-case as the use of AI might not directly translate to improved or more economic treatment, as recently demonstrated for decision-support systems in dermatology, dentistry, and ophthalmology [40]. Towards evaluating medical AI cost-effectiveness, decision analytic modelling [48] could be employed to assess important qualities such as Quality-Adjusted Life Years. Moreover, Wolff et al. suggested that the AI cost-effectiveness in healthcare can be improved by considering also initial investment and operational costs, and by comparing to alternative options for achieving the same impact [123]. Finally, evaluation frameworks should allow for continuous monitoring of the technologies after deployment.

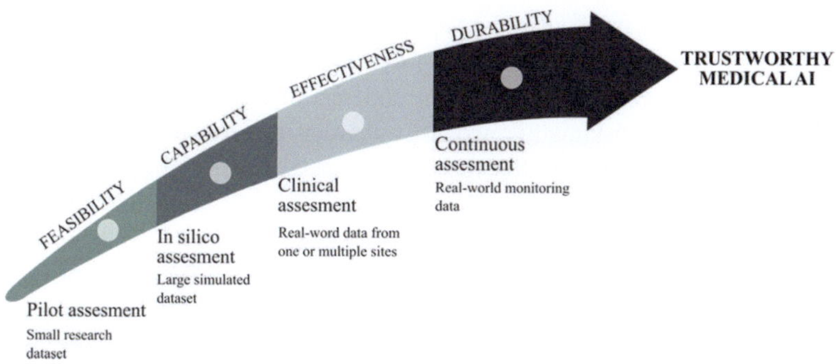

Fig. 4 Multistage evaluation process example [61]. Stages of increasing complexity are proposed for the evaluation of AI algorithms in terms of feasibility, capability, effectiveness and durability

3. *Multistage Evaluation of Increasing Complexity*

A multistage evaluation process of medical AI technologies consisting of stages of increasing complexity allows for minimizing costs and enhancing the quality of the final system deployed in the clinic. The staged process can be divided into four levels (Fig. 4) [61]:

1. Pilot assessment - Feasibility: During this stage the algorithm is evaluated in a controlled environment consisting of small datasets and compared to the state-of-art to demonstrate its feasibility.
2. In silico assessment - Capability: At this stage the real-word performance of the algorithm in terms of accuracy, reliability, and safety is assessed. To simulate real-world conditions, large-scale simulated data are used *to* evaluate *but also* calibrate the AI system. The end-user should be involved to evaluate the simulated conditions and AI-based results. This stage is also known as in-silico validation [117] or virtual clinical trials [1],
3. Clinical assessment—Effectiveness: The effectiveness of the system is *evaluated* during this stage. To this end, the algorithm's performance is assessed in real-world clinical settings including one or multiple sites. The findings should be used to improve the algorithm. Furthermore, it is common that local quality issues are revealed at this stage. These issues should be addressed through collaboration with the local clinical sites.
4. Continuous assessment—Durability: This stage involves the inclusion of mechanisms for continuous monitoring and performance evaluation of the AI technology. Such mechanisms should allow for automatically detecting, reporting, and dealing with errors, and for gathering user feedback. In cases of problems or errors, the system should be adequately updated and tested in a controlled environment before being deployed again in the clinic.

A similar four-level evaluation process was proposed by Park et al. with the difference that a clinical setting is used in both the second and third level, while each evaluation level is focused on addressing a specific challenge or risk, i.e. safety, effectiveness, usability and efficacy [92].

4. *Promotion of external validation using real-word datasets by independententities.*

External validation, as opposed to internal validation, refers to the process of evaluating an algorithm using independent datasets. Internal validation can lead to overoptimistic estimations of model performance. For example, in the medical imaging field, a recent study on the evaluation of 86 image-based deep learning diagnostic AI algorithms demonstrated that most algorithms present a degradation in performance when applied to external datasets [130]. However, in the same field, until recently, only 6% of research works used an external validation cohort as revealed by a systematic review considering 516 studies [55]. Similar discrepancies in performance were observed in other clinical domains. For example, the promising, according to internal validation, COVID-19 mortality prediction tool proposed by Yan et al. [128] failed to demonstrate similar performance (even after re-calibration), when validated externally [8].

Therefore, validation by means of external datasets is imperative and it has been suggested as a key part of the lifecycle of medical AI software development [61, 91]. Datasets for external validation should cover geographical and population variability, while originating from multiple clinical sites to ensure generalization and robustness to diverse acquisition protocols and devices across sites and countries. Given the failures of highly performing AI-based medical solutions, it has been argued that validation datasets should also include real-word data, as opposed to curated data for research purposes, and prospective data [22]. It should be mentioned that the US Food and Drug Administration (FDA) requires validation using prospective data for the final model evaluation.

Lastly, towards ensuring objective and high-quality evaluation of medical AI systems, external validation should be performed by independent third-party evaluators. Such third-party evaluators could include clinical research organisations, research laboratories, or independent institutions. These entities will be responsible for developing and maintaining reference standard data sets and ensuring an AI solution is validated in terms of all important aspects, i.e. accuracy, reliability, fairness and usability, before deployment to the clinic.

5. *Compliance with standardized guidelines for reporting the AI evaluation*

To avoid AI failures in the clinic and their potential devastating effects, it is essential not only to include a thorough and independent multistage evaluation, but also to transparently document and report the developed technologies and their validation process. Toward this, the TRIPOD-AI (Transparent Reporting of a multivariable prediction model for Individual Prognosis Or Diagnosis—artificial intelligence) guideline is currently being developed by an international consortium to allow assessment of potential bias and applicability of diagnostic and prognostic studies involving AI [19]. It is worth mentioning that the TRIBOD-AI is an extension of the TRIPOD guideline [20], consisting of 22 elements to evaluate regression-based predictive models, and the PROBAST (Prediction model study Risk Of Bias Assessment Tool) [123] tool costing of 20 questions organized into four domains, participants, predictors, outcome, and analysis.

Another example of reporting guidelines specific for the rapidly evolving medical AI field is the CONSORT-AI. CONSORT-AI stands for Consolidated Standards of Reporting Trials–Artificial Intelligence and, as its name implies, was proposed as a reporting guideline for clinical trials evaluating AI-based interventions. It is an extension of the CONSORT 2020 guidelines for reporting randomized clinical trials. The CONSORT-AI guidelines comprises 14 items specific to AI, such as intended use, handling of inputs and outputs of the AI intervention, human–AI interaction, impact on clinical practice etc., to be reported along with the original CONSORT 2020 elements. The latter include elements such as title, trial design, participants, interventions, outcomes and sample size.

MINIMAR (MINimum Information for Medical AI Reporting) was proposed in 2020 to feed into the aforementioned initiatives and further stimulate discussion [47]. The proposal involves elements to assess clinical predictive models in terms of (1) study population and setting, (2) training data demographics, (3) model architecture, and (4) model evaluation, optimization, and validation. Assessment of these aspects is critical towards enhancing the understanding, interpretation and critical appraising of AI-based studies.

1.2.3 Regulatory Aspects

The field of medical AI is growing fast, and the current regulatory frameworks do not sufficiently account for the specific challenges of the healthcare domain. For example, in Europe, the available regulatory frameworks, such as the 2017/745 Medical Devices Regulations (MDR) and the 2017/746 In Vitro Diagnostic Medical Devices Regulation (IVDR), were established in 2017 when medical AI was still very new. Hence, they fail to address AI-related risks derived from later developments, such as continuous learning, or risks identified more recently, such as algorithmic biases.

The first proposal for medical AI risk assessment was developed by the German Data Ethics Commission [36]. The proposal involved a "criticality pyramid" comprising five levels of risks/criticality (1: Zero or negligible potential for harm; 2: Some potential for harm; 3: Regular or significant potential for harm; 4: Serious potential for harm; 5: Untenable potential for harm) and suggested an adapted testing or regulatory system depending on the risk level.

Similarly, the European Commission (EC) recently proposed a three-level risk-based classification system of AI tools: (1) unacceptable risk, (2) high risk, and (3) low or minimal risk [26]. The first category comprises tools that contradict the EU principles and should be prohibited. In the second category belong tools that are high-risk but can be adopted if they comply with a list of requirements and obligations such as high-quality training/testing data, documentation and traceability, transparency, human oversight, accuracy, and robustness. Furthermore, special mention is made to AI systems that (1) interact with people, (2) involve emotional or biometric recognition, or (3) generate or manipulate data ("deep fakes"). Such tools have additional transparency obligations, i.e., they must inform the user that is interacting with the AI system and, in the case of "deep fakes", the user should be informed that original content has been manipulated or generated by AI. The last category is that of low-risk tools that have no mandatory obligations but are encouraged to comply with the requirements and obligations of high-risk tools.

Despite the importance of the EC risk-based approach for AI systems evaluation, the proposal presents some limitations. First, the regulation is not focused on medical AI, but rather suggests that AI-based medical devices should be considered high-risk due to the associated safety and privacy risks. This indiscriminatory approach will inevitably lead to unnecessary delays in the adoption of systems that are actually low-risk. Furthermore, the proposal, as opposed to MDR and IVDR, does not cope with specific challenges and risk of AI in the healthcare domain. Lastly, it fails to address AI aspects such as continuous learning. Thus, further improvements in the current regulatory frameworks and a more staged classification of medical AI systems are essential.

The requests for novel regulatory frameworks do not only originate from Europe, as detailed in the previous section, but are worldwide; from United States [4, 45], Japan [17, 88] and China [100]. Recently, the FDA issued the Artificial Intelligence and Machine Learning (ML) Software as a Medical Device Action Plan [116], which advocates for patient-centered methods, specialized rules for medical AI, and appropriate machine learning techniques.

1.3 Summary and Discussion

AI is expected to offer solutions in a wide spectrum of problems in the healthcare domain; risk prediction and disease stratification, diagnosis, therapeutics, patient management, follow up, and administration [46]. This enormous potential has led to an era of exponentially growing medical AI research. Nonetheless, only a limited number of medical AI solutions has reached the clinic. It is worth noting that between 2015 and 2020 only a total of 222 in the USA and 240 in Europe devices based on AI/ML technologies were approved [85]. A key obstacle in the deployment of medical AI in the clinic are the potential risks associated with AI technologies, particularly in the healthcare domain. In an effort to help advance the field, we identified and, hereby, outlined the main risks and challenges associated with medical AI. Furthermore, we discussed mitigation strategies and generic approaches to overcome these issues towards achieving trustworthy solutions and ensuring the widespread use of these promising technologies in the clinic.

In brief, among the main reasons for limited trust and acceptance of AI-based solutions in the clinic, we identified the prospect of patient harm caused by failures of the AI technologies, such as those observed when a system is deployed in novel environments, i.e. different populations than those used for training, for example populations from different centers and/or different geographic locations. Additional risks for patient harm are posed by the currently limited understanding of the way the AI solutions work and reach a decision. Moreover, we identified as one of the most widely discussed issues associated with medical AI the potential security and privacy issues. These include cyber-attacks, adversarial attacks, but also data re-purposing and potential system malfunctions, such as digitalized systems going offline. Another important concern is the lack of transparency which is closely linked to the currently limited explainability and traceability of the tools. Other aspects that constitute major risks for medical AI are difficulties in defining accountability among the involved subjects. AI sex/gender/age/geographic/racial/socieconomic bias is also considered a crucial risk in medical AI as it can exacerbate existing inequalities. Additional obstacles to the deployment of the AI solutions in the clinic include data heterogeneity across sites and countries, concerns regarding the endangerment of the clinician-patient relationship, and difficulties in the integration of novel tools with the currently used electronic health systems and medical practices.

Although challenging, these risks can be addressed with appropriate mitigation strategies. In this work, we outlined approaches for each type of risk, such as adoption of federated solutions to deal with privacy concerns, development of traceability tools to monitor the use of medical AI, systematic training with balanced and representative groups to avoid bias, to name a few. Furthermore, we detailed approaches to minimize risks and increase the overall trustworthiness of medical AI systems. These are mostly related to the evaluation process and how to report it, as well as the continuous monitoring of the tools. More precisely, we discussed current available guidelines for self-assessing the trustworthiness of AI systems in a standardized manner. Among them, the recent FUTURE-AI guideline stands outs thanks to its detailed self-assessment list that covers all major healthcare-specific risks, and thanks to its adaptable and dynamic nature. Combining such guidelines with reporting guidelines for assessing and communicating the design and results from research studies (e.g. TRIPOD-AI, CONSORT-AI, MINIMAR) can further ensure the universality of the algorithms. We also hereby highlighted the need for standardized definition of the clinical tasks to be performed and for evaluation processes that consist of multiple stages of increased complexity and are performed by independent parties using metrics beyond accuracy. Lastly, we briefly discussed the current gaps in regulatory frameworks, particularly in Europe.

The risk mitigation measures and approaches presented in this work comply and complement the recent work of a group of experts who proposed seven areas for improvement to successfully address concerns regarding medical AI and promote wider clinical adoption [63, 64]. The areas are summarized in Fig. 5. In brief, one of the main areas of improvement is the extension of current regulatory frameworks and codes of practice to establish multi-staged, domain-specific evaluation processes by independent third-party evaluators as detailed in Sect. 1.2.2. The evaluation process should assess the performance of the technologies in terms of robustness, fairness, clinical safety and acceptance, transparency, and traceability.

To account for potential risks and past failures of medical AI tools, a shift towards user-centered [31] and human-centered [126]

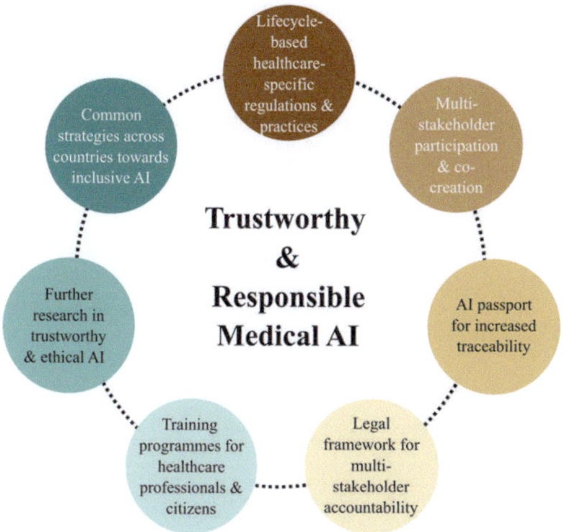

Fig. 5 Recommendations towards trustworthy and responsible AI

approaches for the creation of novel AI tools has been proposed. According to such approaches, the end-users should be involved throughout the lifecycle of the medical AI algorithms, from conceiving the first design to the final validation and long-term use. It should be noted that the user's involvement in the creation of visual interfaces can further enhance the explainability and acceptance of the algorithm's output [7]. Moreover, the additional engagement of other relevant experts, such as biomedical ethicists, apart from AI developers and clinical end-users, can further ensure the improvement of the offered care and patient journey [65]. Co-creation through continuous collaboration of multiple stakeholders, including real-world community members from underrepresented groups, has also the potential to reduce bias and relevant risks leading to more trustworthy AI solutions for healthcare that serve the needs of the clinical end-users and the society.

Another area of improvement is that of increasing the tools' traceability and, therefore, its transparency, as discussed in Sect. 1.1.4. To this end, a global, standardized "AI passport" for all countries and healthcare organizations, has been proposed. The "AI passport" was suggested to inform on at least five crucial aspects of the AI technologies: (1) model information (e.g. architecture, hyperparameters, objective functions, fairness constraints), (2) training data information (e.g. data origin, population, variables, pre-processing), (3) evaluation information (e.g. testing data, metrics, entity performing the evaluation, evaluation metrics and results, identified limitations), (4) usage information (e.g. primary use, secondary use, users, counter-indications, ethical considerations), (5) maintenance information (e.g. last periodic control, identified failures, version number). It is worth mentioning that the last category of information, i.e. the maintenance-related information, is particularly important as AI technologies need to be constantly monitored to ensure early detection of potential data and model drifts [63, 64]. To facilitate the detection and reporting of such issues, the tools should include interfaces for incorporating user feedback, informing the end-user of potential performance drifts, and allow for periodic evaluations. An example "AI passport" according to these guidelines used to assess the trustworthiness of AI systems is provided in Fig. 6.

Another important area for improvement towards developing trustworthy medical AI solutions is the development of frameworks to hold accountable and liable the responsible actor(s) among the involved subjects in case of errors, patient harm or other key ethical concerns such as fairness. A new regulatory body focused on medical AI could be particularly helpful in that direction [57, 115]. Additionally, periodic audits and risk assessments in the entire lifecycle of the AI algorithm from design and development to final deployment and everyday use can help obtain insights into the regulatory needs [98].

Experts highlighted the growing need for the medical curriculum to evolve and incorporate compulsory training on AI technologies to equip future healthcare professionals with the knowledge and skills that will allow them to safely exploit the full potential of AI technologies. At the same time, training of the currently practicing medical doctors by educators from other disciplines, for example, through continuous education programmes [90], can prepare the professionals of today for the changes occurring in clinical practice with the introduction of AI

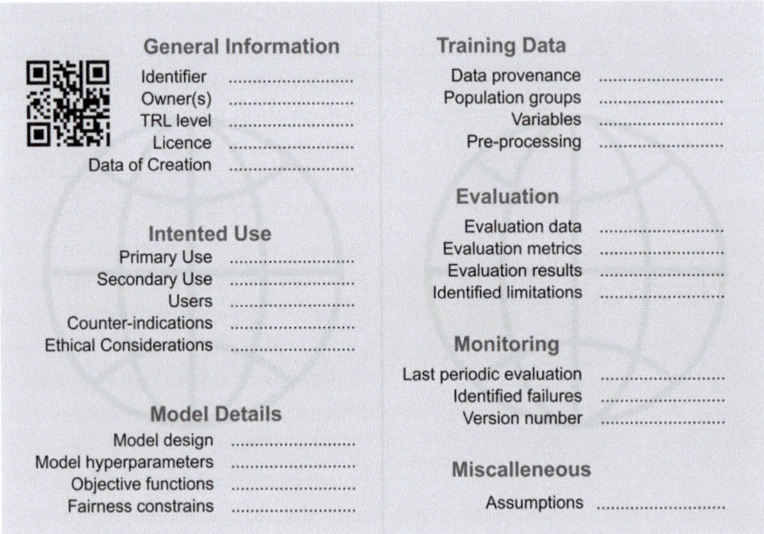

Fig. 6 Example of the recently proposed AI passport that is expected to include information regarding the AI tool, the used model, the training and evaluation process, and related to the continuous monitoring of tool

and reduce the lag in the adoption of trustworthy AI technologies. Apart from increasing the AI-literacy of the healthcare specialists, investing in programs and approaches to increase the AI-literacy of the general public too can ensure safety and optimal use of these promising technologies by increasing public awareness regarding the limitations and risks, particularly of technologies not thoroughly evaluated. This issue has also been discussed in Sect. 1.1.2.

It was suggested to develop common strategies to allow for the development of AI across regions, countries and continents as, currently, inequalities in resources and expertise are resulting in AI innovation being led by high-income countries. This can lead to further aggravation of existing inequalities which, in the healthcare domain, translate to differences in life expectancy, maternal mortality, and other indices of population health across countries. To tackle this challenge, we need investments in training and educational programmes to increase the knowledge, skills, and competencies of future healthcare professionals of emerging countries in the field of AI. Subsequent retention of local AI expertise is also crucial to boost innovation in low- and middle-income countries [3]. Furthermore, apart from human capital, funding of infrastructure programmes to support countries with limited research infrastructures is essential. Common guidelines and regulations to set up inclusive data spaces, such as the long-awaited European Health Data Space [27], can provide access to high quality data to countries with reduced data availability and, therefore, enhance research and innovation opportunities.

Further research for the technical improvement of the solutions is also needed in terms of accuracy, but most importantly, in terms of technical robustness and ethical robustness, i.e. fairness of the algorithms. Towards the latter, in the machine learning field, there exists an increasing number of works focusing on the development of methods and tools to quantify and mitigate bias in AI algorithms [99]; IBM AI Fairness 360 [11]; Microsoft Fairlearn [12], ML Fairness Gym [110], Fairkit [51], among others. Nonetheless, approaches to audit and mitigate for hidden bias, such as bias related to the quality of the labels provided by the healthcare professionals and used to train the systems, remains an open field of research. Another direction for future research involves the development of approaches for enhancing explainability and interpretability. To this end, AI developers should work together with the end-users to ensure that explanations are clear, useful and meaningful for the clinicians. Apart from explainable results, the healthcare professionals should also be informed regarding the level of confidence for the proposed algorithm's output, a relatively new field of study known as uncertainty estimation [58].

Overall, these recommendations jointly with the risk mitigation strategies presented in this chapter pave the path towards addressing current and prospective technical, clinical and socio-ethical issues that emerge from the use of medical AI technologies. By addressing these concerns with reliable solutions and global policies, we can ensure the development of trustworthy systems that can be safely and widely adopted in the daily clinical practice.

References

1. Abadi E, Segars WP, Tsui BMW, Kinahan PE, Bottenus N, Frangi AF, Maidment A, Lo J, Samei E. Virtual clinical trials in medical imaging: a review. J Med Imaging (Bellingham, Wash.). 2020;7(4):042805. https://doi.org/10.1117/1.JMI.7.4.042805
2. Adamson AS, Smith A. Machine learning and health care disparities in dermatology. JAMA Dermatol. 2018;154(11):1247–1248. http://dx.doi.org/10.1001/jamadermatol.2018.2348.
3. Alami H, Rivard L, Lehoux P, Hoffman SJ, Cadeddu SBM, Savoldelli M, Samri MA, Ag Ahmed MA, Fleet R, Fortin J-P. Artificial intelligence in health care: laying the Foundation for responsible, sustainable, and inclusive innovation in low- and middle-income countries. Glob Health. 2020;16(1):52. https://doi.org/10.1186/s12992-020-00584-1.
4. Allen M, Pearn K, Monks T, Bray BD, Everson R, Salmon A, James M, Stein K. Can clinical audits be enhanced by pathway simulation and machine learning? An example from the acute stroke pathway. BMJ Open. 2019;9(9): e028296. https://doi.org/10.1136/bmjopen-2018-028296.
5. Aminololama-Shakeri S, López JE. The doctor-patient relationship with artificial intelligence. AJR Am J Roentgenol. 2019;212(2):308–10. https://doi.org/10.2214/AJR.18.20509.
6. Arora, A. Conceptualising artificial intelligence as a digital healthcare innovation: an introductory review. Med Devices (Auckland, N.Z.). 2020;13:223–30. https://doi.org/10.2147/mder.s262590
7. Barda AJ, Horvat CM, Hochheiser H. A qualitative research framework for the design of user-centered displays of explanations for machine learning model predictions in healthcare. BMC Med Inform Decis Mak. 2020;20(1):257. https://doi.org/10.1186/s12911-020-01276-x.
8. Barish M, Bolourani S, Lau LF, Shah S, Zanos TP. External validation demonstrates limited clinical utility of the interpretable mortality prediction model for patients with COVID-19. Nat Mach Intell. 2021;3(1):25–7. https://doi.org/10.1038/s42256-020-00254-2.
9. Barocas S, Hardt M, Narayanan A. Fairness in machine learning' Nips tutorial, vol. 1. 2017. p. 2. https://fairmlbook.org
10. Bates DW, Levine D, Syrowatka A, Kuznetsova M, Craig KJT, Rui A, Jackson GP, Rhee K. The potential of artificial intelligence to improve patient safety: a scoping review. Npj Digit Med. 2021;4(1):54. https://doi.org/10.1038/s41746-021-00423-6.
11. Bellamy RKE, Dey K, Hind M, Hoffman SC, Houde S, Kannan K, Lohia P, Martino J, Mehta S, Mojsilovic A, Nagar S, Ramamurthy KN, Richards J, Saha D, Sattigeri P, Singh, M, Varshney, KR, Zhang Y. AI fairness 360: an extensible toolkit for detecting and mitigating algorithmic bias. IBM J Res Dev. 2019;63(4/5):4:1–4:15. https://doi.org/10.1147/jrd.2019.2942287
12. Bird S, Dudík M, Edgar R, Horn B, Lutz R, Milan V, Sameki M, Wallach H, Walker K, Design A. Fairlearn: a toolkit for assessing and improving fairness in AI. Microsoft.com. 2020. https://www.microsoft.com/en-us/research/uploads/prod/2020/05/Fairlearn_WhitePaper-2020-09-22.pdf
13. Brooke J. SUS: A "quick and dirty" usability scale. In: Usability evaluation in industry 1st ed. CRC Press; 1996. p. 207–12.
14. Campello VM, Gkontra P, Izquierdo C, Martin-Isla C, Sojoudi A, Full PM, Maier-Hein K, Zhang Y, He Z, Ma J, Parreno M, Albiol A, Kong F, Shadden SC, Acero JC, Sundaresan V, Saber M, Elattar M, Li H, Lekadir K. Multi-centre, multi-vendor and multi-disease cardiac segmentation: the M&Ms challenge. IEEE Trans Med Imaging. 2021;40(12):3543–54. https://doi.org/10.1109/TMI.2021.3090082.
15. Challen R, Denny J, Pitt M, Gompels L, Edwards T, Tsaneva-Atanasova K. Artificial intelligence, bias and clinical safety. BMJ Qual Saf. 2019;28(3):231–7. https://doi.org/10.1136/bmjqs-2018-008370.
16. Ching T, Himmelstein DS, Beaulieu-Jones BK, Kalinin AA, Do BT, Way GP, Ferrero E, Agapow P-M, Zietz M, Hoffman MM, Xie W, Rosen GL, Lengerich BJ, Israeli J, Lanchantin J, Woloszynek S, Carpenter AE, Shrikumar A, Xu J, Greene CS. Opportunities and obstacles for deep learning in biology and medicine. J R Soc Interface. 2018;15(141):20170387. https://doi.org/10.1098/rsif.2017.0387.

17. Chinzei K, Shimizu A, Mori K, Harada K, Takeda H, Hashizume M, Ishizuka M, Kato, N, Kawamori R, Kyo S, Nagata K, Yamane T, Sakuma I, Ohe K, Mitsuishi M. Regulatory science on AI-based medical devices and systems. Adv Biomed Eng 2018;7(0):118–23. https://doi.org/10.14326/abe.7.118
18. Cohen IG. Informed consent and medical artificial intelligence: What to tell the patient? SSRN Electron J. 2020. https://doi.org/10.2139/ssrn.3529576.
19. Collins GS, Dhiman P, Andaur Navarro CL, Ma J, Hooft L, Reitsma JB, Logullo P, Beam AL, Peng L, Van Calster B, van Smeden M, Riley RD, Moons KG. Protocol for development of a reporting guideline (TRIPOD-AI) and risk of bias tool (PROBAST-AI) for diagnostic and prognostic prediction model studies based on artificial intelligence. BMJ Open. 2021;11(7): e048008. https://doi.org/10.1136/bmjopen-2020-048008.
20. Collins GS, Reitsma JB, Altman DG, Moons KGM. Transparent reporting of a multivariable prediction model for individual prognosis or diagnosis (TRIPOD): the TRIPOD Statement. BMC Med. 2015;13(1):1. https://doi.org/10.1186/s12916-014-0241-z.
21. Din NU, Ukoumunne OC, Rubin G, Hamilton W, Carter B, Stapley S, Neal RD. Age and gender variations in cancer diagnostic intervals in 15 cancers: Analysis of data from the UK clinical practice research datalink. PLOS One. 2015;10(5):e0127717. http://dx.doi.org/10.1371/journal.pone.0127717.
22. Domalpally A, Channa R. Real-world validation of artificial intelligence algorithms for ophthalmic imaging. Lancet Digit Health. 2021;3(8):e463–4. https://doi.org/10.1016/S2589-7500(21)00140-0.
23. Doyen S, Dadario NB. 12 plagues of AI in healthcare: a practical guide to current issues with using machine learning in a medical context. Frontiers in Digital Health. 2022;4: 765406. https://doi.org/10.3389/fdgth.2022.765406.
24. Ellahham S, Ellahham N, Simsekler MCE. Application of artificial intelligence in the health care safety context: opportunities and challenges. Am J Med Qual: Off J Am Coll Med Qual. 2020;35(4):341–8. https://doi.org/10.1177/1062860619878515.
25. European Commission, Directorate-General for Communications Networks, Content and Technology. The Assessment List for Trustworthy Artificial Intelligence (ALTAI) for self assessment. Publications Office. 2020. https://doi.org/10.2759/002360
26. European Commission. Proposal for a Regulation laying down harmonised rules on Artificial Intelligence (Artificial Intelligence Act) and amending certain Union legislative acts. (n.d.). Europeansources.Info. 2021. Available 4 Aug 2022 from https://www.europeansources.info/record/proposal-for-a-regulation-laying-down-harmonised-rules-on-artificial-intelligence-artificial-intelligence-act-and-amending-certain-union-legislative-acts/
27. European Health Data Space. Public health. n.d. Available 4 Aug 2022, from https://health.ec.europa.eu/ehealth-digital-health-and-care/european-health-data-space_en
28. De Fauw J, Ledsam JR, Romera-Paredes B, Nikolov S, Tomasev N, Blackwell S, Askham H, Glorot X, O'Donoghue B, Visentin D, van den Driessche G, Lakshminarayanan B, Meyer C, Mackinder F, Bouton S, Ayoub K, Chopra R, King D, Karthikesalingam A, Ronneberger O. Clinically applicable deep learning for diagnosis and referral in retinal disease. Nat Med. 2018;24(9):1342–50. https://doi.org/10.1038/s41591-018-0107-6.
29. Ferryman K, Pitcan M. Fairness in precision medicine. 2018. https://datasociety.net/library/fairness-in-precision-medicine/
30. Fihn SD, Saria S, Mendonça E, Hain S, Matheny M, Shah N, Liu H, Auerbach A. Deploying AI in clinical settings. In artificial intelligence in health care: the hope, the hype, the promise, the peril. In: Matheny M, Israni ST, Ahmed M, Whicher D, editors. Washington, DC: National Academy of Medicine; 2019.
31. Filice RW, Ratwani RM. The case for user-centered artificial intelligence in radiology. Radiology Artificial Intelligence. 2020;2(3): e190095. https://doi.org/10.1148/ryai.2020190095.
32. Finlayson SG, Bowers JD, Ito J, Zittrain JL, Beam AL, Kohane IS. Adversarial attacks on medical machine learning. Science (New York, N.Y.). 2019;363(6433):1287–89. https://doi.org/10.1126/science.aaw4399
33. Floyd BJ. Problems in accurate medical diagnosis of depression in female patients. Social Sci Medicine. 1997;44(3):403–412. http://dx.doi.org/10.1016/s0277-9536(96)00159-1.
34. Freeman K, Dinnes J, Chuchu N, Takwoingi Y, Bayliss SE, Matin RN, Jain A, Walter FM, Williams HC, Deeks JJ. Algorithm based smartphone apps to assess risk of skin cancer in adults: systematic review of diagnostic accuracy studies. BMJ (Clin Res Ed). 2020;368: m127. https://doi.org/10.1136/bmj.m127.
35. Gerke S, Minssen T, Cohen G. Ethical and legal challenges of artificial intelligence-driven healthcare. In: Artificial intelligence in healthcare. Elsevier; 2020. p. 295–36.
36. German Data Ethics Commission, Opinion of the Data Ethics Commission. 2019. https://www.bmi.bund.de/SharedDocs/downloads/EN/themen/it-digital-policy/datenethikkommission-abschlussgutachten-lang.pdf?__blob=publicationFile&v=4
37. Ghassemi M, Oakden-Rayner L, Beam AL. The false hope of current approaches to explainable artificial intelligence in health care. Lancet Digit Health. 2021;3(11):e745–50. https://doi.org/10.1016/S2589-7500(21)00208-9.

38. Gillespie N, Lockey S, Curtis C. Trust in artificial Intelligence: a five country study. The University of Queensland and KPMG; 2021. https://doi.org/10.14264/e34bfa3
39. Gillies RJ, Kinahan PE, Hricak H. Radiomics: images are more than pictures, they are data. Radiology. 2016;278(2):563–77. https://doi.org/10.1148/radiol.2015151169.
40. Gomez Rossi J, Rojas-Perilla N, Krois J, Schwendicke F. Cost-effectiveness of artificial intelligence as a decision-support system applied to the detection and grading of melanoma, dental caries, and diabetic retinopathy. JAMA Netw Open. 2022;5(3): e220269. https://doi.org/10.1001/jamanetworkopen.2022.0269.
41. Guo J, Li B. The application of medical artificial intelligence technology in rural areas of developing countries. Health Equity. 2018;2(1):174–81. https://doi.org/10.1089/heq.2018.0037.
42. Guo J, Li B The application of medical artificial intelligence technology in rural areas of developing countries. In: Health equity, vol. 2, Issue 1. Mary Ann Liebert Inc.; 2018. p. 174–81. https://doi.org/10.1089/heq.2018.0037
43. Haibe-Kains B, Adam GA, Hosny A, Khodakarami F, Massive Analysis Quality Control (MAQC) Society Board of Directors Shraddha Thakkar 35 Kusko Rebecca 36 Sansone Susanna-Assunta 37 Tong Weida 35 Wolfinger Russ D. 38 Mason Christopher E. 39 Jones Wendell 40 Dopazo Joaquin 41 Furlanello Cesare 42, Waldron L, Wang B, McIntosh C, Goldenberg A, Kundaje A, Greene CS, Broderick T, Hoffman M. M, Leek JT, Korthauer K, Huber W, Brazma A, Pineau J, Tibshirani R, Hastie T, Ioannidis JPA, Quackenbush J, Aerts HJWL. Transparency and reproducibility in artificial intelligence. Nature. 2020;586(7829):E14–E16. https://doi.org/10.1038/s41586-020-2766-y.
44. Harned Z, Lungren MP, Rajpurkar P. Machine vision, medical AI, and malpractice. Compar Polit Econ: Regul eJ. 2019. https://jolt.law.harvard.edu/digest/machine-vision-medical-ai-and-malpractice
45. Harvey HB, Gowda V. How the FDA regulates AI. Acad Radiology. 2020;27(1):58–61. http://dx.doi.org/10.1016/j.acra.2019.09.017.
46. He J, Baxter SL, Xu J, Xu J, Zhou X, Zhang K. The practical implementation of artificial intelligence technologies in medicine. Nat Med. 2019;25(1):30–6. https://doi.org/10.1038/s41591-018-0307-0.
47. Hernandez-Boussard T, Bozkurt S, Ioannidis JPA, Shah NH. MINIMAR (MINimum Information for Medical AI Reporting): Developing reporting standards for artificial intelligence in health care. J Am Med Inf Assoc: JAMIA. 2020;27(12):2011–5. https://doi.org/10.1093/jamia/ocaa088.
48. Hill NR, Sandler B, Mokgokong R, Lister S, Ward T, Boyce R, Farooqui U, Gordon J. Cost-effectiveness of targeted screening for the identification of patients with atrial fibrillation: evaluation of a machine learning risk prediction algorithm. J Med Econ. 2020;23(4):386–93. https://doi.org/10.1080/13696998.2019.1706543.
49. Hocking L, Parks S, Altenhofer M, Gunashekar S. Reuse of health data by the European pharmaceutical industry: current practice and implications for the future. RAND Corporation. 2019. https://doi.org/10.7249/RR3247.
50. Hoffman KM, Trawalter S, Axt JR, Oliver MN. Racial bias in pain assessment and treatment recommendations, and false beliefs about biological differences between blacks and whites. Proc Natl Acad Sci USA. 2016;113(16):4296–301. https://doi.org/10.1073/pnas.1516047113.
51. Johnson B, Bartola J, Angell R, Keith K, Witty S, Giguere SJ, Brun Y. Fairkit, fairkit, on the wall, who's the fairest of them all? Supporting data scientists in training fair models. 2020. https://doi.org/10.48550/ARXIV.2012.09951
52. Karimi D, Dou H, Warfield SK, Gholipour A. Deep learning with noisy labels: Exploring techniques and remedies in medical image analysis. Med Image Anal. 2020;65(101759): 101759. https://doi.org/10.1016/j.media.2020.101759.
53. Kaushal A, Altman R, Langlotz C. Geographic distribution of US cohorts used to train deep learning algorithms. JAMA: J Am Med Assoc 2020;324(12):1212–13. https://doi.org/10.1001/jama.2020.12067
54. Kiener M. '"You may be hacked" and other things doctors should tell you'. The Conversation. 3 November 2020. https://theconversation.com/you-may-be-hacked-and-other-things-doctors-should-tell-you-148946
55. Kim DW, Jang HY, Kim KW, Shin Y, Park SH. Design characteristics of studies reporting the performance of artificial intelligence algorithms for diagnostic analysis of medical images: Results from recently published papers. Korean J Radioly: Off J Korean Radiol Soc. 2019;20(3):405–10. https://doi.org/10.3348/kjr.2019.0025.
56. Klonoff DC. Cybersecurity for connected diabetes devices. J Diabetes Sci Technol. 2015;9(5):1143–7. https://doi.org/10.1177/1932296815583334.
57. Koene A, Clifton C, Hatada Y, Webb H, Richardson R. A governance framework for algorithmic accountability and transparency. EPRS, European Parliament; 2019. https://www.europarl.europa.eu/thinktank/en/document/EPRS_STU(2019)624262
58. Kompa B, Snoek J, Beam AL. Second opinion needed: communicating uncertainty in medical machine learning. Npj Digit Med. 2021;4(1):4. https://doi.org/10.1038/s41746-020-00367-3.
59. Koops B-J. The concept of function creep. Law Innov Technol. 2021;13(1):29–56. https://doi.org/10.1080/17579961.2021.1898299.
60. Langlotz CP, Allen B, Erickson BJ, Kalpathy-Cramer J, Bigelow K, Cook TS, Flanders AE, Lungren MP, Mendelson DS, Rudie JD, Wang G,

Kandarpa K. A roadmap for foundational research on artificial intelligence in medical imaging: From the 2018 NIH/RSNA/ACR/the academy workshop. Radiology. 2019;291(3):781–91. https://doi.org/10.1148/radiol.2019190613.
61. Larson DB, Harvey H, Rubin DL, Irani N, Tse JR, Langlotz CP. Regulatory frameworks for development and evaluation of artificial intelligence-based diagnostic imaging algorithms: summary and recommendations. J Am Coll Radiol: JACR. 2021;18(3 Pt A):413–24. https://doi.org/10.1016/j.jacr.2020.09.060
62. Lehne M, Sass J, Essenwanger A, Schepers J, Thun S. Why digital medicine depends on interoperability. Npj Digit Med. 2019;2(1):79. https://doi.org/10.1038/s41746-019-0158-1.
63. Lekadir K et al. 'FUTURE-AI: best practices for trustworthy AI in medicine'. 2022. www.future-ai.org
64. Lekadir K, Quaglio G, Tselioudis Garmendia A, Gallin C. Artificial intelligence in healthcare: applications, risks, and ethical and societal impacts. (n.d.). Europa.Eu.; 2022. https://www.europarl.europa.eu/thinktank/en/document/EPRS_STU(2022)729512
65. Leone D, Schiavone F, Appio FP, Chiao B. How does artificial intelligence enable and enhance value co-creation in industrial markets? An exploratory case study in the healthcare ecosystem. J Bus Res. 2021;129:849–59. https://doi.org/10.1016/j.jbusres.2020.11.008.
66. Leslie D, Mazumder A, Peppin A, Wolters MK, Hagerty A. Does "AI" stand for augmenting inequality in the era of covid-19 healthcare? BMJ (Clinical Research Ed). 2021;372: n304. https://doi.org/10.1136/bmj.n304.
67. Lewis JR. The system usability scale: Past, present, and future. Int J Hum-Comput Interact. 2018;34(7):577–90. https://doi.org/10.1080/10447318.2018.1455307.
68. Li Y, Vasconcelos N. REPAIR: Removing representation bias by dataset resampling. In: 2019 IEEE/CVF conference on computer vision and pattern recognition (CVPR); 2019. https://doi.org/10.1109/CVPR.2019.00980
69. Linardatos P, Papastefanopoulos V, Kotsiantis S. Explainable AI: a review of machine learning interpretability methods. Entropy (Basel, Switzerland). 2020;23(1):18. https://doi.org/10.3390/e23010018.
70. Liu X, Cruz Rivera S, Moher D, Calvert MJ, Denniston AK, SPIRIT-AI and CONSORT-AI Working Group. Reporting guidelines for clinical trial reports for interventions involving artificial intelligence: the CONSORT-AI extension. Nat Med 2020;26(9):1364–1374. https://doi.org/10.1038/s41591-020-1034-x
71. Lyratzopoulos G, Abel GA, McPhail S, Neal RD, Rubin GP. Gender inequalities in the promptness of diagnosis of bladder and renal cancer after symptomatic presentation: evidence from secondary analysis of an English primary care audit survey. BMJ Open. 2013;3(6):e002861. http://dx.doi.org/10.1136/bmjopen-2013-002861.
72. Mackey TK, Nayyar G. Digital danger: a review of the global public health, patient safety and cybersecurity threats posed by illicit online pharmacies. Br Med Bull. 2016;118(1):110–26. https://doi.org/10.1093/bmb/ldw016.
73. Maliha G, Gerke S, Cohen IG, Parikh RB. Artificial intelligence and liability in medicine: balancing safety and innovation. Milbank Q. 2021;99(3):629–47. https://doi.org/10.1111/1468-0009.12504.
74. Manne R, Kantheti SC. Application of artificial intelligence in healthcare: chances and challenges. Curr J Appl Sci Technol. 2021;40(6):78–89. https://doi.org/10.9734/cjast/2021/v40i631320.
75. Matheny ME, Whicher D, Thadaney Israni S. Artificial intelligence in health care: A report from the national academy of medicine: a report from the national academy of medicine. JAMA: J Am Med Assoc 2020;323(6):509–10. https://doi.org/10.1001/jama.2019.21579
76. McCarthy J, Hayes PJ. Some philosophical problems from the standpoint of artificial intelligence. In: Readings in artificial intelligence. Elsevier; 1981. p. 431–50.
77. McKeown A, Mourby M, Harrison P, Walker S, Sheehan M, Singh I. Ethical issues in consent for the reuse of data in health data platforms. Sci Eng Ethics. 2021;27(1):9. https://doi.org/10.1007/s11948-021-00282-0.
78. McKinney SM, Sieniek M, Godbole V, Godwin J, Antropova N, Ashrafian H, Back T, Chesus M, Corrado GS, Darzi A, Etemadi M, Garcia-Vicente F, Gilbert FJ, Halling-Brown M, Hassabis D, Jansen S, Karthikesalingam A, Kelly CJ, King D, Shetty S. International evaluation of an AI system for breast cancer screening. Nature. 2020;577(7788):89–94. https://doi.org/10.1038/s41586-019-1799-6.
79. Meskó B, Görög M. A short guide for medical professionals in the era of artificial intelligence. Npj Digital Medicine. 2020;3(1):126. https://doi.org/10.1038/s41746-020-00333-z.
80. Mikolajczyk A, Grochowski M. Data augmentation for improving deep learning in image classification problem. In: 2018 International interdisciplinary Ph.D. workshop (IIPhDW). IEEE; 2018. https://doi.org/10.1109/iiphdw.2018.8388338
81. Mikolajczyk A, Grochowski M. Data augmentation for improving deep learning in image classification problem. In: 2018 International interdisciplinary Ph.D. workshop (IIPhDW); 2018. https://doi.org/10.1109/iiphdw.2018.8388338
82. Mongan J, Moy L, Kahn CE Jr. Checklist for artificial intelligence in medical imaging (CLAIM): A guide for authors and reviewers. Radiol Artif Intell. 2020;2(2): e200029. https://doi.org/10.1148/ryai.2020200029.

83. Mora-Cantallops M, Sánchez-Alonso S, García-Barriocanal E, Sicilia M-A. Traceability for trustworthy AI: a review of models and tools. Big Data Cogn Comput. 2021;5(2):20. https://doi.org/10.3390/bdcc5020020.
84. Morley J, Floridi L. An ethically mindful approach to AI for health care. Lancet. 2020;395(10220):254–5. https://doi.org/10.1016/S0140-6736(19)32975-7.
85. Muehlematter UJ, Daniore P, Vokinger KN. Approval of artificial intelligence and machine learning-based medical devices in the USA and Europe (2015–20): a comparative analysis. Lancet Digit Health. 2021;3(3):e195–203. https://doi.org/10.1016/S2589-7500(20)30292-2.
86. Nagendran M, Chen Y, Lovejoy CA, Gordon AC, Komorowski M, Harvey H, Topol EJ, Ioannidis JPA, Collins GS, Maruthappu M. Artificial intelligence versus clinicians: systematic review of design, reporting standards, and claims of deep learning studies. BMJ (Clin Res Ed). 2020;368: m689. https://doi.org/10.1136/bmj.m689.
87. Obermeyer Z, Powers B, Vogeli C, Mullainathan S. Dissecting racial bias in an algorithm used to manage the health of populations. Science (New York, N.Y.). 2019;366(6464):447–453. https://doi.org/10.1126/science.aax2342
88. Ota N, Tachibana K, Kusakabe T, Sanada S, Kondoh M. A concept for a Japanese regulatory framework for emerging medical devices with frequently modified behavior: a regulatory concept for innovation. Clin Transl Sci. 2020;13(5):877–9. https://doi.org/10.1111/cts.12784.
89. Panch T, Mattie H, Atun R. Artificial intelligence and algorithmic bias: implications for health systems. J Glob Health. 2019;9(2): 010318. https://doi.org/10.7189/jogh.09.020318.
90. Paranjape K, Schinkel M, Nannan Panday R, Car J, Nanayakkara P. Introducing artificial intelligence training in medical education. JMIR Med Educ. 2019;5(2): e16048. https://doi.org/10.2196/16048.
91. Park SH, Han K. Methodologic guide for evaluating clinical performance and effect of artificial intelligence technology for medical diagnosis and prediction. Radiology. 2018;286(3):800–9. https://doi.org/10.1148/radiol.2017171920.
92. Park Y, Jackson GP, Foreman MA, Gruen D, Hu J, Das AK. Evaluating artificial intelligence in medicine: phases of clinical research. JAMIA Open. 2020;3(3):326–31. https://doi.org/10.1093/jamiaopen/ooaa033.
93. Pinto A, Pinto F, Faggian A, Rubini G, Caranci F, Macarini L, Genovese EA, Brunese L (2013) Sources of error in emergency ultrasonography. Crit Ultrasound J 2013;5 Suppl 1(S1):S1. https://doi.org/10.1186/2036-7902-5-S1-S1
94. Quaglio G, Pirona A, Esposito G, Karapiperis T, Brand H, Dom G, Bertinato L, Montanari L, Kiefer F, Carrà G. Knowledge and utilization of technology-based interventions for substance use disorders: an exploratory study among health professionals in the European Union. Drugs (Abingdon, England). 2018;26(5):437–46. https://doi.org/10.1080/09687637.2018.1475549.
95. Raji ID, Smart A, White RN, Mitchell M, Gebru T, Hutchinson B, Smith-Loud J, Theron D, Barnes P. Closing the AI accountability gap: defining an end-to-end framework for internal algorithmic auditing. In: Proceedings of the 2020 conference on fairness, accountability, and transparency; 2020. https://doi.org/10.1145/3351095.3372873
96. Rajkomar A, Hardt M, Howell MD, Corrado G, Chin MH. Ensuring fairness in machine learning to advance health equity. Ann Intern Med. 2018;169(12):866–72. https://doi.org/10.7326/M18-1990.
97. Reddy S, Rogers W, Makinen V-P, Coiera E, Brown P, Wenzel M, Weicken E, Ansari S, Mathur P, Casey A, Kelly B. Evaluation framework to guide implementation of AI systems into healthcare settings. BMJ Health Care Inf 2021; 28(1). https://doi.org/10.1136/bmjhci-2021-100444
98. Reisman D, Schultz J, Crawford K, Whittaker M. A practical framework for public agency accountability. Ainowinstitute.org. n.d. Available 3 Aug 2022, from https://ainowinstitute.org/aiareport2018.pdf
99. Richardson B, Gilbert JE. A framework for fairness: A systematic review of existing fair AI solutions. 2021. arXiv [cs.AI]. http://arxiv.org/abs/2112.05700.
100. Roberts H, Cowls J, Morley J, Taddeo M, Wang V, Floridi L. The Chinese approach to artificial intelligence: an analysis of policy, ethics, and regulation. AI Soc. 2021;36(1):59–77. https://doi.org/10.1007/s00146-020-00992-2.
101. Samulowitz A, Gremyr I, Eriksson E, Hensing G. "brave men" and "emotional women": A theory-guided literature review on gender bias in health care and gendered norms towards patients with chronic pain. Journal de La Societe Canadienne Pour Le Traitement de La Douleur (Pain Res Manag). 2018;2018:1–14. https://doi.org/10.1155/2018/6358624.
102. Scheetz J, Rothschild P, McGuinness M, Hadoux X, Soyer HP, Janda M, Condon JJJ, Oakden-Rayner L, Palmer LJ, Keel S, van Wijngaarden P. A survey of clinicians on the use of artificial intelligence in ophthalmology, dermatology, radiology and radiation oncology. Sci Rep. 2021;11(1):5193. https://doi.org/10.1038/s41598-021-84698-5.
103. Scott I, Carter S, Coiera E. Clinician checklist for assessing suitability of machine learning applications in healthcare. BMJ Health Care Inf. 2021;28(1): e100251. https://doi.org/10.1136/bmjhci-2020-100251.
104. Seyyed-Kalantari L, Liu G, McDermott M, Chen IY, Ghassemi M. CheXclusion: Fairness gaps in deep chest X-ray classifiers. Biocomputing 2021. 2020. https://doi.org/10.1142/9789811232701_0022

105. Shin EK, Mahajan R, Akbilgic O, Shaban-Nejad A. Sociomarkers and biomarkers: predictive modeling in identifying pediatric asthma patients at risk of hospital revisits. Npj Digit Med. 2018;1(1):50. https://doi.org/10.1038/s41746-018-0056-y.
106. Shortliffe EH, Sepúlveda MJ (2018) Clinical decision support in the era of artificial intelligence. JAMA: J Am Med Assoc 2018;320(21):2199–200. https://doi.org/10.1001/jama.2018.17163
107. Sipola T, Kokkonen T. One-pixel attacks against medical imaging: a conceptual framework. In: Advances in intelligent systems and computing. Springer; 2021. p. 197–03. https://doi.org/10.1007/978-3-030-72657-7_19
108. Sit C, Srinivasan R, Amlani A, Muthuswamy K, Azam A, Monzon L, Poon DS. Attitudes and perceptions of UK medical students towards artificial intelligence and radiology: a multicentre survey. Insights into Imaging. 2020;11(1). https://doi.org/10.1186/s13244-019-0830-7.
109. Smith H. Clinical AI: opacity, accountability, responsibility and liability. AI Society. 2021;36(2):535–545. http://dx.doi.org/10.1007/s00146-020-01019-6.
110. Srinivasan H. ML-fairness-gym: A tool for exploring long-term impacts of machine learning systems. Googleblog.com. 2020. https://ai.googleblog.com/2020/02/ml-fairness-gym-tool-for-exploring-long.html.
111. Stylianou N, Fackrell R, Vasilakis C. Are medical outliers associated with worse patient outcomes? A retrospective study within a regional NHS hospital using routine data. BMJ Open. 2017;7(5): e015676. https://doi.org/10.1136/bmjopen-2016-015676.
112. Subbaswamy A, Saria S. From development to deployment: dataset shift, causality, and shift-stable models in health AI. Biostatistics (Oxford, England). 2020;21(2):345–52. https://doi.org/10.1093/biostatistics/kxz041.
113. Tanguay-Sela M, Benrimoh D, Perlman K, Israel S, Mehltretter J, Armstrong C, Fratila R, Parikh S, Karp J, Heller K, Vahia I, Blumberger D, Karama S, Vigod S, Myhr G, Martins R, Rollins C, Popescu C, Lundrigan E, Margolese H. Evaluating the usability and impact of an artificial intelligence-powered clinical decision support system for depression treatment. Biol Psychiat. 2020;87(9):S171. https://doi.org/10.1016/j.biopsych.2020.02.451.
114. Tulk Jesso S, Kelliher A, Sanghavi H, Martin T, Henrickson Parker S. Inclusion of clinicians in the development and evaluation of clinical artificial intelligence tools: A systematic literature review. Front Psychol. 2022;13: 830345. https://doi.org/10.3389/fpsyg.2022.830345.
115. Tutt A. An FDA for algorithms. SSRN Electron J. 2016. https://doi.org/10.2139/ssrn.2747994.
116. U.S. Food and Drug Administration (FDA). Artificial intelligence/machine learning (AI/ML)-based software as a medical device (SaMD) action plan; 2021.
117. Viceconti M, Pappalardo F, Rodriguez B, Horner M, Bischoff J, Musuamba Tshinanu F. In silico trials: verification, validation and uncertainty quantification of predictive models used in the regulatory evaluation of biomedical products. Methods (San Diego, Calif.). 2021;185:120–27. https://doi.org/10.1016/j.ymeth.2020.01.011
118. Vokinger KN, Feuerriegel S, Kesselheim AS. Continual learning in medical devices: FDA's action plan and beyond. Lancet Digit Health. 2021;3(6):e337–8. https://doi.org/10.1016/S2589-7500(21)00076-5.
119. Vokinger KN, Feuerriegel S, Kesselheim AS. Mitigating bias in machine learning for medicine. Commun Med. 2021;1(1):25. https://doi.org/10.1038/s43856-021-00028-w.
120. Wager TD, Woo C-W. Imaging biomarkers and biotypes for depression. Nat Med. 2017;23(1):16–7. https://doi.org/10.1038/nm.4264.
121. Westergaard D, Moseley P, Sørup FKH, Baldi P, Brunak S. Population-wide analysis of differences in disease progression patterns in men and women. Nat Commun. 2019;10(1):666. https://doi.org/10.1038/s41467-019-08475-9.
122. Whitby B. Automating medicine the ethical way. In: Machine medical ethics. Springer; 2015. p. 223–32.
123. Wolff RF, Moons KGM, Riley RD, Whiting PF, Westwood M, Collins GS, Reitsma JB, Kleijnen J, Mallett S, PROBAST Group†. PROBAST: a tool to assess the risk of bias and applicability of prediction model studies. Ann Intern Med. 2019;170(1):51–58. https://doi.org/10.7326/M18-1376
124. World Health Organization (WHO). Ethics and governance of artificial intelligence for health: WHO guidance. 2021. https://www.who.int/publications/i/item/9789240029200
125. Xivuri K, Twinomurinzi H. A systematic review of fairness in artificial intelligence algorithms. In: Responsible AI and analytics for an ethical and inclusive digitized society. Springer; 2021. p. 271–284. https://doi.org/10.1007/978-3-030-85447-8_24
126. Xu W. Toward human-centered AI: a perspective from human-computer interaction. Interactions. 2019;26(4):42–6. https://doi.org/10.1145/3328485.
127. Xu H, Ma Y, Liu H-C, Deb D, Liu H, Tang J-L, Jain AK. Adversarial attacks and defenses in images, graphs and text: a review. Int J Autom Comput. 2020;17(2):151–78. https://doi.org/10.1007/s11633-019-1211-x.
128. Yan L, Zhang H-T, Goncalves J, Xiao Y, Wang M, Guo Y, Sun C, Tang X, Jing L, Zhang M, Huang X, Xiao Y, Cao H, Chen Y, Ren T, Wang F, Xiao Y, Huang S, Tan X, Yuan Y. An interpretable mortality prediction model for COVID-19 patients. Nat Mach Intell. 2020;2(5):283–8. https://doi.org/10.1038/s42256-020-0180-7.
129. Yu K-H, Kohane IS. Framing the challenges of artificial intelligence in medicine. BMJ Qual

Saf. 2019;28(3):238–41. https://doi.org/10.1136/bmjqs-2018-008551.

130. Yu AC, Mohajer B, Eng J. External validation of deep learning algorithms for radiologic diagnosis: a systematic review. Radiol Artif Intell. 2022;4(3): e210064. https://doi.org/10.1148/ryai.210064.

131. Zech JR, Badgeley MA, Liu M, Costa AB, Titano JJ, Oermann EK. Variable generalization performance of a deep learning model to detect pneumonia in chest radiographs: a cross-sectional study. PLoS Med. 2018;15(11): e1002683. https://doi.org/10.1371/journal.pmed.1002683.

132. Zhang BH, Lemoine B, Mitchell M. Mitigating unwanted biases with adversarial learning. In: Proceedings of the 2018 AAAI/ACM conference on AI, ethics, and society; 2018.

MIX
Papier aus verantwortungsvollen Quellen
Paper from responsible sources
FSC® C105338

If you have any concerns about our products,
you can contact us on
ProductSafety@springernature.com

In case Publisher is established outside the EU,
the EU authorized representative is:
Springer Nature Customer Service Center GmbH
Europaplatz 3, 69115 Heidelberg, Germany

Printed by Libri Plureos GmbH
in Hamburg, Germany